SOURCEBOOK OF PHONOLOGICAL AWARENESS ACTIVITIES

VOLUME II
CHILDREN'S CORE LITERATURE

SOURCEBOOK OF PHONOLOGICAL AWARENESS ACTIVITIES

VOLUME II
CHILDREN'S CORE LITERATURE

Candace L. Goldsworthy, Ph.D.
Department of Speech Pathology and Audiology
California State University, Sacramento
Partner, Speech-Language Learning Associates
Sacramento, California

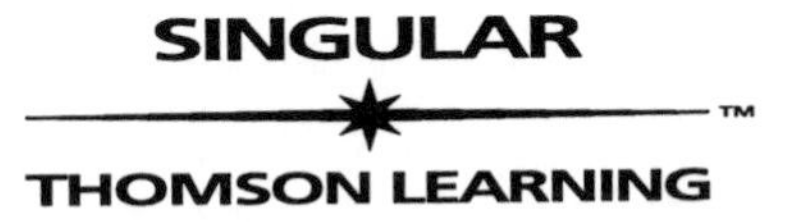

Africa • Australia • Canada • Denmark • Japan • Mexico • New Zealand • Philippines
Puerto Rico • Singapore • Spain • United Kingdom • United States

MW

NOTICE TO THE READER

Publisher does not warrant or guarantee any of the products described herein or perform any independent analysis in connection with any of the product information contained herein. Publisher does not assume, and expressly disclaims, any obligation to obtain and include information other than that provided to it by the manufacturer.

The reader is expressly warned to consider and adopt all safety precautions that might be indicated by the activities herein and to avoid all potential hazards. By following the instructions contained herein, the reader willingly assumes all risks in connection with such instructions.

The Publisher makes no representation or warranties of any kind, including but not limited to, the warranties of fitness for particular purpose or merchantability, nor are any such representations implied with respect to the material set forth herein, and the publisher takes no responsibility with respect to such material. The publisher shall not be liable for any special, consequential, or exemplary damages resulting, in whole or part, from the readers' use of, or reliance upon, this material.

Printed in the Canada
2 3 4 5 6 XXX 03 02 01

For more information, contact Singular Publishing Group, 401 West "A" Street, Suite 325 San Diego, CA 92101-7904; or find us on the World Wide Web at http://www.singpub.com

Library of Congress Cataloging-in-Publication Data:

Goldsworthy, Candace L.
Sourcebook of phonological awareness activities: children's core literature/ Candace L. Goldsworthy.
p. cm.
ISBN 0-7693-0090-1
1. Reading disability. 2. Reading—Remedial teaching. 3. English language—Phonetics—Study and teaching (Preschool). 4. English language—Phonetics—Study and teaching (Elementary). 5. Speech therapy for children. 6. Language acquisition. I. Title.
[DNLM: 1. Speech Therapy—methods. 2. Phonetics. 3. Awareness. 4. Literature. WL 340.2 G624s 1998]
LB1050.5.G66 1998
371.91'44—dc21
DNLM/DLC
for Library of Congress 98-18159
CIP

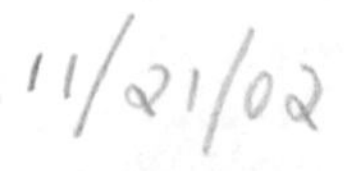

CONTENTS

PREFACE

It's been almost 20 years since I presented my first workshop on the role of the speech-language specialist in developmental reading problems. At that time I was convinced that speech-language specialists had a role in working with these students, but I had not yet clearly defined the role in my mind. The more I worked with students and their families, the more convinced I became that speech-language specialists can contribute immeasurably to the team of professionals working with students who have reading problems. Over the years, my earlier "hunch" was increasingly validated primarily because of the following:

- Research continued to demonstrate that written language problems stem from earlier oral language problems.
- Evidence emerged from speech-language specialists showing that many preschool and kindergarten children with oral language impairment were dismissed from speech therapy caseloads after reaching their targeted oral language goals, only to be *relabeled* later as reading disabled.
- The increasing numbers of students not identified as having early oral language problems but presenting reading, writing, and spelling problems in second, third, and fourth grades. These students fell through the cracks because their early symptoms were not severe enough for them to qualify for remedial/tutorial services.
- The identification of phonological awareness as critical to successful acquisition of reading and spelling.

In *Developmental Reading Disabilities: A Language Based Treatment Approach* (Goldsworthy, 1996), a rationale for the speech-language specialists' role in assessing and treating developmental reading problems is presented. Included in that text is a suggested hierarchical phonological awareness training program, beginning with the word level, then transitioning to the syllable level and finally to the phoneme level. The primary purpose of phonological awareness training is to anchor children in the sound system of English to help get students ready to map the graphemic system onto a phonological system, a necessary step for successful reading acquisition.

One source of effective phonological awareness training materials should include activities with vocabulary from books that children may be hearing read to them or that they are reading in their homes or classrooms. To that end, the *Sourcebook of Phonological Awareness Training: Children's Classic Literature* (Goldsworthy, 1998) and now this *Sourcebook of Phonological Awareness Training: Children's Core Literature* include numerous phonological awareness activities integrating the language of children's classic and core literature. Vocabulary from these rich literature sources was selected for use with phonological awareness activities at the word, syllable, and phoneme levels. These materials are intended for use with preschool and elementary-aged children to facilitate their journey into reading acquisition. My hope is that these books will provide a rich source of phonological awareness training materials for teachers, speech-language specialists, reading specialists, resource specialists, parents, grandparents, and other individuals working with children.

ACKNOWLEDGMENTS

Many valuable suggestions have been given to me over the past few years as to what works in therapy rooms and classrooms as we work together with children needing phonological awareness training. I thank my friends, colleagues, and the clients I work with for specific suggestions on how to modify the activities included in this book. Thanks also to friends who make suggestions on which books to include and willingly loan their books, especially Margaret Addicott. And to Stacey Jorgensen, my sincerest thanks. I would not have met deadline without your data input.

CHAPTER

INTRODUCTION

In the past 5 years, the term "phonological awareness" has become a household term. *Sourcebook of Phonological Awareness Activities: Children's Classic Literature* (Goldsworthy, 1998) was written to provide materials for use in phonological awareness training. The response to the phonological awareness sourcebook VOL. I has been so positive that soon after its release the next step became quite clear. Write another one! *Sourcebook of Phonological Awareness Activities Volume II: Children's Core Literature* was written in response to the ever-increasing demand for more training materials. Like the first phonological awareness sourcebook, the intent of Volume II is to provide innovative materials linked to children's literature rather than to provide decontextualized materials with no relevance to literature children are reading or that is read to them.

Books included in Sourcebook II are *Blueberries for Sal, Corduroy, Happy Birthday, Moon, Harry and the Terrible Whatzit, Harry the Dirty Dog, Stone Soup, The Hungry Thing, The Little Red Hen, The Three Little Pigs, The Snowy Day,* and *The Very Hungry Caterpillar.* These books were selected because they are on a number of core reading lists for children in preschool through third grade. Furthermore, a variety of various children's authors is expected to be more useful to parents and educators than the work of just one author. Based on positive feedback from readers of the earlier book, the following sections modified for inclusion in this book are:

- Phonological awareness definitions
- Linkage between phonological awareness and reading
- Phonological awareness skill development

WHAT IS PHONOLOGICAL AWARENESS?

In their text on applied phonology, Hodson and Edwards (1997) defined the terms:

phonological processing: using phonological information to process oral and written language.

phonological representation: stored knowledge about what a word sounds like (sufficient to recognize it when heard) and how to discriminate it from similar sounding words.

phonological processing difficulties: problems with phonological input (auditory processing), lexical representation, and/or phonological output speech.

phonological deviations: broad simplifications (e.g., stopping, cluster reduction) that adversely affect intelligibility (p. 230).

Stackhouse (1997) defined ***phonological awareness*** as "the ability to reflect on and manipulate the structure of an utterance (e.g., into words, syllables, or sounds) as distinct from its meaning" (p. 157). Snow, Burns, and Griffin (1998) explained that, when this awareness extends to understanding that words can be divided into a sequence of phonemes, "this finer-grained sensitivity is termed ***phonemic awareness***" (p. 51).

WHAT IS THE LINK BETWEEN PHONOLOGICAL AWARENESS AND READING?

During the development of speech, a child progresses through a series of stages. Articulatory gestures become integrated into automatic phonetic routines as the child practices producing speech (Stackhouse, 1997). Consequently, the phonologic code becomes a more efficient means for encoding and retrieving structures in verbal working memory. As phonemes begin to emerge as definite forms, the child becomes aware of them as structures in and of themselves. Becoming aware of these structures is critical for the language learner to develop strong, efficient phonological representations. A child comes to appreciate that phonemes can be "played with" as if they were mental toys. Words can be broken into parts; syllables and sounds within syllables can be added, deleted, and/or moved around in words. Becoming aware of phonemes-as-structures provides a solid foundation onto which a language learner can build. That is, the learner can add another layer of language, namely, a visual representation. A strongly stored phonological system allows a novice reader to have a much easier time mapping a visual, graphemic system onto it. Stated differently, the phonological code forms the foundation onto which the graphemic system will be laid. Phonological processing should naturally lead the way to phonological awareness with the child's exposure to print facilitating this developing phonological awareness. Frith (1986) maintained that the more proficient the novice reader is at accessing stored phonological word representations, the easier it is for that reader to isolate individual phonemes. This, in turn, helps the reader learn to "crack the code" between phonemes and graphemes, the "core subskill in learning to read" (Farnham-Diggory, 1990). Moats, Furry, and Brownell (1998) cited reviews documenting phonological awareness as "the best predictor of learning to read in English between kindergarten and second grade" (p. 21). According to Moats et al. (1998), phonological awareness is unrelated to intelligence or listening comprehension—that is, children at any level of intelligence and/or listening comprehension may have difficulty with phonological awareness. According to the primary literacy standards (1999) of the National Center on Education and the Economy, "children who readily develop phonemic awareness in kindergarten probably will learn to read easily" (p. 52).

PHONOLOGICAL AWARENESS SKILL DEVELOPMENT

Lance, Swanson, and Peterson (1997) explained that because phonological awareness involves numerous cognitive abilities related to the child's understanding of the segmental nature of English, "several different levels of phonological knowledge exist (i.e., synthesis, analysis, implicit, and explicit), and different tasks are employed to assess phonological awareness on different levels, e.g., phoneme blending, phoneme segmentation, phoneme deletion, multisyllabic word production, etc." (p. 1002).

Signs of emerging phonological awareness appear during the preschool years in most normally developing children. According to Snow et al. (1998), even 2- and 3-year-olds occasionally correct speech errors and "play" with speech sounds, "e.g., 'pancakes, cancakes, canpakes'" (p. 51). Perfetti (1991), Goldsworthy (1996), Stackhouse (1997), Snow et al. (1998), and Moats et al. (1998) have presented developmental perspectives for the emergence of phonological awareness skills in children. The following list provides current information about developmental progression of phonological awareness.

At 3 years of age, children are usually able to:

- Recognize that two words rhyme (emerging) (Snow et al., 1998).
- Recognize alliteration (words beginning with the same first sound), such as, "Mommy, Michele, they're the same."
- Recite known rhymes, for example, Jack and Jill (Moats et al., 1998).
- Produce rhyme by pattern, for example, give the word "cat" as a rhyming word for "hat."

At 4 years of age, children are usually able to:

- Segment syllables, such as, know there are two parts to the word "cowboy."
- Count the number of syllables in words (50% of 4-year-olds can do this) (Moats et al., 1998).

At 5 years of age, children are usually able to:

- Count syllables in words (90% of 5-year-olds can do this) (Moats et al., 1998).
- Count phonemes within words (less than 50% of 5-year-olds can do this) (Moats et al., 1998).

At 6 years of age, children are usually able to:

- Match initial consonants in words, such as recognize that "shoe" and "sheep" begin with the same first sound.

- Blend two-to-three phonemes, for example, recognize that the sounds /d/ /o/ /g/ form the word "dog."
- Count phonemes within words (70% of 6-year-olds can do this) (Moats et al., 1998).
- Divide words by onset (first consonant or blend) and rime (rest of the word), for example, can divide the word "stop" into /st/ /op/.

At 7 years of age, children are usually able to:

- Blend phonemes to form words.
- Segment three-to-four phonemes within words.
- Spell phonetically.
- Delete phonemes from words, such as, omit the /t/ sound in the word "cat."

The primary literacy standards (1999) of the National Center on Education and the Economy suggest that specific phonemic awareness goals be met by the end of kindergarten:

- Produce rhyming words.
- Recognize pairs of rhyming words.
- Isolate initial consonants in single-syllable words, for example, /t/ is the first sound in "top."
- Identify the onset (speech sounds before a vowel) and rime (vowel and what follows) in a one-syllable word, for example, /k/ is the onset and (-at) is the rime in the word "cat."
- Begin to fully segment sounds in a one-syllable word, such as /k/ /a/ /t/.
- Blend onsets /k/ and rimes (-at) to form words (cat).
- Begin to blend separate spoken phonemes (sounds) into one-syllable words, for example, /k/ /a/ /t/ is "cat" (p. 54).

The same primary literacy standards (1999) suggest that specific phonemic awareness goals be met by the end of first grade:

- Segment the sounds in a word by saying each sound aloud, for example, /k/ /a/ /t/.
- Blend separated spoken phonemes (sounds) into meaningful words (p. 96).
- The standards specifically state that "by the end of the year, first-grade students' phonemic awareness should be consolidated fully. They should be able to demonstrate, without difficulty, all the skills and knowledge expected at the end of kindergarten" (p. 96).

The California State Department of Education language arts content standards (1998) suggest specific phonemic awareness goals for kindergarten:

1.7. Track (move sequentially from sound to sound) and represent the number, sameness/difference, and order of two and three isolated phonemes (e.g., /f, s, th/, /j, d, j/).

1.8. Track (move sequentially from sound to sound) and represent changes in simple syllables and words with two and three sounds as one sound is added, substituted, omitted, shifted, or repeated (vowel-consonant, consonant-vowel, or consonant-vowel-consonant)
1.9. Blend vowel–consonant sounds orally to make words or syllables.
1.10. Identify and produce rhyming words in response to an oral prompt.
1.11. Distinguish orally stated one-syllable words and separate into beginning or ending sounds.
1.12. Track auditorily each word in a sentence and each syllable in a word.
1.13. Count the number of sounds in syllables and syllables in words.

The California State Department of Education language arts content standards (1998) suggest specific phonemic awareness goals for first grade:

1.4. Distinguish initial, medial, and final sounds in single-syllable words.
1.5. Distinguish long and short vowel sounds in orally stated single-syllable words (bit/bite).
1.6. Create and state a series of rhyming words, including consonant blends.
1.7. Add, delete, or change target sounds in order to change words (e.g., change cow to how; pan to an).
1.8. Blend two-to-four phonemes into a recognizable word (e.g., /c/a/t/ = cat; /f/l/a/t/ = flat).
1.9. Segment single-syllable words into their components (e.g., /c/a/t/ = cat; /s/p/l/a/t/ = splat; /r/i/ch/ = rich) (p. 86).

The remainder of this book has been organized for maximum usefulness. Chapter 2 provides suggested teaching instructions and correction procedures. Chapters 3–13 offer phonological awareness activities for the children's books featured in this volume. An appendix for suggested record keeping is at the end of the book.

CHAPTER 2

HOW THE MATERIALS ARE ARRANGED

From the activities suggested in *Developmental Reading Disabilities: A Language Based Treatment Approach* (Goldsworthy, 1996), 36 were selected for use in this book. Five activities are at the **word** level, 6 at the **syllable** level, and 25 at the **phoneme** level. Because there is a developmental progression of phonological awareness activities, users are encouraged to begin with the word level if the student needs to begin there and progress to the syllable and finally to the phoneme level. Activities included in each of the three levels have been arranged according to difficulty. For instance, some of the activities included at the **phoneme** level include lower level activities such as rhyming in patterns to higher, more explicit level activities, including providing initial and final sounds in words, segmenting sounds in syllables, replacing sounds within words, phoneme switching (switching the first two phonemes in words, such as, "feed me" becomes "meed fee"), and finally pig latin. It is suggested that a user begin with the first activity level under each category and move through the activities in the suggested sequence. However, as with other developmental sequences, children will vary in their acquisition of phonological awareness and consequently demonstrate skills for more difficult activities and have problems with what are considered more basic activities. Phonological awareness activities included in *Volume II* are listed below. Individual speech sounds, not alphabet letters, are placed between / /. Because phonetic notation is not generally used in this book, most vowel sounds are described as long or short for example, /long A/, /short U/. The user should pronounce the vowel sound and not describe, such as, don't say "long A," or "short U." Rather, provide the actual sounds.

PHONOLOGICAL AWARENESS ACTIVITIES AT THE WORD LEVEL

1. Counting words.

What to say to the student: "We're going to count words."
EXAMPLE: "How many words do you hear in this sentence (or phrase)? 'her bear.'" (2)

2. Identifying missing word from list.

What to say to the student: "Listen to the words I say. I'll say them again. You tell me which word I leave out."
EXAMPLE: "Listen to the words I say: 'tin, crow, pail.' I'll say them again. Tell me which one I leave out: 'tin, pail.'" (crow)

3. Identifying missing word in phrase or sentence.

What to say to the student: "Listen to the sentence I read. Tell me which word is missing the second time I read the sentence."
EXAMPLE: "' He was a big fat caterpillar.' Listen again and tell me which word I leave out. 'He was a big fat ____ .'" (caterpillar)

4. Supplying missing word as adult reads.

What to say to the student: "I want you to help me read the story. You fill in the words I leave out."
EXAMPLE: "Blueberries for ____." (Sal)

5. Rearranging words.

What to say to the student: "I'll say some words out of order. You put them in the right order so they make sense."
EXAMPLE: "'size right.' Put those words in the right order." (right size)

PHONOLOGICAL AWARENESS ACTIVITIES AT THE SYLLABLE LEVEL

1. Syllable counting.

What to say to the student: "We're going to count syllables (or parts) of words."
EXAMPLE: "How many syllables do you hear in '_____'?" (stimulus word) (e.g., "How many syllables in 'bear'?") (1)

2. Initial syllable deleting.

What to say to the student: "We're going to leave out syllables (or parts of words)."
EXAMPLE: "Say '_____.'" (stimulus word) "Say it again without '_____.'" (stimulus syllable) (e.g., "Say 'mouthful' without 'mouth.'") (ful)

3. Final syllable deleting.

What to say to the student: "We're going to leave out syllables (or parts of words)."
EXAMPLE: "Say '_____.'" (stimulus word) "Say it again without '_____.'" (stimulus syllable) (e.g., "Say 'around' without 'round.'") (a)

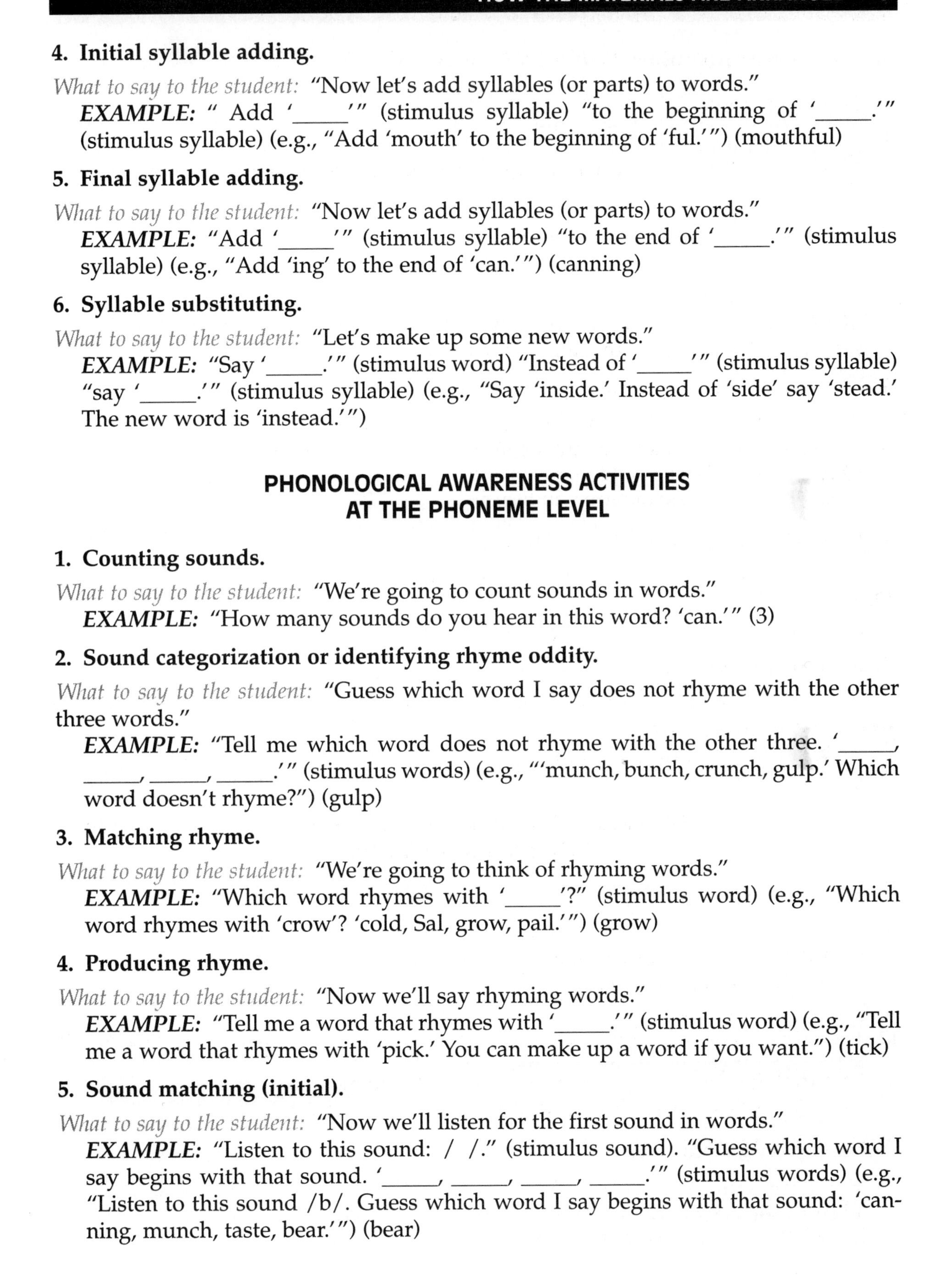

4. Initial syllable adding.

What to say to the student: "Now let's add syllables (or parts) to words."

EXAMPLE: " Add '_____'" (stimulus syllable) "to the beginning of '_____.'" (stimulus syllable) (e.g., "Add 'mouth' to the beginning of 'ful.'") (mouthful)

5. Final syllable adding.

What to say to the student: "Now let's add syllables (or parts) to words."

EXAMPLE: "Add '_____'" (stimulus syllable) "to the end of '_____.'" (stimulus syllable) (e.g., "Add 'ing' to the end of 'can.'") (canning)

6. Syllable substituting.

What to say to the student: "Let's make up some new words."

EXAMPLE: "Say '_____.'" (stimulus word) "Instead of '_____'" (stimulus syllable) "say '_____.'" (stimulus syllable) (e.g., "Say 'inside.' Instead of 'side' say 'stead.' The new word is 'instead.'")

PHONOLOGICAL AWARENESS ACTIVITIES AT THE PHONEME LEVEL

1. Counting sounds.

What to say to the student: "We're going to count sounds in words."

EXAMPLE: "How many sounds do you hear in this word? 'can.'" (3)

2. Sound categorization or identifying rhyme oddity.

What to say to the student: "Guess which word I say does not rhyme with the other three words."

EXAMPLE: "Tell me which word does not rhyme with the other three. '_____, _____, _____, _____.'" (stimulus words) (e.g., "'munch, bunch, crunch, gulp.' Which word doesn't rhyme?") (gulp)

3. Matching rhyme.

What to say to the student: "We're going to think of rhyming words."

EXAMPLE: "Which word rhymes with '_____'?" (stimulus word) (e.g., "Which word rhymes with 'crow'? 'cold, Sal, grow, pail.'") (grow)

4. Producing rhyme.

What to say to the student: "Now we'll say rhyming words."

EXAMPLE: "Tell me a word that rhymes with '_____.'" (stimulus word) (e.g., "Tell me a word that rhymes with 'pick.' You can make up a word if you want.") (tick)

5. Sound matching (initial).

What to say to the student: "Now we'll listen for the first sound in words."

EXAMPLE: "Listen to this sound: / /." (stimulus sound). "Guess which word I say begins with that sound. '_____, _____, _____, _____.'" (stimulus words) (e.g., "Listen to this sound /b/. Guess which word I say begins with that sound: 'canning, munch, taste, bear.'") (bear)

6. Sound matching (final).

What to say to the student: "Now we'll listen for the last sound in words."

EXAMPLE: "Listen to this sound: / /" (stimulus sound). "Guess which word I say ends with that sound. '_____, _____, _____, _____.'" (stimulus words) (e.g., "Listen to this sound /n/. Guess which word I say ends with that sound: 'berry, tin, with, pail.'") (tin)

7. Identifying initial sound in words.

What to say to the student: "I'll say a word two times. Tell me what sound is missing. '_____, _______.'" (stimulus words)

EXAMPLE: "What sound do you hear in '_____'" (stimulus word) "that is missing in '_____'?" (stimulus word) (e.g., "What sound do you hear in 'time,' that is missing in 'I'm'?") (/t/)

8. Identifying final sound in words.

What to say to the student: "I'll say a word two times. Tell me what sound is missing. '______,' '_______.'" (stimulus words)

EXAMPLE: "What sound do you hear in '_____'" (stimulus word) "that is missing in '_____'?" (stimulus word) (e.g., "What sound do you hear in 'time,' that is missing in 'tie'?") (/m/)

9. Segmenting initial sound in words.

What to say to the student: "Listen to the word I say and tell me the first sound you hear."

EXAMPLE: "What's the first sound in '_____'?" (stimulus word) (e.g., "What's the first sound in 'berry'?" (/b/)

10. Segmenting final sound in words.

What to say to the student: "Listen to the word I say and tell me the last sound you hear."

EXAMPLE: "What's the last sound in the word '_____'?" (stimulus word) (e.g., "What's the last sound in the word 'took'?") (/k/)

11. Generating words from the story beginning with a particular sound.

What to say to the student: "Let's think of words from the story that start with certain sounds."

EXAMPLE: "Tell me a word from the story that starts with / /." (stimulus sound) (e.g., "the sound /p/.") (partridge)

12. Blending sounds in monosyllabic words divided into onset-rime beginning with two consonant cluster + rime.

What to say to the student: "Now we'll put sounds together to make words."

EXAMPLE: "Put these sounds together to make a word (/ / + / /)." (stimulus sounds) "What's the word?" (e.g., "gr + ow: What's the word?") (grow)

13. Blending sounds in monosyllabic words divided into onset-rime beginning with single consonant + rime.

What to say to the student: "Let's put sounds together to make words."

EXAMPLE: "Put these sounds together to make a word (/ / + / /)." (stimulus sounds) "What's the word?" (e.g., "/d/ + ay: what's the word?") (day)

14. Blending sounds to form a monosyllabic word beginning with a continuant sound.

What to say to the student: "We'll put sounds together to make words."
EXAMPLE: "Put these sounds together to make a word (/ / + / / + / /)." (stimulus sounds) (e.g., "/m/ /long A/ /k/.") (make)

15. Blending sounds to form a monosyllabic word beginning with a noncontinuant sound.

What to say to the student: "We'll put sounds together to make words."
EXAMPLE: "Put these sounds together to make a word (/ / + / / + / /)." (stimulus sounds) (e.g., "/p/ /long A/ /l/.") (pail)

16. Substituting initial sound in words.

What to say to the student: "We're going to change the beginning/first sound in words."
EXAMPLE: "Say '_____.'" (stimulus word) "Instead of / /" (stimulus sound) "say / /." (stimulus sound) (e.g., "Say 'bear.' Instead of /b/ say /ch/. What's your new word?") (chair)

17. Substituting final sound in words.

What to say to the student: "We're going to change the ending/last sound in words."
EXAMPLE: "Say '_____.'" (stimulus word) "Instead of / /" (stimulus sound) "say / /." (stimulus sound) (e.g., "Say 'ate.' Instead of /t/ say /m/. What's your new word?") (aim)

18. Segmenting middle sound in monosyllabic words.

What to say to the student: "Tell me the middle sound in the word I say."
EXAMPLE: "What's the middle sound in the word '_____'?" (stimulus word) (e.g., "What's the middle sound in the word 'feet'?") (/long E/)

19. Substituting middle sound in words.

What to say to the student: "We're going to change the middle sound in words."
EXAMPLE: "Say '_____.'" (stimulus word) "Instead of / /" (stimulus sound) "say / /." (stimulus sound) (e.g., "Say 'Sal.' Instead of /short A/ say /long E/. What's your new word?") (seal)

20. Identifying all sounds in monosyllabic words.

What to say to the student: "Now tell me all the sounds you hear in the word I say."
EXAMPLE: "What sounds do you hear in the word '_____'?" (stimulus word) (e.g., "What sounds do you hear in the word 'Sal'?") (/s/ /short A/ /l/)

21. Deleting sounds within words.

What to say to the student: "We're going to leave out sounds in words."
EXAMPLE: "Say '_____'" (stimulus word) "without / /." (stimulus sound) (e.g., "Say 'grains' without /r/.") (gains)

22. Substituting consonant in words having a two-sound cluster.

What to say to the student: "We're going to substitute sounds in words."

EXAMPLE: "Say '_____.'" (stimulus word) "Instead of / /" (stimulus sound) "say / /" (stimulus sound) (e.g., "Say 'climb.' Instead of /l/ say /r/.") (crime)

23. Phoneme reversing.

What to say to the student: "We're going to say words backward."

EXAMPLE: "Say the word '_____'" (stimulus word) "backward." (e.g., "If we say 'gulp' backward, the word is 'plug.'")

24. Phoneme switching.

What to say to the student: "We're going to switch the first sounds in two words."

EXAMPLE: "Switch the first sounds in '_____' and '_____.'" (stimulus words) (e.g., "Switch the first sounds in 'sat down.'") (dat sown)

25. Pig latin.

What to say to the student: "We're going to talk in a secret language using words from the story. In pig latin, you take off the first sound of a word, put it at the end of the word, and add a long A sound."

EXAMPLE: "Say 'moon' in pig latin." (oonmay)

As mentioned in Chapter 1, the intent of the materials in this book is to promote phonological awareness activities by incorporating the richness of children's literature. To that end, 11 children's books were selected for use: *Blueberries for Sal; Corduroy; Happy Birthday, Moon; Harry and the Terrible Whatzi; Harry the Dirty Dog; Stone Soup; The Hungry Thing; The Little Red Hen; The Three Little Pigs; The Snowy Day;* and *The Very Hungry Caterpillar*. Vocabulary was selected from these stories and used as stimulus items. Each of the 36 activities is repeated for all 11 stories, but individualized with the vocabulary specific to each story. The purpose is twofold: to integrate phonological awareness activities into children's literature and to acquaint students with the vocabulary of these classic tales. Because the selected activities represent many critical word-, syllable-, and phoneme-level phonological awareness abilities, the redundancy of their inclusion for each story is believed to be important. As students become familiar with what is being requested, for example, "Now let's leave one syllable out of words," their phonological awareness abilities will be strengthened as they simultaneously enjoy the stories and learn new vocabulary and semantic-syntactic constructions. One version of each child's book was used for vocabulary sources. Users of this book are encouraged to use the vocabulary from these versions or integrate vocabulary from other story versions into activities included in this book.

WHAT IS INCLUDED IN EACH ACTIVITY

Four items are included in each of the 36 activities.

1. **What to say to the student and an example.** For instance, Activity 1: Counting Words under Phonological Awareness Activities at the Word Level for *Harry the Dirty Dog*:

What to say to the student: "We're going to count words."
EXAMPLE: "How many words do you hear in this sentence (or phrase)? 'He played tag.'"

2. **The correct answer in parentheses: (3)**
3. **A NOTE for suggested use:**

> **NOTE:** *Use pictured items and/or manipulatives if necessary. Use any of the following stimulus phrases or sentences and/or others you select from the story. Correct answers are in parentheses.*

4. **Ten stimulus items with correct answers in parentheses:**

Stimulus items:

piggy bank (2)
he played dead (3)
he slid down (3)
Harry wagged his tail (4)
white dog with black spots (5)
scrub brush (2)
a white dog (3)
he ran back home (4)
he took the brush (4)
up the stairs he dashed (5)

HOW TO USE THESE MATERIALS

It is recommended that materials be coordinated with corresponding activities of parents and/or teachers. For instance, a unit that includes *Blueberries for Sal* might be selected and introduced, with the parent or teacher reading aloud either the version suggested for use with this sourcebook or another edition. It is recommended that the story be read to and discussed with students at least three times and that the students be able to retell the story in sequence. Younger children are not expected to retell the story with as much detail as older students. Language activities, such as flannel board presentations and hand puppet role plays, can be used to facilitate a student's use of vocabulary in the stories before introducing the corresponding phonological awareness activities.

Ten examples are provided for each of the 36 activities. Many more examples can be added per activity by employing different vocabulary words from each story. The number 10 was selected for ease in computing percent accuracy of a student's responses. It is usually assumed that if a student demonstrates proficiency with a language activity at the 80% accuracy level during two consecutive days, the student has mastered that particular step. For accurate determination of a student's progress at a certain level and also for accurate ongoing outcome performance data, 10 examples per activity was believed to be a clinically sound number.

SUGGESTED TEACHING STEPS AND CORRECTION PROCEDURES

The following suggestions are provided for use in introducing activities and in correcting student errors. These suggestions are meant as general guidelines. The user is encouraged to move through the sequence of teaching and/or correction steps in the order in which they are presented here. Please add other teaching/correction steps that you find useful with your students. The suggested teaching steps and correction procedures are only outlined here and are not repeated with the corresponding activities in the rest of the book. Users are encouraged to review this section before introducing activities.

PHONOLOGICAL AWARENESS ACTIVITIES AT THE WORD LEVEL

1. Counting words.

What to say to the student: "We're going to count words."

EXAMPLE: "How many words do you hear in this sentence (or phrase)? 'He played tag.'" (3)

TEACHING STEPS:

1. Place manipulatives or pictured items from the book in front of the student. For instance, put 1 wooden block or plastic chip in front of the student and say: "This stands for a word. I'll say the word 'dog,' and you point to the block/chip and tell me how many words you hear."
2. Repeat Step 1 with pictured objects from the story, such as pictures of a pail and a bear from *Blueberries for Sal.* Point to the pictured pail and say "pail." Point to the pictured bear and say "bear." Then point to the pictured pail and say "one," then to the pictured bear and say "two. There are two words."
3. Repeat Step 2 without pictures.
4. If the student is correct, reinforce by saying: "Good, you counted the words."
5. Repeat Steps 2–4 with 3, 4, and 5 words.

CORRECTION PROCEDURES:

1. If unable to do this activity with manipulatives or pictures from the story, the student may need more experience with counting in sequence and one-to-one correspondence. This may be achieved by providing many instances of placing 1, 2, and 3 blocks in front of the student. Ask the student to touch each block as you say "block"(using 1 block), or "block, block" (using 2 blocks), or "block, block, block" (using 3 blocks).
2. Ask the student to point to each block again and to count "1," or "1, 2," or "1, 2, 3." In each instance, ask the student "how many words?"
3. If the student is correct, reinforce by saying: "Good, you counted the words."
4. If the student is incorrect, provide more experiences with counting and provide the written number symbol above the objects to help the student

keep the correct number in memory while responding to your question: "How many words?"

5. Repeat Steps 1–3 with pictured objects.
6. Repeat Steps 1–3 with 4 and 5 objects.
7. Repeat activity without manipulatives.

2. Identifying missing word from list.

What to say to the student: "Listen to the words I say. I'll say them again. You tell me which word I leave out."

EXAMPLE: "Listen to the words I say: 'tub, dirty, house.' I'll say them again. Tell me which one I leave out: 'tub, house.'" (dirty)

TEACHING STEPS:

1. Place 2 pictures in front of the student (e.g., girl and wolf.) Say: "I'll say two words: 'girl, wolf.'"
2. Say: "Now I'll leave one word out." Remove the pictured 'girl.' Say: "Guess which one I leave out: 'wolf.' Which word is missing?" (girl).
3. If the student is correct, reinforce by saying: "Nice job, you told me which word is missing."
4. Repeat activity without manipulatives.

CORRECTION PROCEDURES:

1. If unable to do this activity with manipulatives from the story, the student may need instruction on dealing with "what's missing" before this activity. This can be achieved by placing an object in front of the student. Request that the object be named. Remove the object saying: "(object name) is missing." Immediately ask the student to name the missing object.
2. Repeat Step 1 with different objects.
3. Now place 1 red block and 1 blue block in front of the student and say: "I'll say two words: 'red' and 'blue.'" Point to each block as you say each word.
4. Say: "Now I'll leave one word out." Take away the red block. Say: "Guess which one I leave out: 'blue.' Which word is missing?" (red).
5. Repeat Steps 3–4 using 2 different colored blocks in each example. Vary which block you remove, that is, one time take away the first block and the next time the second block.
6. If the student is correct, reinforce by saying: "Good, you told me which word is missing."
7. Repeat activity without manipulatives (i.e., with words only).

3. Identifying missing word in phrase or sentence.

What to say to the student: "Listen to the sentence I read. Tell me which word is missing the second time I read the sentence."

EXAMPLE: "'He felt tired.' Listen again and tell me which word I leave out. 'He felt ___.'" (tired)

TEACHING STEPS:

1. Place 2 manipulatives (e.g., 2 red wooden blocks) in front of the student.
2. Point to the block on the student's left and say "red."
3. Point to the block on the student's right and say "block."
4. Point to the first block saying "red." Point to the second block and ask: "What word goes with this one?" (block)
5. If the student is correct, reinforce by saying: "OK. You told me the word I left out, the one that is missing."
6. Repeat activity with 3, 4, and 5 blocks and words.
7. Repeat activity without manipulatives.

CORRECTION PROCEDURES:

1. Place 2 objects in front of the student (e.g., a toy car and a toy cat).
2. Remove 1 object (car).
3. Point to the cat and say "car is missing."
4. Ask the student: "Which one is missing?"
5. If the student is correct, reinforce by saying: "Right. You told me which word is missing."
6. Place 1 red block and 1 blue block in front of the student and say: "These blocks stand for words." Point to the red block and say "red;" point to the blue block as you say "blue."
7. Ask the student to point to the first block as you say "red." Ask the student to point to the second block as you say "blue."
8. Point to the first block and ask the student: "What word is this?" (red) Point to the second block and ask the student: "What word is this?" (blue)
9. Say: "I'm only going to say one of the words. You tell me the word that's missing." Point to the red block and say "red." Point to the blue block and ask: "What's this one?" (blue)
10. If the student answers correctly, reinforce by saying: "Right. You said 'blue.' You told me the missing word."
11. If the student answers incorrectly, go through Steps 6–10 with additional examples of 2 blocks or toys.
12. Repeat activity without manipulatives.

4. Supplying missing word as adult reads.

What to say to the student: "I want you to help me read the story. You fill in the words I leave out."

EXAMPLE: "I've always wanted to climb a _____." (mountain)

TEACHING STEPS:

1. Place 2 objects (e.g., cup and shoe) in front of the student. Point to the cup and say "cup." Point to the shoe and say "shoe."
2. Remove the shoe. Point to the cup saying: "cup." Point to where the shoe had been and say "shoe."

3. Repeat Step 2 but after pointing to where the shoe was ask: "What word was this?"
4. Repeat Steps 1–3 with different sets of 2 objects.
5. If the student answers correctly, reinforce by saying: "Nice work, you told me which word is missing."
6. Repeat activity without manipulatives.

CORRECTION PROCEDURES:

1. Place 2 red blocks in front of the student and say: "These blocks stand for words." Point to the first block as you say "red" and point to the second block as you say "block."
2. Ask the student to point to the first block as you say "red." Ask the student to point to the second block as you say "block."
3. Point to the first block and ask the student: "What word is this?" (red) Repeat with the second block. (block)
4. Now tell the student: "I'm only going to say one of the words. You tell me the word that's missing." Point to the first block and say "red." Point to the second block and ask: "What's this one?" (block)
5. If the student answers correctly, reinforce by saying: "Right. You said 'block.' You told me the word I left out, the missing word."
6. If the student answers incorrectly, repeat Steps 1–5 with 2 yellow blocks or toy objects, or 2 blue blocks or toy objects, or 2 green blocks or toy objects.
7. Repeat activity without manipulatives.

5. Rearranging words.

What to say to the student: "I'll say some words out of order. You put them in the right order so that they make sense."

EXAMPLE: "'bank piggy.' Put those words in the right order." (piggy bank)

TEACHING STEPS:

1. Place 2 objects (e.g., key and book in front of the student, with the key on the student's left and the book on the right). Point to the key and say: "key"; point to the book and say: "book."
2. Switch the objects so the book is to the student's left side and the key to the student's right side. Point to the book and say, "book." Point to key and say: "key. I switched the words around. First it was 'key, book,' now it's 'book, key.'"
3. Repeat Steps 1–2 with different sets of two objects or pictures.
4. Repeat activity without manipulatives.
5. If the student answers correctly, reinforce by saying: "Right, you put the words in the right order. Now they make sense."

CORRECTION PROCEDURES:

1. Place 2 objects (e.g., key and book in front of the student, with the key on the student's left and the book on the right). Point to the key and say,

"key"; point to the book and say, "book." Ask the student to name each object.

2. Ask the student to switch the objects around, so the book is to the student's left and the key is to the student's right side.
3. Point to the book asking the student to name it. Point to the key asking the student to name it. Then say: "You switched the words around. First it was 'key, book'; now it's 'book, key.'"
4. Repeat Steps 1–4 with different sets of 2 objects or pictures.
5. Repeat activity without manipulatives. Say 2 words of a familiar phrase (e.g., "Santa Claus"). Then say: "If I switch those words around it's 'Claus Santa.'"
6. Repeat Step 5 with another familiar phrase (e.g., "Birthday Happy"). Ask the student to "put the words in the right order."
7. If the student answers correctly, reinforce by saying: "Good. You're switching the words around so they make sense."

PHONOLOGICAL AWARENESS ACTIVITIES AT THE SYLLABLE LEVEL

1. Syllable counting.

What to say to the student: "We're going to count syllables (or parts) of words."

EXAMPLE: "How many syllables do you hear in 'noodles'?" (2)

TEACHING STEPS:

1. Place 1 wooden block or plastic chip in front of the student.
2. Point to the block/chip saying: "This stands for a word. I'll say the word 'dog,' and you point to the block/chip and tell me how many parts you hear."
3. If the student is correct, reinforce by saying: "Yes, you told me that there is 1 part or syllable."
4. Place 2 blocks/chips in front of the student and say: "These stand for two word parts, or syllables. Listen, 'dog—ee,'" pointing to the first block/chip as you say 'dog,' and to the second block/chip as you say 'ee.' There are two parts, or syllables."
5. Say: "I'll say 'dog,' and you point to the block and say 'one.' Then I'll say 'ee,' and you point to the second block and say 'two.' How many syllables in 'doggy'?"
6. If the student is correct, reinforce by saying: "Yes, you told me that there are 2 parts, or syllables."
7. Repeat activity without manipulatives.

CORRECTION PROCEDURES:

1. Show the student how some things are parts of a whole. For instance, using a child's puzzle, have the student remove 1 piece as you say: "That is

one part of the puzzle." Repeat this step several times with the puzzle. Then explain that a syllable is a part of a word, as a puzzle piece is part of the puzzle.

2. Place 2 pictures (representing the 2 parts of a compound word) in front of the student, such as cup and cake.
3. Write the number 1 below the pictured cup and the number 2 below the pictured cake. Then say: "There are two syllables in the word 'cupcake.'" Ask the student: "How many syllables in the word 'cupcake'?"
4. If the student answers correctly, reinforce by saying: "Good, you counted the syllables."
5. Repeat Steps 2–4 with additional compound words and pictures.
6. Repeat Steps 2–4 with 3- and 4-syllable words.
7. Repeat Steps 2–4 without pictured items.
8. Repeat activity without manipulatives.

2. Initial syllable deleting.

What to say to the student: "We're going to leave out syllables (or parts of words)."
EXAMPLE: "Say '_____.'" (stimulus word) "Say it again without '_____.'" (stimulus syllable) (e.g., "Say 'besides.' Say it again without 'be.'") (sides)

TEACHING STEPS:

1. Place 2 pictures, such as cow and boy in front of the student. Point to the pictured cow to the student's left as you say, "cow." Point to the pictured boy to the student's right as you say, "boy."
2. Take the pictured cow away and say: "When I take the word 'cow' away from 'cowboy' the part that's left is 'boy.'"
3. Repeat Steps 1–2 with another compound word and 2 pictures (e.g., cupcake). Take away the pictured cup saying: "Say 'cupcake' without 'cup.' Which part is left?"
4. If the student is correct, reinforce by saying: "Good, you told me 'cake' is left; you told me which syllable is left when you take the first one away."
5. Repeat activity without pictures.

CORRECTION PROCEDURES:

1. Place 2 colored blocks or plastic chips in front of the student (e.g., a green one and a red one). Make sure the color names have only 1 syllable each (e.g., red, brown, green, pink, white, etc.).
2. If you have placed the red block/chip to the left of the student and the blue block/chip to the right of the student, take away the red block and say: "Blue is left."
3. Repeat Steps 1–2. Ask the student: "Which one is left?"
4. If correct, reinforce the student for naming the remaining part, or syllable.
5. Repeat Steps 1–4 a number of times changing the color of the blocks/chips.

6. Repeat activity with 2 small toys (e.g., bus and dog), again making sure that each word's name has only 1 syllable.
7. Repeat activity with pictured compound or words, for example, cupcake, armchair, rainbow, baseball, and so on.
8. Ask the student to take the first part away and "Name the part that's left,"such as "cake," "chair," "bow," "ball," and so on as the student removes each.
9. If the student is correct, reinforce for naming the part or syllable that's left.
10. Repeat activity without manipulatives.

3. Final syllable deleting.

What to say to the student: "We're going to leave out syllables (or parts of words)." ***EXAMPLE:*** "Say '_____.'" (stimulus word) "Say it again without '_____.'" (stimulus syllable) (e.g., "Say 'evening' without '-ing.'") (even)

TEACHING STEPS:

1. Place 2 pictures (e.g., of a cow and a boy) in front of the student. Point to the pictured cow on the student's left as you say, "cow." Point to the pictured boy to the student's right as you say, "boy."
2. Take the pictured boy away and say: "When I take the word 'boy' away from 'cowboy' the part that's left is 'cow.'"
3. Repeat Steps 1–2 with another pictured compound word (e.g., horsefly). Ask the student to "Say 'horsefly' without 'fly.' Which part is left?"
4. If the student is correct, reinforce by saying: "Good, you told me which part, or syllable is left."
5. Repeat activity without manipulatives.

CORRECTION PROCEDURES:

1. Place 2 colored blocks or plastic chips in front of the student, such as a green one and a red one. Make sure the color names have 1 syllable each (e.g., red, brown, green, pink, white, etc.)
2. If you have placed the green block/chip to the left of the student and the red block/chip to the right of the student, take away the red block/chip and say: "When we take red away, green is left."
3. Repeat Steps 1–2. Each time you take away the block/chip on the student's right say: "You tell me which one is left."
4. Repeat Steps 1–3 a number of times changing the color of the blocks/chips.
5. Repeat Steps 1–3 with 2 small toys, such as a bus and a dog, again making sure that each word's name has only 1 syllable.
6. Repeat activity with pictures of compound words (e.g., "cupcake," "armchair," "rainbow," "baseball," etc.)
7. Ask the student to take the last part away and name the syllable that's left (e.g., "cup," "arm," "rain," "base") as each is removed.
8. If correct, reinforce the student for naming the part, or syllable that is left.
9. Repeat activity without manipulatives.

4. Initial syllable adding.

What to say to the student: "Now let's add syllables (or parts) to words."

EXAMPLE: " Add '_____'" (stimulus syllable) "to the beginning of '_____.'" (stimulus syllable) (e.g., "Add 'on' to the beginning of 'to.'") (onto)

TEACHING STEPS:

1. Place 2 pictures (e.g., tooth and brush) in front of the student.
2. Say: "If you add 'tooth' to the beginning of 'brush,' what new word is it?"
3. If the student is correct, reinforce by saying: "Good, you added 'tooth' to the beginning of 'brush' and made a new word, 'toothbrush.'"
4. Repeat Steps 1–3 with other compound words and pictures (e.g., blue + bird).
5. Repeat activity without manipulatives.

CORRECTION PROCEDURES:

1. Place 3 pictures in front of the student (e.g., pictured tooth, brush, and toothbrush).
2. Explain to the student that we can put two word parts (or syllables) together to make a new word.
3. Say: "tooth" as you move the pictured tooth in front of the student. Say "brush" as you move the pictured brush in front of the student, making sure the tooth is on the left side of brush.
4. Point to pictured toothbrush saying: "When I add 'tooth' to the beginning of 'brush,' the new word is 'toothbrush.'"
5. Provide more pictured compound words or objects (e.g., cupcake, armchair, rainbow, baseball). In each instance ask the student to add "_____" (first syllable) to "_____" (second syllable). Ask the student to name the new word.
6. If the student is correct, reinforce by saying: "Good, you added '_____' (first syllable) to the beginning of '_____' (second syllable) and made a new word '_____.'"
7. Repeat activity without manipulatives.

5. Final syllable adding.

What to say to the student: "Now let's add syllables (or parts) to words."

EXAMPLE: "Add '_____'" (stimulus syllable) "to the end of '_____'" (stimulus syllable) (e.g., "Add 'ment' to the end of 'depart.'") (department).

TEACHING STEPS:

1. Place 2 pictures (e.g., butter and fly) in front of the student.
2. Say: "If we add 'fly' to the end of 'butter,' what new word is it?"
3. If the student is correct, reinforce by saying: "Good, you added 'fly' to the end of 'butter' and made a new word 'butterfly.'"
4. Repeat Steps 1–3 with other compound words and pictures (e.g., "wheel"+ "chair").

5. Repeat Steps 1–3 with 3- and 4-word syllable words.
6. Repeat activity without manipulatives.

CORRECTION PROCEDURES:

1. Place 3 pictures in front of the student (e.g., pictured dragon, fly, and dragonfly.)
2. Explain to the student that: "We can put 2 word parts (or syllables) together to make a new word."
3. Say "fly" as you move the pictured fly in front of the student.
4. Say "dragon" as you move the pictured dragon in front of the student making sure it's to the student's left side.
5. Point to the pictured dragonfly, saying: "When I add 'fly' to the end of 'dragon,' the new word is 'dragonfly.'"
6. Provide more pictured compound words or objects representing them (e.g., rainbow, baseball). In each instance ask the student to add "_____" (second syllable) to "_____" (first syllable). Ask the student to name the new word.
7. If the student is correct, reinforce by saying: "Good, you added '_____' (second syllable) to the end of '_____ ,'" (first syllable) "and made a new word '_____.'"
8. Repeat activity with 3- and 4-word syllable words.
9. Repeat activity without manipulatives.

6. Syllable substituting.

What to say to the student: "Let's make up some new words."

EXAMPLE: "Say '_____.'" (stimulus word) "Instead of '_____'" (stimulus syllable) "say '_____.'" (stimulus syllable) (e.g., "Say 'buying.' Instead of '-ing' say '-er.' The new word is 'buyer.'")

TEACHING STEPS:

1. Place 2 pictures (e.g., tooth and brush next to each other (tooth to left of brush) in front of the student and say: "toothbrush."
2. Place a picture of 'hair' (e.g., a black and white picture of a child where his or her hair is colored in or has an arrow pointing to it) next to the pictures of tooth and brush.
3. Replace the pictured tooth with the pictured hair, saying: "If I take 'tooth' away and put in 'hair,' the new word is 'hairbrush.'"
4. Repeat Steps 1–3 with other compound words and pictures (e.g., black + bird). In each instance, have the student name the first compound word and then the compound word that results when you substitute one syllable with an alternative.
5. If the student is correct, reinforce by saying: "Good, you changed part of the word and made up a new word."
6. Repeat activity without manipulatives.

CORRECTION PROCEDURES:

1. Place 2 red blocks/chips in front of the student saying: "red" as you point to the first block/chip and "red" as you point to the second block/chip.
2. Replace the second red block/chip with a blue block/chip. Say "red" as you point to the first block/chip and "blue" as you point to the second block/chip.
3. Repeat Steps 1–2 several times, replacing the first OR second block/chip with a different colored block/chip. Point to each block/chip naming only the color.
4. Repeat Steps 1–3, asking the student to name the color of the blocks/chips.
5. If the student is correct, reinforce by saying: "Good, you changed part of the word and made up a new word."
6. Repeat Teaching Steps 1–6 for this activity.

PHONOLOGICAL AWARENESS ACTIVITIES AT THE PHONEME LEVEL

1. Counting sounds.

What to say to the student: "We're going to count sounds in words."
EXAMPLE: "How many sounds do you hear in this word 'dog'?" (3)

TEACHING STEPS:

1. Place a picture from the story in front of the student (e.g., dog.) Place 3 wooden blocks or plastic chips below the pictured dog.
2. Point to each of the manipulatives and say: "These stand for the sounds in the word 'dog.'" Say the sounds separately as you point to each of the 3 blocks/chips: "/d/ /ah/ /g/ 'dog.' Three sounds in the word 'dog.'"
3. Say: "I'll say the word 'dog,' and you point to the blocks/chips and tell me how many sounds you hear in the word."
4. If the student is correct, reinforce by saying: "Good, you told me how many sounds in the word."
5. Repeat activity with additional monosyllabic words with 4, 5, and 6 sounds.
6. Repeat activity without manipulatives.

CORRECTION PROCEDURES:

1. If unable to do this activity with manipulatives or pictures from the story, the student may need more experience with counting in sequence and one-to-one correspondence. This may be achieved through providing many instances of placing 1, 2, and 3 blocks/chips in front of the student. Using the pictured dog, ask the student to touch each block as you say /d/, or /d/ /ah/, or /d/ /ah/ /g/.
2. Ask the student to point to each block/chip again as you count, "one," or "one, two," or "one, two, three." Each time ask: "How many sounds?"

3. If the student is correct, reinforce by saying: "Good, you counted the sounds."
4. If the student is incorrect, provide more experiences with counting and write the numeral above the objects to help the student keep each number in memory while responding to your question: "How many sounds?"
5. Repeat Steps 1–3 asking the student to draw lines for each sound heard as you say a word. Drawing lines replaces counting blocks/chips. You say a word (e.g., "cat,") and the student draws a separate line for each sound heard in the word, and then the student can count the number of lines, in this case, 3.
6. Repeat activity with additional monosyllabic words.
7. Repeat activity without manipulatives.

2. Sound categorization or identifying rhyme oddity.

What to say to the student: "Guess which word I say does not rhyme with the other three words."

EXAMPLE: "Tell me which word does not rhyme with the other three. '_____, _____, _____, _____.'" (stimulus words) (e.g., "brown, down, both, crown. Which word doesn't rhyme?") (both)

TEACHING STEPS:

1. Place 4 pictured items in front of the student (e.g., pictures of blink, overalls, sink, wink (from *Corduroy*).
2. Name the pictures and ask the student "Which word does not rhyme with the other three?"
3. If the student is correct, reinforce by saying: "Right, you told me the word that doesn't rhyme with the others."
4. Repeat activity without pictures.

CORRECTION PROCEDURES:

1. Place 2 pictured items in front of the student (e.g., pictures of blink and wink from *Corduroy*).
2. Name the 2 pictures and say: "These words rhyme."
3. Repeat Steps 1–2 with 2 additional pictured rhyming items from the story and ask: "Do these rhyme?"
4. If the student is correct, reinforce by saying: "Right, you told me the word that doesn't rhyme."
5. If incorrect, place 2 pictured nonrhyming items in front of the student (e.g., pictures of button and overalls from *Corduroy*).
6. Name the 2 pictures and say: "These words don't rhyme."
7. Place 2 pictured items in front of the student (e.g., pictures of sink and overalls from *Corduroy*).
8. Name the 2 pictures and ask the student if these 2 words rhyme.
9. If the student is correct, reinforce by saying: "Good, you told me they don't rhyme."

10. Repeat activity with 2 words until the student is successful at this level.
11. Repeat activity with 3 words until the student is successful at this level.
12. Repeat activity with 4 words until the student is successful at this level.
13. Repeat activity without pictures.

3. Matching rhyme.

What to say to the student: "We're going to think of rhyming words."

EXAMPLE: "Which word rhymes with '_____'?" (stimulus word) (e.g., "Which word rhymes with 'button'? 'bed, mutton, quite, bang.'" (mutton)

TEACHING STEPS:

1. Place 5 pictured items from the story, two of which rhyme (e.g., plum, pie, green, thumb, sausage from *The Very Hungry Caterpillar*) in front of the student.
2. Name 1 of the rhyming pictures (e.g., "plum") and ask the student: "Which of these words rhymes with 'plum': 'pie, green, thumb, sausage'?"
3. If the student is correct, reinforce by saying: "Right, you told said 'thumb' rhymes with 'plum.'"

CORRECTION PROCEDURES:

1. Place 2 rhyming pictured items from the story in front of the student (e.g., plum and thumb.) Say: "These words rhyme."
2. Place the 2 pictured items in front of the student again and ask: "Do these words rhyme?"
3. Repeat Step 2 with different sets of 2 pictures each.
4. If the student is correct, reinforce by saying: "Right, you told me those words rhyme with each other.
5. Place 2 pictured items that from the story that do not rhyme in front of the student (e.g., plum and pie.) Say: "These words do not rhyme."
6. Repeat Step 5 and ask the student: "Do these words rhyme?"
7. Repeat Steps 5–6 with different sets of 2 pictures each.
8. If the student is correct, reinforce by saying: "Right, you told me those words do not rhyme."
9. Repeat activity with 3, 4, then 5 words.
10. Repeat activity without manipulativess.

4. Producing rhyme.

What to say to the student: "Now we'll say rhyming words."

EXAMPLE: "Tell me a word that rhymes with '_____.'" (stimulus word) (e.g., "Tell me a word that rhymes with 'saved.' You can make up a word if you want.") (paved)

TEACHING STEPS:

1. Name 1 word from the story (e.g., "plum" from *The Very Hungry Caterpillar*).

2. Say: "Tell me a word that rhymes with 'plum.' It's okay if you make up a word."
3. If the student is correct, reinforce by saying: "Yes, you told me a word that rhymes with 'plum.'"

CORRECTION PROCEDURES:

1. Place 2 pictured items in front of the student (e.g., plum and thumb) and ask: "Do these words rhyme?"
2. If the student is correct, reinforce by saying: "Right, you said 'thumb' rhymes with 'plum.'"
3. Leave the 2 pictures in front of the student and say: "Tell me a word that rhymes with 'plum,'" and point to the picture of thumb.
4. If the student is correct, reinforce by saying: "Right, you told said 'thumb' rhymes with 'plum.'"
5. Place 2 pictures of words that do not rhyme (e.g., plum and pie) in front of the student. Say: "'plum' 'pie.' These words do not rhyme."
6. Leave the pictured plum and add another pictured item from the story that does not rhyme with plum (e.g., orange.) Ask: "Does 'plum' rhyme with 'orange'?"
7. If the student is correct, reinforce by saying: "Right, you told me these words do not rhyme."
8. Repeat activity using other words and pictured items from the story.
9. Repeat teaching Steps 1–3.

5. Sound matching (initial).

What to say to the student: "Now we'll listen for the first sound in words."

EXAMPLE: "Listen to this sound: / /." (stimulus sound). "Guess which word I say begins with that sound. '_____, _____, _____, _____.'" (stimulus words) (e.g., "Listen to this sound /w/. Guess which word I say begins with that sound: heard, button, cried, wondered.") (wondered)

TEACHING STEPS:

1. Say the beginning sound of 1 of the words from the story (e.g., /m/.)
2. Name 4 words from the story, 1 of which begins with /m/ (e.g., "king, bread, meat, fire" (from *Stone Soup*).
3. Say: "Tell me which word begins with /m/."
4. If the student is correct, reinforce saying: "Okay, you said 'meat' begins with /m/."

CORRECTION PROCEDURES:

1. Place 2 pictured items in front of the student (e.g., king and meat from *Stone Soup*). Say: "The first sound in 'king' is /k/. Tell me the first sound in 'king.'"
2. If the student is correct, reinforce by saying: "Right, you said the first sound in 'king' is /k/."
3. Ask the student: "Does 'king' begin with /m/?"

4. If the student is correct, reinforce by saying: "Good, you said that 'king' does not begin with /m/."
5. Repeat Step 1 asking the student: "What's the first sound in 'meat'?"
6. If the student is correct, reinforce by saying: "Right, you said the first sound in 'meat' is /m/."
7. Repeat Steps 1–6 with other 2-word pairs from the story.
8. Repeat Steps 1–6 with other 3-word, then 4-word pairs from the story.
9. Repeat activity without pictures.

6. Sound matching (final).

What to say to the student: "Now we'll listen for the last sound in words."

EXAMPLE: "Listen to this sound: / /" (stimulus sound). "Guess which word I say ends with that sound '_____, _____, _____, _____.'" (stimulus words) (e.g., "Listen to this sound: /r/. Guess which word I say ends with that sound: counted, friend, customer, Lisa.") (customer)

TEACHING STEPS:

1. Say the final sound of one of the words from the story (e.g., /z/.)
2. Name 4 words from the story, 1 of which ends with /z/ (e.g., "garden, snooze, warm, red" from *The Little Red Hen*).
3. Ask: "Which word ends with /z/?"
4. If the student is correct, reinforce by saying: "Good, you said 'snooze' ends with /z/."

CORRECTION PROCEDURES:

1. Place 2 pictured items in front of the student (e.g., red and snooze from *The Little Red Hen*). Say: "The last sound in 'snooze' is /z/. Tell me the last sound in 'snooze.'"
2. If the student is correct, reinforce by saying: "Right, you said the last or ending sound in 'snooze' is /z/."
3. Ask the student: "Does /snooze/ end with /t/?"
4. If the student is correct, reinforce by saying: "Right. You said that 'snooze' does not end with /t/."
5. Repeat Steps 1–4 asking: "What is the last sound in 'red'?"
6. If the student is correct, reinforce by saying: "Right, you said the last sound in 'red' is /d/."
7. Repeat Steps 1–6 with other 2-word pairs from the story.
8. Repeat Steps 1–6 with other 3-word, then 4-word pairs from the story.
9. Repeat activity without pictures.

7. Identifying initial sound in words.

What to say to the student: "I'll say a word two times. Tell me what sound is missing the second time. '_______, _______.'" (stimulus words)

EXAMPLE: "What sound do you hear in '_____'" (stimulus word) "that is missing in '_____'?" (stimulus word) (e.g., "What sound do you hear in 'gate,' that is missing in '-ate'?" (/g/)

TEACHING STEPS:

1. Choose 1 word from the story that can have 1 sound removed to form a real or nonreal word, (e.g., "grain," "rain.")
2. Say "grain, -rain. What sound in 'grain' is missing in 'rain'?"
3. If the student is correct, reinforce by saying: "Good you said /g/ is the missing sound in 'rain.'"

CORRECTION PROCEDURES:

1. Place 2 pictured items in front of the student (e.g., grain and rain from *The Little Red Hen*).
2. Place 4 wooden blocks or plastic chips under the pictured grain and 3 blocks/chips under the pictured rain.
3. Say: "/g/ /r/ /long A/ /n/," as you point to each of the blocks/chips under grain.
4. Say: "/r / /long A/ /n/" as you point to each of the blocks under rain.
5. Say: "Which sound in 'grain'" pointing to the block/chip that represents /g/, "is missing in 'rain'?" as you point to the picture of rain.
6. If the student is correct, reinforce by saying: "Right, you said that /g/ is the sound in 'grain' that is missing in 'rain.'"
7. Repeat activity with other sets of two words from the story.
8. Repeat activity without manipulatives.

8. Identifying final sound in words.

What to say to the student: "I'll say a word two times. Tell me what sound is missing the second time. '_______, _______.'" (stimulus words)

EXAMPLE: "What sound do you hear in '_____'" (stimulus word) "that is missing in '_____'?" (stimulus word) (e.g., "What sound do you hear in 'soup' that is missing in 'Sue'?") (/p/)

TEACHING STEPS:

1. Choose 1 word from the story that can have 1 sound removed to form a real or nonreal word, (e.g., "Soup," "Sue.")
2. Say: "soup, Sue. What sound in 'soup' is missing in 'Sue'?"
3. If the student is correct, reinforce by saying: "Good you said /p/ is the missing sound in 'Sue.'"

CORRECTION PROCEDURES:

1. Place 2 pictured items in front of the student (e.g., brown and brow from *Corduroy*).
2. Place 4 wooden blocks or plastic chips under the pictured brown and 3 blocks/chips under the pictured brow.
3. Say: "/b/ /r/ /ow/ /n/" as you point to each of the blocks/chips under the brown picture.
4. Say: "/b/ /r/ /ow/" as you point to each of the blocks/chips under the brow picture.

5. Say: "Which sound in 'brown'" (pointing to the block or chip that represents /n/), "is missing in 'brow'?" as you point to the picture of brow.
6. If the student is correct, reinforce by saying: "Right, you said that /n/ is the sound in 'brown' that is missing in 'brow.'"
7. Repeat activity without manipulatives.

9. Segmenting initial sound in words.

What to say to the student: "Listen to the word I say and tell me the first sound you hear.

EXAMPLE: "What's the first sound in '_____'?" (stimulus word) (e.g., "What's the first sound in 'button'?") (/b/)

TEACHING STEPS:

1. Say: "Listen for the first sound in the word I say."
2. Say 1 word from the story (e.g., "dog"). Say: "What is the first sound in that word?"
3. If the student is correct, reinforce by saying: "Yes, /d/ is the first sound in 'dog.'"

CORRECTION PROCEDURES:

1. Place a picture of a dog in front of the student.
2. Place 3 wooden blocks or plastic chips beneath the pictured dog.
3. Say each sound of the word, dog, as you point to each block/chip (i.e., "/d/ /ah/ /g/.")
4. Point to the first block/chip again and say: "/d/ is the first sound in 'dog.'"
5. Repeat Steps 1–3. Point to the first block/chip again and ask: "What is the first sound in 'dog'?"
6. If the student is correct, reinforce by saying: "Right, you said the first sound in 'dog' is /d/."
7. Repeat activity with other pictured items from the story.
8. Repeat activity without manipulatives.

10. Segmenting final sound in words.

What to say to the student: "Listen to the word I say and tell me the last sound you hear.

EXAMPLE: "What's the last sound in the word '_____'?" (stimulus word) (e.g., "What's the last sound in the word 'lamp'?") (/p/)

TEACHING STEPS:

1. Say "Listen for the last sound in the word I say."
2. Say one word from the story (e.g., "lamp"). Say: "What is the last sound in that word?"
3. If the student is correct, reinforce by saying: "Yes, /p/ is the last sound in 'lamp.'"

CORRECTION PROCEDURES:

1. Place a picture of a lamp in front of the student.
2. Place 4 wooden blocks or plastic chips beneath the pictured lamp.
3. Say each sound of the word, "lamp," as you point to each block/chip (i.e., "/l/ /short A/ /m/ /p/").
4. Point to the last block/chip again and say "/p/ is the last sound in 'lamp.'"
5. Repeat Steps 1–3. Point to the last block/chip again and ask: "What is the last sound in 'lamp'?"
6. If the student is correct, reinforce by saying: "Right, you said the last sound in 'lamp' is /p/."
7. Repeat activity with other pictured items from the story.
8. Repeat activity without manipulatives.

11. Generating words from the story beginning with a particular sound.

What to say to the student: "Let's think of words **from the story** that start/begin with certain sounds."

EXAMPLE: "Tell me a word from the story that starts/begins with / /" (stimulus sound) (e.g., "the sound /p/.") (pig)

TEACHING STEPS:

1. Say "Listen to this sound: /p/. 'Pig' begins with that sound. Tell me another word from the story that starts with that sound."
2. If the student is correct, reinforce by saying: "Yes, 'path' begins with a /p/ sound."

CORRECTION PROCEDURES:

1. Place 2 pictures in front of the student, each beginning with /p/ (e.g., pig and pot from *The Three Little Pigs*).
2. Place 3 wooden blocks or plastic chips beneath the pictured pig.
3. Say each sound of the word, "pig," as you point to each block/chip (i.e., "/p/ /short I/ /g/").
4. Then point to the first block/chip again and say: "The first sound in 'pig' is /p/. What's the first sound?"
5. If the student is correct, reinforce by saying: "Right, you said the first sound in 'pig' is /p/."
6. Then ask: "What's the first sound in 'pot'?"
7. Repeat activity with blocks/chips and other pictured items from the story.
8. Repeat activity without manipulatives.

12. Blending sounds in monosyllabic words divided into onset-rime beginning with two consonant cluster + rime.

What to say to the student: "Now we'll put sounds together to make words."

EXAMPLE: "Put these sounds together to make a word (/ / + / /)." (stimulus sounds) "What's the word?" (e.g., "bl + ink: What's the word?") (blink)

TEACHING STEPS:

1. Say the first 2-consonant cluster of a 1-syllable word, then the rest of the 1-syllable word (e.g., "bl" + "ink").
2. Ask the student: "What word is it when you put those parts together?"
3. If the student is correct, reinforce by saying: "Right. When you put 'bl' with 'ink' the word is 'blink.'"

CORRECTION PROCEDURES:

1. Select a word from the story beginning with a 2-consonant blend (e.g., "cheese" from *The Very Hungry Caterpillar*). Copy a picture of cheese from the story and cut the picture in half.
2. Point to the left half of the pictured cheese and say /ch/. Point to the right half of the pictured cheese and say "eese."
3. Move the 2 halves together and say "cheese."
4. Repeat Steps 1–3 asking the student to "Say the word parts (i.e., /ch/ and "eese.")
5. Place 2 wooden blocks or plastic chips in front of the student.
6. Point to the block/chip on the student's left and say: "This is /ch/." Point to the block/chip on the student's right and say: "This is 'eese.'"
7. Then move the 2 blocks/chips together and say: "When we put these together the word is 'cheese.'"
8. Repeat Steps 5–6 asking the student: "What do each of these say: /ch/ 'eese?'"
9. If the student is correct, reinforce by saying: "Good, you told me this block says /ch/ and this one says 'eese.'"
10. Move the blocks/chips together and ask: "When we put the parts together, what's the word?"
11. If the student is correct, reinforce by saying: "Right, you said that when you put /ch/ and 'eese' together the word is 'cheese.'"
12. Repeat activity with other 1-syllable words from the story beginning with 2-consonant blends.
13. Repeat activity without manipulatives.

13. Blending sounds in monosyllabic words divided into onset-rime beginning with single consonant + rime.

What to say to the student: "Let's put sounds together to make words."
EXAMPLE: "Put these sounds together to make a word (/ / + / /)." (stimulus sounds) "What's the word?" (e.g., "/d/ + 'og': what's the word?") (dog)

TEACHING STEPS:

1. Say the first single-consonant of a 1-syllable word, then the rest of the word (e.g., /d/ "og").
2. Say: "When you put those sounds together the word is 'dog.'"
3. Repeat Step 1 with another word from the story beginning with a single consonant (e.g., /k/ "at.") Ask: "What word is it?"
4. If the student is correct, reinforce by saying: "Right. When you put /k/ with 'at' the word is 'cat.'"

CORRECTION PROCEDURES:

1. Select a word from the story beginning with a single consonant (e.g., "dog" from *Hairy The Dirty Dog*). Copy a picture of a dog from the story and cut the picture in half.
2. Point to the left half of the pictured dog and say /d/. Point to the right half of the pictured dog and say "og."
3. Move the 2 halves together and say "dog."
4. Repeat Steps 1–3 asking the student to say the word parts (i.e., /d/ and "og.")
5. Place 2 wooden blocks or plastic chips in front of the student.
6. Point to the block/chip on the student's left and say: "This is /d/." Point to the block/chip on the student's right and say: "This is 'og.'"
7. Then move the 2 blocks/chips together and say: "When we put these together the word is 'dog.'"
8. Repeat Steps 5–6 asking the student: "What do each of these say?"
9. If the student is correct, say: "Good, you told me this block says /d/ and this one says 'og'" (as you point to each of the blocks/chips).
10. Point to the blocks/chips and ask: "When we put the parts together, what's the word?"
11. If the student is correct, reinforce by saying: "Right, you said that when you put /d/ and 'og' together the word is 'dog.'"
12. Repeat activity with other 1-syllable words from the story beginning with single consonant sounds.
13. Repeat activity without manipulatives.

14. Blending sounds to form a monosyllabic word beginning with a continuant sound.

What to say to the student: "We'll put sounds together to make words."
EXAMPLE: "Put these sounds together to make a word (/ / + / / + / /)." (stimulus sounds) (e.g., "/n/ /long I/ /t/"). (night)

TEACHING STEPS:

1. Say each sound in a 1-syllable word from the story (e.g., /n/ /long I/ /t/).
2. Say: "When you put those sounds together the word is 'night.'"
3. Repeat Step 1 with another word from the story beginning with a single consonant (e.g., /m/ /oo/ /n/). Ask: "What word is it?"
4. If the student is correct, reinforce by saying: "Right. When you put /m/ /oo/ /n/ together, the word is 'moon.'"

CORRECTION PROCEDURES:

1. Select a word from the story beginning with a continuant sound (e.g., /m/, /n/, /s/, /z/, /r/, /f/, /h/, /l/, /v/, /w/, /sh/, /voiceless th/, /voiced th/, or /j/ as in yellow, e.g., "Sal" from *Blueberries for Sal*). Copy a picture of Sal from the story and cut the picture in thirds.

2. Point to the left 1/3 of the pictured Sal and say /s/. Point to the middle 1/3 of the picture and say /short A/. Point to the right 1/3 of the pictured Sal and say /l/.
3. Move the 3 parts of the picture together and say "Sal."
4. Repeat Steps 1–3 asking the student to say the sounds (i.e., /s/ /short A/ /l/).
5. Place 3 wooden blocks or plastic chips in front of the student.
6. Point to the block/chip on the student's left and say: "This is /s/." Point to the middle block/chip and say: "This is /short A/." Point to the block/chip on the student's right and say: "This is /l/."
7. Then move the 3 blocks/chips together and say: "When we put these together the word is 'Sal.'"
8. Repeat Step 5 asking the student: "What do each of these say?"
9. If the student is correct, reinforce by saying: "Good. You told me what each sound is."
10. Say: "Move the blocks together and tell me the word."
11. If the student is correct, say: "Good, you told me when we move the sounds /s/ /short A/ /l/ together, the word is 'Sal.'"
12. Repeat activity with other 1-syllable words from the story beginning with continuant sounds.
13. Repeat activity without manipulatives.

15. Blending sounds to form a monosyllabic word beginning with a noncontinuant sound.

What to say to the student: "We'll put sounds together to make words."

EXAMPLE: "Put these sounds together to make a word (/ / + / / + / /)." (stimulus sounds) (e.g., "/p/ /short I/ /k/.") (pick)

TEACHING STEPS:

1. Say each sound in a 1-syllable word from the story (e.g., /p/ /short I/ /k/.)
2. Say: "When you put those sounds together the word is 'pick.'"
3. Repeat Step 1 with another word from the story beginning with a single consonant (e.g., /k/ /long I/ /t/.)
4. Ask: "What word is it when you put those sounds together?"
5. If the student is correct, reinforce by saying: "Right. When you put /k/ /long I/ /t/ together, the word is 'kite.'"

CORRECTION PROCEDURES:

1. Select a word from the story beginning with a noncontinuant sound (e.g., /p/, /b/, /t/, /d/, /k/, /g/, /ch/, /dz/ as in jelly; e.g., " pig" from *The Three Little Pigs*). Copy a picture of pig from the story and cut the picture in thirds.
2. Point to the left 1/3 of the pictured pig and say /p/. Point to the middle 1/3 of the picture and say /short I/. Point to the right 1/3 of the pictured pig and say /g/.

3. Move the 3 parts of the picture together and say "pig."
4. Repeat Steps 1–3 asking the student to say the sounds (i.e., /p/ /short I/ /g/.)
5. Place 3 wooden blocks or plastic chips in front of the student.
6. Point to the block/chip on the student's left and say: "This is /p/." Point to the middle block/chip and say: "This is /short I/." Point to the block/chip on the student's right and say: "This is /g/."
7. Then move the 3 blocks/chips together and say: "When we put these together the word is 'pig.'"
8. Repeat Step 5 asking the student: "What do each of these say?"
9. If the student is correct, reinforce by saying: "Good. You told me what each sound is."
10. Say: "Move the blocks together and tell me the word."
11. If the student is correct, say: "Good, you told me when we move the sounds /p/ /short I/ /g/ together, the word is 'pig.'"
12. Repeat activity with other 1-syllable words from the story beginning with noncontinuant sounds.
13. Repeat activity without manipulatives.

16. Substituting initial sound in words.

What to say to the student: "We're going to change beginning/first sounds in words."
EXAMPLE: "Say '_____.'" (stimulus word) "Instead of / /" (stimulus sound) "say / /." (stimulus sound) (e.g., "Say 'cat.' Instead of /k/ say /s/. What's your new word?") (sat)

TEACHING STEPS:

1. Place 3 wooden blocks or plastic chips next to each other in front of the student.
2. Say /k/ as you point to the first block/chip; /short A/ as you point to the middle block/chip, and /t/ as you point to the third block/chip. Motion to the blocks/chips and say: "This says 'cat.'"
3. Replace the first wooden block/chip with a different color block/chip and say: "/s/. Now this says 'sat.'"
4. Say /s/ as you point to the first block/chip, /short A/ as you point to the middle block/chip, and /t/ as you point to the third block/chip. Motion to the blocks and ask: "What word do these sounds make?"
5. If the student is correct, reinforce by saying: "Good, you changed the first sound in 'cat,' /k/ to /s/ and now the word is 'sat.'"
6. Repeat activity without manipulatives.

CORRECTION PROCEDURES:

1. Place 2 red blocks/chips in front of the student, saying: "red" as you point to the first block/chip and "red" as you point to the second block/chip.

2. Replace the first red block/chip with a blue block/chip saying "blue" as you point to the first block and "red" as you point to the second block. Then say: "I changed the first part."
3. Repeat Step 2 several times replacing the first colored block/chip with a different colored block/chip than the one with which you started. In each instance, have the student name the color of the first block and "red" as you point to the second block/chip.
4. If the student is correct, reinforce by saying: "Good, you changed the first part."
5. Place 2 blocks/chips in front of the student. Instead of saying the color of the blocks/chips, say /k/ as you point to the first block/chip and /long A/ as you point to the second block/chip.
6. Replace the first block/chip and say /d/ as you point to it and /long A/ as you point to the second block/chip. Say: "I changed the first sound of the word."
7. Repeat Steps 5–6 changing the first sound as you point to the first block/chip, and /long A/ as you point to the second block/chip. Have the student tell you what the new word is each time. Reinforce by saying: "Good, you changed the first part."
8. Repeat activity with other 1-syllable words from the story.
9. Repeat activity without manipulatives.

17. Substituting final sound in words.

What to say to the student: "We're going to change ending/last sounds in words. ***EXAMPLE:*** "Say '_____.'" (stimulus word) "Instead of / /" (stimulus sound) "say / /." (stimulus sound) (e.g., "Say 'night.' Instead of /t/ say /n/. What's your new word?") (nine)

TEACHING STEPS:

1. Place 3 wooden blocks or plastic chips next to each other in front of the student.
2. Say /d/ as you point to the first block/chip, /short O/ as you point to the middle block, and /g/ as you point to the third block. Motion to the blocks and say: "This says 'dog.'"
3. Replace the third block/chip with a different color block/chip and say: "/k/. Now this says 'dock.'"
4. Say /d/ as you point to the first block/chip, /short O/ as you point to the middle block/chip, and /k/ as you point to the third block/chip. Motion to the blocks and ask: "What word do these sounds make?"
5. If the student is correct, reinforce by saying: "Good, you changed the last sound in 'dog,' /g/ to /k/ and now the word is 'dock.'"
6. Repeat activity without manipulatives.

CORRECTION PROCEDURES:

1. Place 2 red blocks/chips in front of the student, saying "red" as you point to the first block/chip and "red" as you point to the second block/chip.

2. Replace the second block/chip with a blue block/chip saying: "red" as you point to the first block/chip and "blue" as you point to the second block/chip. Then say: "I changed the last part."
3. Repeat Step 2 several times replacing the second colored block/chip with a different colored block/chip than the one with which you started. In each instance, have the student name the first block/chip "red" and the name of the color of the second block/chip as you point to it.
4. If the student is correct, reinforce by saying: "Good, you changed the last part."
5. Place 2 blocks/chips in front of the student. Instead of saying the color of the blocks/chips, say /k/ as you point to the first block/chip and /long A/ as you point to the second block/chip.
6. Replace the second block/chip and say /k/ as you point to the first block/chip and /long E/ as you point to the second block/chip. Say: "I changed the last sound of the word."
7. Repeat Steps 5–6 changing the last (second) sound as you point to the second block/chip, and /k/ as you point to the first block/chip. Have the student tell you what the new word is each time. Reinforce by saying: "Good, you changed the last part."
8. Repeat activity with other 1-syllable words from the story.
9. Repeat activity without manipulatives.

18. Segmenting middle sound in monosyllabic words.

What to say to the student: "Tell me the middle sound in the word I say."

EXAMPLE: "What's the middle sound in the word '_____'?" (stimulus word) (e.g., "What's the middle sound in the word 'hug'?") (/short U/)

TEACHING STEPS:

1. Place a pictured item from the story (e.g., "moon" from *Happy Birthday, Moon*) and 3 wooden blocks or plastic chips next to each other in front of the student.
2. Say /m/ as you point to the first block/chip, /oo/ as you point to the middle block/chip, and /n/ as you point to the third block/chip.
3. Ask: "What is the middle sound in 'moon'?"
4. If the student is correct, reinforce by saying: "Yes, /oo/ is the middle sound in 'moon.'"

CORRECTION PROCEDURES:

1. Place a picture of a moon from *Happy Birthday, Moon* in front of the student.
2. Place 3 wooden blocks or plastic chips beneath the pictured moon.
3. Say each sound of the word as you point to each block/chip (i.e., /m/ /oo/ /n/).
4. Point to the first block/chip again and ask the student: "What is the first sound?"
5. If the student is correct, reinforce by saying: "Right, you said the first sound in 'moon' is /m/."

6. Repeat Step 4, pointing to the second and third blocks and reinforcing the student saying: "Good, you said the middle sound in 'moon' is /oo/ and the last sound in 'moon' is /n/."
7. Ask: "What's the middle sound in 'moon'?"
8. Repeat activity with other 1-syllable words and pictures from the story.
9. Repeat activity without manipulatives.

19. Substituting middle sound in words.

What to say to the student: "We're going to change the middle sound in words."
EXAMPLE: "Say '_____.'" (stimulus word) "Instead of / /" (stimulus sound) "say / /." (stimulus sound) (e.g., "Say 'flop.' Instead of /ah/ say /short I/. What's your new word?") (flip)

TEACHING STEPS:

1. Place 3 wooden blocks or plastic chips next to each other in front of the student.
2. Say /d/ as you point to the first block/chip, /ah/ as you point to the middle block/chip, and /g/ as you point to the third block/chip. Motion to the blocks/chips and say: "This says 'dog.'"
3. Replace the middle block/chip with a different color block/chip and say /short I/.
4. Say /d/ as you point to the first block/chip, /short I/ as you point to the middle block/chip, and /g/ as you point to the third block/chip. Motion to the blocks and ask: "What word do these sounds make"?
5. If the student is correct, reinforce by saying: "Good, you changed the middle sound in 'dog'; /ah/ to /short I/ and now the word is 'dig.'"
6. Repeat activity without manipulatives.

CORRECTION PROCEDURES:

1. Place 3 red blocks/chips in front of the student saying "red" as you point to the first block/chip, "red" as you point to the second block/chip, and "red" as you point to the third block/chip.
2. Replace the second block/chip with a blue block/chip saying: "red" as you point to the first block/chip, "blue" as you point to the second block/chip, and "red" as you point to the third block/chip. Then say: "I changed the middle part."
3. Repeat Steps 1–2. In Step 2 ask the student: "What do you change the middle one to?"
4. If the student is correct, reinforce by saying: "Good, you changed the middle part."
5. Place 2 pictures from the story in front of the student (e.g., pail and pill: pail from *Blueberries for Sal*).
6. Place 3 wooden blocks or plastic chips in front of the student. Instead of saying the color of the blocks/chips, say /p/ as you point to the first block/chip, /long A/ as you point to the second block/chip, and /l/ as you point to the third block/chip. Point to the pictured pail then point to the blocks/chips and say "pail."

7. Point to the pictured pill and replace the second block/chip with a different color block/chip. Say /p/ as you point to the first block/chip, /short I/ as you point to the second block/chip, and /l/ as you point to the third block/chip. Say: "I changed the middle sound of the word."
8. Repeat Steps 5–7 several times changing the middle (second) sound as you point to the second block/chip. Have the student tell you what the new word is each time. Reinforce by saying: "Good, you changed the middle part of the word."
9. Repeat activity with other 1-syllable words from the story.
10. Repeat activity without manipulatives.

20. Identifying all sounds in monosyllabic words.

What to say to the student: "Now tell me all the sounds you hear in the word I say."
EXAMPLE: "What sounds do you hear in the word '_____'?" (stimulus word) (e.g., "What sounds do you hear in the word 'gave'?") (/g/ /long A/ /v/)

TEACHING STEPS:

1. Place 3 wooden blocks or plastic chips next to each other in front of the student. Say: "Each of these blocks/chips stands for one sound in a word."
2. Say: "gave." Say /g/ as you point to the first block/chip, /long A/ as you point to the middle block/chip, and /v/ as you point to the third block/chip. Motion to the blocks/chips and say: "This says 'gave.'"
3. Place 3 blocks/chips in front of the student. Say another monosyllabic word from the story, beginning and ending with consonants and a vowel sound in the middle.
4. Ask the student to tell you the sounds in the word you say.
5. If the student is correct, reinforce by saying: "Good, you told me what sounds are in the word."
6. Repeat activity without manipulatives.

CORRECTION PROCEDURES:

1. Place a picture of a hen (from *The Little Red Hen*) in front of the student.
2. Place 3 wooden blocks or plastic chips beneath the pictured hen.
3. Say each sound of the word "hen" as you point to each block/chip (i.e., /h/ /short E/ /n/.)
4. Then point to the pictured hen again and ask the student: "What sounds do you hear in the word 'hen'?"
5. If the student is correct, reinforce by saying: "Yes, the sounds in 'hen' are /h/ /short E/ /n/."
6. Repeat activity with blocks/chips and other 1-syllable words and pictures from the story.
7. Repeat activity without manipulatives.

21. Deleting sounds within words.

What to say to the student: "We're going to leave out sounds in words."

EXAMPLE: "Say '_____'" (stimulus word) "without / /." (stimulus sound) (e.g., "Say 'grains' without /r/.") (gains) Say: "The word that was left, 'gains,' is a real word. Sometimes the word won't be a real word."

TEACHING STEPS:

1. Place 4 wooden blocks or plastic chips next to each other in front of the student. Say: /g/ as you point to the first block/chip, /r/ as you point to the second block/chip, /long A/ as you point to the next block/chip and /n/ as you point to the fourth block/chip. Motion to the blocks/chips and say: "This says 'grain'" (from *The Little Red Hen*) as you motion to the blocks/chips.
2. Remove the second block/chip and say: "Now this says 'gain.'"
3. Replace the second block/chip and ask: "What is the word"? (grain)
4. Remove the second block/chip and ask: "Now what's the word"?
5. If the student is correct, reinforce by saying: "Good, when we take /r/ from 'grain,' the word is 'gain.'"
6. Repeat activity without manipulatives.

CORRECTION PROCEDURES:

1. Place 2 red blocks/chips in front of the student, saying: "red" as you point to each of them.
2. Place a green block/chip between the 2 red blocks/chips and say "red" as you point to the first red block/chip, "green" as you point to the middle block/chip, and "red" as you point to the second red block/chip.
3. Remove the green block/chip and say: "When I take out the green block I have 'red' 'red,'" as you point to each of the 2 red blocks/chips.
4. Repeat Step 1–3 several times with different colored blocks/chips always keeping the first and third blocks/chips the same color and different than the second block/chip. In each instance, say: "Name the color of the 3 blocks." And each time you remove the second block/chip say: "Name the 2 remaining blocks/chips."
5. Repeat activity with 4 blocks/chips. Keep the first, third, and fourth blocks the same color. The second block should be a different color. Ask the student to name the colored blocks/chips (e.g., "red, blue, red, red"). Then remove the blue block and have the student name the remaining blocks. (red, red, red.)
6. Place 4 blocks/chips in front of the student. Instead of saying the color of the blocks/chips, say /g/ as you point to the first block/chip, /r/ as you point to the second block/chip, /long A/ as you point to the third block/chip, and /n/ as you point to the fourth block/chip.
7. Remove the second block/chip. Ask: "What sound did I take away"? (/r/) Then ask: "What word is this now"? (gain)
8. If the student is correct, reinforce by saying: "Good, when we take /r/ from 'grain,' the word is 'gain.'"
9. Repeat activity with 1-syllable words, (4 sounds each) from the story. Continue to use blocks/chips to represent the sounds of the words.
10. Repeat activity without manipulatives.

22. Substituting consonant in words having a two-sound cluster.

What to say to the student: "We're going to substitute sounds in words."

EXAMPLE: "Say '_____'" (stimulus word). "Instead of / /" (stimulus sound) "say / /" (stimulus sound) (e.g., "Say 'climb.' Instead of /l/ say /r/.") (crime). "Sometimes the new word will be a made up word."

TEACHING STEPS:

1. Say 1 word from the story (e.g., "store" from *Corduroy*).
2. Draw 4 lines and say: "The sounds in 'store' are /s/ /t/ /long O/ /r/" as you point to each of the lines.
3. Say: "Now I'll change one of the sounds." Circle the second line and say: "/n/. I changed /t/ to /n/. The new word is 'snore.'"
4. Erase the circled line. Point to the lines and say "store." Circle the second line and say "/n/. I changed /t/ to /n/. What's the new word?"
5. If the student is correct, reinforce by saying: "Yes. When you change /t/ to /n/ the new word is 'snore.'"
6. Repeat activity with other 1-syllable words from the story.
7. Repeat activity without drawn lines.

CORRECTION PROCEDURES:

1. Say 2 words: "store, snore."
2. Place 2 pictures in front of the student: store (from *Corduroy*) and snore (e.g., a picture of a person sleeping.)
3. Place 5 wooden blocks or plastic chips in front of the student.
4. Say: "The sounds in 'store' are /s/ /t/ /long O/ /r/" as you point to each of the blocks/chips under the pictured store.
5. Replace the second block/chip with a different colored block/chip.
6. Say: "I switched /t/ to /n/. Now the word is 'snore.'" Point to the pictured "snore."
7. Replace the exchanged block/chip with the original one representing /t/. Ask: "What was the first word"?
8. If the student is correct, reinforce by saying: "Right, this word is 'store,'" as you point to the pictured store.
9. Reinsert the block/chip representing /n/ and ask: "What's the word now"? (snore)
10. If the student is correct, reinforce by saying: "Good. We switched /t/ to /n/. The word changed from 'store' to 'snore.'"
11. Repeat activity with blocks/chips, pictures and other 1-syllable words from the story.
12. Repeat activity without manipulatives.

23. Phoneme reversing.

What to say to the student: "We're going to say words backward."

EXAMPLE: "Say the word '_____'" (stimulus word) "backward." (e.g., "Say 'bed' backward.") (deb)

TEACHING STEPS:

1. Say 1 word from the story, (e.g., "bed"). Ask: "What sounds do you hear in that word"?
2. If the student is correct, reinforce by saying: "Yes, the sounds in 'bed' are /b/ /short E/ /d/."
3. Say: "Now I'll say those same sounds in the reverse order, or backward. Listen: 'deb.'"
4. Say: "I'll say another word from the story and I want you to say the sounds in the word in the reverse order." Present another word from the story and say: "Say the sounds in the reverse order. Say the word backward."
5. If the student is correct, say: "Good, you said the word backward."

CORRECTION PROCEDURES:

1. Place 2 pictures in front of the student: a 10 and a net.
2. Place 3 different colored wooden blocks or plastic chips beneath the pictured 10.
3. Say each sound of the word "ten," as you point to each block/chip (i.e., as you say /t/ point to the red block/chip, as you say /short E/ point to the green block/chip and as you say /n/ point to the blue block/chip).
4. Point to the pictured net and switch the order of the blocks/chips putting them under the pictured net, (i.e., the blue block/chip is under the /n/, the green block/chip is under the /short E/, and the red block/chip is under the /t/).
5. Say: "If we switch the sounds in 'ten' around, the new word is 'net.'"
6. Present other 1-syllable words from the story with the correct number of blocks/chips under each. Ask the student to reverse the sounds and blocks/chips in each word.
7. If the student is correct, reinforce by saying: "Yes, when you reverse the sounds in the word, it makes a new word. You can say the word backward."
8. Repeat activity without manipulatives.

24. Phoneme switching.

What to say to the student: "We're going to switch the first sounds in 2 words."
EXAMPLE: "Switch the first sounds in '_____' and '_____.'" (stimulus words) (e.g., "Switch the first sounds in 'her dog.'") (der hog)

TEACHING STEPS:

1. Say 2 words from the story (e.g., "her dog.") Say: "What beginning sounds do you hear in those words"?
2. If the student is correct, reinforce by saying: "Yes, the first sound in 'her' is /h/ and the first sound in 'dog' is /d/."
3. Say: "When we switch the first sounds in the 2 words it's 'der hog.'"
4. Repeat Steps 1–2 with 2 more words (e.g., "red hen.") Tell the student to: "Switch the first sounds. What are the words now"? (head ren)
5. If the student is correct, reinforce by saying: "Great. You switched the first sounds so that 'red hen' became 'head ren.'"

CORRECTION PROCEDURES:

1. Place 2 pictures in front of the student (e.g., bear and hat from *Happy Birthday, Moon*).
2. Place 3 wooden blocks or plastic chips beneath picture. The first block/chip under the picture is different from the others (e.g., a black block/chip under the bear and an orange block/chip under the hat.) The next 2 blocks/chips under each picture should be the same in color but not black or orange. (e.g., under the bear there is 1 black block/chip and 2 red blocks/chips. Under the hat there is 1 orange block/chip followed by 2 red blocks/chips.
3. Say each sound of the word "bear" (i.e., /b/ /long A/ /r/) as you point to each block/chip under the pictured bear, and say each sound of the word "hat" (i.e., /h/ /short A/ /t/) as you point to the pictured hat.
4. Say: "If we reverse the first sounds in 'bear' and 'hat,'" (as you switch the black and orange blocks/chips) "the new words are 'hair' 'bat.'"
5. Repeat Steps 2–4. Ask the student what the new words are when you reverse the first sounds.
6. If the student is correct, reinforce by saying: "Yes, when you reverse the first sounds in the words, the new words are 'hair' 'bat.'"
7. Repeat activity with other sets of 2 one-syllable words.
5. Repeat activity without manipulatives.

25. Pig latin.

What to say to the student: "We're going to talk in a secret language using words from the story. In pig latin, you take off the first sound of a word, put it at the end of the word, and add a long A sound."

EXAMPLE: "Say chest in pig latin." (estchay)

TEACHING STEPS:

1. Say 1 word from the story (e.g., "rice").
2. Say: "When we take the first sound off the word 'rice,' the new word is 'ice.'"
3. Say: "If we put the /r/ at the end of 'ice,' the word is 'icer.'"
4. Say: "Now if we add /long A/ sound to the end of 'icer' the word is 'ice-ray.' This is how we talk in pig latin."
5. Say: "Say 'rice' in pig latin."
6. If the student is correct, reinforce by saying: "Nice work. You can talk in pig latin."

CORRECTION PROCEDURES:

1. Place 3 wooden blocks or plastic chips in front of the student.
2. Place a picture of a cat in front of the student and move 2 of the blocks/chips under the pictured cat, saying: "This is /k/" as you point to the block/chip on the student's left. Say: "This is 'at'" as you point to the block/chip on the student's right.

3. Move the first block/chip to the right of the second block/chip and say: "Now this says 'atk.'"
4. Move the third block/chip to the right of the block representing /k/ and say: "/long A/. Now this says 'atkay.'"
5. Repeat Step 2 asking the student to tell you what the 2 blocks stand for. (/k/ "at")
6. Repeat Step 3 asking the student to tell you what the new word is when you move the first block/chip to the right of the second block/chip. ("atk")
7. Repeat Step 4 asking the student to say what the new word is.
8. If the student is correct, reinforce by saying: "Great, you said the new word is 'atkay.' You can talk in pig latin.
9. Repeat activity with other pictured 1-syllable words from the story and colored blocks/chips."
10. Repeat activity without manipulatives.

SOME SPECIFIC SUGGESTIONS FOR USE WITH MATERIALS

Begin at the level where your student performs below the 80%–100% accuracy level. If your student can already correctly perform activities at the word level, begin activities at the syllable level. Or if the student demonstrates errors on some of the syllable level activities, begin with them and move into phonemic level activities.

It is extremely important for the user of these materials to give the sound the letters make rather than giving the letter names when presenting all the activities. The sound system of our language is what phonological awareness training is about, not teaching students names of alphabet letters. For example, when asking the student to provide words from the story beginning with /b/, be sure to give the sound /b/ and not the alphabet letter name [B]. With the exception of /dz/ (as in jelly), alphabetic letters were used rather than the phonetic symbols typically employed by speech-language specialists. Likewise, the descriptors "long" and "short" instead of phonetic symbols indicate vowel sounds. In many instances, the way a word sounds is presented for ease of presentation instead of the correct spelling, for example: "Add 'possess' to the ending '–shun'" (rather than "-sion").

If your student is not yet able to count objects, select other activities at the word level to increase phonological awareness abilities as the student is learning how to count and one-to-one correspondence.

If your student uses another word instead of the one listed or the one you're thinking of in the "fill in missing word" activity, you can suggest that the student think of a word from the story. For instance, one item under activity 2 at the word level (Supplying Words As Adult Reads) included under *Stone Soup*: "Came back with big _____ of meat." The correct answer is "chunks." If the student answers "bites," ask the student to think about the words from the story. Pictured items from the book may be used to assist the student in recall of the specific vocabulary item intended. If additional prompting does not cue the student to provide the intended response, the response "bites" should be considered correct. The purpose of the activity is to increase the student's ability to supply a missing word, not correct recall of specific vocabulary items. If the student's response is totally incorrect, then additional readings of the story and exposure to the vocabulary should be undertaken prior to specific work on phonological awareness activities.

If your student cannot add syllables (e.g., add "cow" to the end of "boy") or delete syllables (e.g., say "cowboy" without "boy"), use 2 pictures (e.g., a cow and a boy) to help illustrate the example. In training the student to add pictures, show the picture of a cow and have the student name the picture. Then add the picture of the boy to the right of cow and ask your student to put the 2 words together to make a new word, for example, "cowboy." In training your student to delete a syllable, show both pictures, with the pictured boy to the right of the pictured cow. Then take away 1 of the pictures, for example, the boy, and ask your student to tell you "What's left"?

If your student cannot correctly respond to an item involving counting words, syllables, or phonemes, add in manipulatives (e.g., plastic or wooden blocks, square pieces of paper, etc.) so the student has something concrete to count. Or have the student draw lines (___ ___ ___) or slash marks (/ / /) to represent each word, syllable, or phoneme in the stimulus word you say. Only use such manipulatives when necessary. If the student can perform the activity without the use of manipulatives, then present the activity stimulus items without them.

If your student is having trouble with blending syllables (e.g., "cow" + "boy") or phonemes (/k/ /ae/ /t/) to form a word, use plastic or wooden blocks or plastic cubes that snap together as you add a syllable or sounds together to form words.

If your student adds voicing to sounds when saying them after you, for example, /kuh/ (with voice) rather than /k/ (voiceless), tell him or her to "turn voice off," or "no voice." It's important that our students play with the sounds in isolation as much as possible.

If your student's memory is a factor in following directions during phonological awareness activities, simplify the direction. For instance, FIRST DIRECTION: "We're going to leave out syllables, or parts of words. Say 'cowboy.' Now say it again without 'cow.' What's left"? SECOND DIRECTION: "Let's drop syllables. Say 'cowboy' without 'cow.'"

If you need to increase or decrease the number of items for any given activity, do so. Use the vocabulary listed for the story or any other vocabulary from the story version you use. Add or delete items, depending on students' memory.

Always begin each activity with training on words not included in the stimulus items listed for the activity if you are using those stimulus items to count for student's performance level.

CHAPTER

PHONOLOGICAL AWARENESS ACTIVITIES TO USE WITH *BLUEBERRIES FOR SAL*

Text version used for selection of stimulus items:

McCloskey, R. (1981). *Blueberries for Sal.* New York: Puffin Books.

PHONOLOGICAL AWARENESS ACTIVITIES AT THE WORD LEVEL

1. Counting words.

What to say to the student: "We're going to count words."

EXAMPLE: "How many words do you hear in this sentence (or phrase) 'her bear'?" (2)

> *NOTE: Use pictured items and/or manipulatives if necessary. Use any of the following stimulus phrases or sentences and/or others you select from the story. Correct answers are in parentheses.*

Stimulus items:

sat down (2)

can them (2)

all mixed up (3)

right up close (3)

he could reach (3)

out of her pail (4)

he heard a noise (4)

put them in her pail (5)

we must store up food (5)

that kind of a noise (5)

2. Identifying missing word from list.

What to say to the student: "Listen to the words I say. I'll say them again. You tell me which word I leave out."

EXAMPLE: "Listen to the words I say: 'tin, crow, pail.' I'll say them again. Tell me which one I leave out: 'tin, pail.'" (crow)

> ***NOTE:*** *Use pictured items and/or manipulatives if necessary. Use any of the following stimulus words and/or others you select from the story. Correct answers are in parentheses.*

Stimulus set #1	Stimulus set #2
day, pail	day (pail)
child, berries	berries (child)
lips, mother, hunt	lips, hunt (mother)
ate, picked, bear	ate bear (picked)
munch, people, stopped	people, stopped (munch)
hard, kuplink, taste	hard, taste (kuplink)
turned, gulp, clump, feet	turned, clump, feet (gulp)
middle, gasp, bottom, bear	gasp, bottom, bear (middle)
swallow, dropped, mean, down	swallow, dropped, down (mean)
stump, winter, crow, eat	stump, winter, crow (eat)

3. Identifying missing word in phrase or sentence.

What to say to the student: "Listen to the sentence I read. Tell me which word is missing the second time I read the sentence."

EXAMPLE: "'Store up food.' Listen again and tell me which word I leave out. 'Store ____ food.'" (up)

> *NOTE: Use pictured items and/or manipulatives, if necessary. Use any of the following stimulus sentences and/or others you select from the story. Correct answers are in parentheses.*

Stimulus items:

Next winter. Next _____. (winter)

Little Bear. ____ Bear. (Little)

Blueberries for Sal. Blueberries for ______. (Sal)

Clump of bushes. Clump of ______. (bushes)

All four blueberries. All ____ blueberries. (four)

That is my mother. That is _____ mother. (my)

Followed behind his mother. Followed behind his _____. (mother)

She peeked into her pail. She _____ into her pail. (peeked)

This is not my child. This is _____ my child. (not)

I'm talking to the moon. I'm _____ to the moon. (talking)

4. Supplying missing word as adult reads.

What to say to the student: "I want you to help me read the story. You fill in the word I leave out."

EXAMPLE: "Blueberries for ____." (Sal)

> *NOTE: Use pictured items and/or manipulatives, if necessary. Use any of the following stimulus sentences and/or others you select from the story. Correct answers are in parentheses.*

Stimulus items:

She heard a _____. (noise)

Grow big and _____. (fat)

Choking on a mouthful of _____. (berries)

You are not Little _____. (Sal or Bear)

Kuplink! The _____ dropped into the pail. (berries)

He sat in a clump of _____ . (bushes)

That surely is my _____. (mother)

On the other side of Blueberry _____ . (Hill)

Little Bear sat munching and licking his _____. (lips)

We will have _____ for winter. (food or berries)

5. Rearranging words.

What to say to the student: "I'll say some words out of order. You put them in the right order so they make sense."

EXAMPLE: "'winter long.' Put those words in the right order." (long winter)

NOTE: Use pictured items and/or manipulatives, if necessary. Use any of the following stimulus words and/or others you select from the story. Correct answers are in parentheses. This word-level activity can be more difficult than some of the syllable- or phoneme-level activities because of the memory load. If your students are only able to deal with two or three words to be rearranged, add more two- and three-word samples from the story and omit the four-word level until a later time.

Stimulus items:

Hill Blueberry (Blueberry Hill)

crow mother (mother crow)

along hustle (hustle along)

pail tin little (little tin pail)

walked slowly she (she walked slowly)

lips his licking (licking his lips)

bears of shy (shy of bears)

fat grow and big (grow big and fat)

Sal for Little look (look for Little Sal)

spilled the almost pail (almost spilled the pail)

PHONOLOGICAL AWARENESS ACTIVITIES AT THE SYLLABLE LEVEL

1. Syllable counting.

What to say to the student: "We're going to count syllables (or parts) of words."
EXAMPLE: "How many syllables do you hear in '_____'?" (stimulus word) (e.g., "How many syllables in 'bear'?") (1)

> *NOTE: Use pictured items and/or manipulatives, if necessary. Use any of the of the following stimulus words and/or others you select from the story. Use any group of 10 stimulus items you select per teaching set.*

Stimulus items:

One-syllable words: pail, peek, pick, pull, put, back, bear, big, brought, but, take, taste, time, tin, to, took, turn, day, down, drove, came, can, catch, caw, close, clump, cold, could, crow, kept, gasp, get, go, gone, grow, gulp, just, make, mean, mix, more, munch, must, my, know, next, not, now, said, Sal, sat, seen, side, small, so, sound, spill, store, stump, earth, reach, rest, right, rock, run, far, fast, feet, few, find, flew, food, for, from, full, one, walk, wants, was, way, we, went, were, where, will, with, she, shy, thought, three, through, that, the, them, then, they, there, though, you, yours, all, and, as, ate, eat, I, in, is, off, old, on, out, own, up

Two-syllable words: paddle, partridge, people, person, picking, putting, because, behind, berries, besides, bottom, bushes, tired, tramping, didn't, canning, cover, kuplank, kuplink, kuplunk, quickly, garumpf, goodness, child, children, choking, many, middle, mistake, mother, mouthful, moving, nowhere, saying, single, sitting, slowly, storing, struggle, swallow, really, follow, hadn't, handful, hunted, hurried, hustle, hustling, licking, little, very, walking, wanted, winter, without, surely, thinking, along, among, around, away, eaten, eating, enough, even, inside, instead, other, over

Three-syllable words: possibly, blueberry, together, tremendous, already, another

2. Initial syllable deleting.

What to say to the student: "We're going to leave out syllables (or parts of words)."
EXAMPLE: "Say '_____.'" (stimulus word) "Say it again without '_____.'" (stimulus syllable) (e.g., "Say 'mouthful' without 'mouth.'") (ful)

NOTE: *Use pictured items and/or manipulatives if necessary. Use any of the following stimulus words and/or others you select from the story. Correct answers are in parentheses.*

Stimulus items:

"Say handful without hand." (ful)

"Say nowhere without no." (where)

"Say goodness without good." (ness)

"Say partridge without part." (ridge)

"Say blueberry without blue." (berry)

"Say garumpf without gar." (umpf)

"Say children without chill." (dren)

"Say kuplank without kuh-." (plank)

"Say already without all." (ready)

"Say instead without in." (stead)

3. Final syllable deleting.

What to say to the student: "We're going to leave out syllables (or parts of words)." *EXAMPLE:* "Say '_____.'" (stimulus word) "Say it again without '_____.'" (stimulus syllable) (e.g., "Say 'around' without 'round.'") (a)

NOTE: *Use pictured items and/or manipulatives if necessary. Use any of the following stimulus words and/or others you select from the story. Correct answers are in parentheses.*

Stimulus items:

"Say bottom without um." (bought)

"Say person without son." (purr)

"Say besides without sides." (be)

"Say mouthful without -ful." (mouth)

"Say goodness without -ness." (good)

"Say mistake without take." (mis)

"Say licking without -ing." (lick)

"Say garumpf without -umpf." (gar)

"Say inside without side." (in)

"Say surely without lee." (sure)

4. Initial syllable adding.

What to say to the student: "Now let's add syllables (or parts) to words."
EXAMPLE: " Add '_____' " (stimulus syllable) "to the beginning of '_____.' " (stimulus syllable) (e.g., "Add 'mouth' to the beginning of 'ful.' ") (mouthful)

> ***NOTE:*** *Use pictured items and/or manipulatives if necessary. Use any of the following stimulus words and/or others you select from the story. Correct answers are in parentheses.*

Stimulus items:

"Add part to the beginning of ridge." (partridge)

"Add be to the beginning of sides." (besides)

"Add good to the beginning of -ness." (goodness)

"Add mis- to the beginning of take." (mistake)

"Add lick the beginning of -ing." (licking)

"Add no to the beginning of where." (nowhere)

"Add en- to the beginning of tire." (entire)

"Add fall to the beginning of oh." (follow)

"Add sure to the beginning of lee." (surely)

"Add choke to the beginning of -ing." (choking)

5. Final syllable adding.

What to say to the student: "Now let's add syllables (or parts) to words."
EXAMPLE: "Add '_____' " (stimulus syllable) "to the end of '_____.' " (stimulus syllable) (e.g., "Add 'ing' to the end of 'can.' ") (canning)

> ***NOTE:*** *Use pictured items and/or manipulatives if necessary. Use any of the following stimulus words and/or others you select from the story. Correct answers are in parentheses.*

Stimulus items:

"Add where to the end of no." (nowhere)

"Add sides to the end of be." (besides)

"Add full to the end of hand." (handful)

"Add ridge the end of part." (partridge)

"Add lee to the end of sure." (surely)

"Add -oh to the end of swall-." (swallow)

"Add -plunk to the end of kuh-." (kuplunk)

"Add –ren to the end of chilled." (children)

"Add out to the end of with." (without)

"Add round to the end of a." (around)

6. Syllable substituting.

What to say to the student: "Let's make up some new words."

EXAMPLE: "Say '_____.'" (stimulus word) "Instead of '_____'" (stimulus syllable) "say '_____.'" (stimulus syllable) (e.g., "Say 'inside.' Instead of 'side' say 'stead.' The new word is 'instead.'")

> ***NOTE:*** *Use pictured items and/or manipulatives if necessary. Use any of the following stimulus words and/or others you select from the story. Correct answers are in parentheses.*

Stimulus items:

"Say blueberry. Instead of blue say straw." (strawberry)

"Say without. Instead of with say look." (look out)

"Say kuplink. Instead of plink say plunk." (kuplunk)

"Say choking. Instead of choke say move." (moving)

"Say goodness. Instead of -ness say bye." (goodbye)

"Say handful. Instead of ful say shake." (handshake)

"Say inside. Instead of in say be." (beside)

"Say behind. Instead of hind say low." (below)

"Say follow. Instead of oh say down." (fall down)

"Say struggle. Instead of strug- say gig-." (giggle)

PHONOLOGICAL AWARENESS ACTIVITIES AT THE PHONEME LEVEL

1. Counting sounds.

What to say to the student: "We're going to count sounds in words."

EXAMPLE: "How many sounds do you hear in this word? 'can.'" (3)

> ***NOTE:*** *Use pictured items and/or manipulatives if necessary. Use any of the following stimulus words and/or others you select from the story. Be sure to give the letter sound and not the letter name. Use any group of 10 stimulus items you select per teaching set.*

Stimulus words with two sounds: to, day, caw, go, my, so, earth, he, we, she, shy, they, though, all, as, ate, eat, in, is, off, on, own, up

Stimulus words with three sounds: pail, pick, put, back, bear, big, but, take, time, tin, took, came, can, could, get, gone, make, mean, not, reach, said, Sal, sat, seen, side, right, rock, run, feet, food, had, hill, home, like, with, three, that, then, and, eaten

Stimulus words with four sounds: peeked, picked, backed, brought, taste, tired, drop, drove, close, cold, kept, kind, gasp, grow, gulp, child, choke, just, many, munch, must, small, sound, spill, reached, rest, fast, find, from, hold, hunt, lips, lots, want, went, enough

Stimulus words with five sounds: mixed, paddled, because, didn't, dropped, clump, gasped, slowly, spilled, stopped, stump, followed, hadn't, hunted, wanted, wants, along, among

2. Sound categorization or identifying rhyme oddity.

What to say to the student: "Guess which word I say does not rhyme with the other three words."

EXAMPLE: "Tell me which word does not rhyme with the other three. '_____, _____, _____, _____.'" (stimulus words) (e.g., "munch, bunch, crunch, gulp. Which word doesn't rhyme?") (gulp)

> ***NOTE:*** *Use pictured items if necessary. Use any of the following stimulus words and/or others you select from the story. Correct answers are in parentheses.*

Stimulus items:

pail, day, tail, fail (day)

clump, berry, cherry, carry (clump)

more, store, down, four (down)

hook, look, cook, tin (tin)

pal, Sal, bear, Al (bear)

lick, shy, tick, kick (shy)

feet, hill, bill, chill (feet)

mother, brother, other, crow (crow)

taste, thought, fought, taught (taste)

choke, coke, oak, kuplank (kuplank)

3. Matching rhyme.

What to say to the student: "We're going to think of rhyming words."
EXAMPLE: "Which word rhymes with '_____'?" (stimulus word) (e.g., "Which word rhymes with 'crow:' 'cold, Sal, grow, own'?") (grow)

> ***NOTE:*** *Use pictured items if necessary. Use any of the following stimulus words and/or others you select from the story. Correct answers are in parentheses.*

Stimulus items:

hill: brought, picked, bill, turned (bill)

dropped: hurried, chopped, lots, food (chopped)

surely: berries, bottom, peeked, curly (curly)

hustle: heard, rustle, ahead, then (rustle)

thinking: sinking, winter, yours, all (sinking)

middle: garumpf, eaten, fiddle, without (fiddle)

tired: feet, fired, trampling, back (fired)

gasp: catch, besides, dropped, clasp (clasp)

canning: fanning, pail, mother, partridge (fanning)

tramping: bear, caw, camping, berry (camping)

4. Producing rhyme.

What to say to the student: "Now we'll say rhyming words."
EXAMPLE: "Tell me a word that rhymes with '_____.'" (stimulus word) (e.g., "Tell me a word that rhymes with 'pick.' You can make up a word if you want.") (tick)

> *NOTE: Use pictured items if necessary. Use any of the following stimulus words and/or others you select from the story (i.e., you say a word from the list below) and the student is to think of a rhyming word. Use any group of 10 stimulus items you select per teaching set.*

Stimulus items:

/p/: padded, pail, peek, pick, picking, pulled, put

/b/: back, bear, berries, berry, big, brought, but

/t/: take, taste, time, tin, tired, to, took, tramped, tramping, turned

/d/: day, down, dropped, drove

/k/: came, can, catch, caw, close, clump, cold, could, crow, kept, kind, quick

/g/: gasp, get, go, gone, grow, gulp

/ch/: child, choking

/dz/: (as 1st sound in jelly): just

/m/: make, many, mean, middle, mix, more, mother, moving, munch, must, my

/n/: knew, next, noise, not, now

/s/: said, Sal, sat, saying, seen, side, single, sitting, slow, small, so, sound, spill, standing, start, stop, store, stump, swallow

/f/: far, fast, feet, few, find, flew, follow, food, for, from, full

/v/: very

/h/: had, he, heard, her, hill, hold, home, hunt, hurry, hustle, whole

/r/: earth, reach, really, rest, right, rock, run

/l/: large, licking, like, lips, little, long, look, lots

/w/, /wh/: one, walking, want, was, way, we, went, were, what, where, will, winter, with

/sh/: she, shy, surely

/voiceless th/: thinking, thought, three, through

/voiced th/: that, the, them, they, there, though

/y/ (as 1st sound in yellow): you, yours

vowels: all, and, as, ate, eat, eaten, even, I, in, off, old, on, out, over, own, up

5. Sound matching (initial).

What to say to the student: "Now we'll listen for the first sound in words."
EXAMPLE: "Listen to this sound: / /." (stimulus sound). "Guess which word I say begins with that sound: '_____, _____, _____, _____.'" (stimulus words) (e.g., "Listen to this sound /b/. Guess which word I say begins with that sound: 'canning, munch, taste, bear.'") (bear)

> *NOTE: Give letter sound not letter name. Use pictured items if necessary. Use any of the following stimulus words and/or others you select from the story. Correct answers are in parentheses.*

Stimulus items:

/g/: this, pulled, garumpf, mouthful (garumpf)

/voiceless th/: eaten, hustling, tin, thought (thought)

/s/: swallow, hill, mother, along (swallow)

/n/: people, didn't, kept, nowhere (nowhere)

/f/: turned, blueberries, far, ate (far)

/t/: tramped, winter, munch, whole (tramped)

/b/: where, bushes, licking, partridge (bushes)

/sh/: lips, surely, handful, Sal (surely)

/k/: covered, mixed, other, gasped (covered)

/ch/: possibly, day, though, choking (choking)

6. Sound matching (final).

What to say to the student: "Now we'll listen for the last sound in words."
EXAMPLE: "Listen to this sound: / /" (stimulus sound). "Guess which word I say ends with that sound '_____, _____, _____, _____.'" (stimulus words) (e.g., "Listen to this sound /n/. Guess which word I say ends with that sound: 'berry, tin, with, pail.'" (tin)

NOTE: Give letter sound not letter name. Use pictured items if necessary. Use any of the following stimulus words and/or others you select from the story. Correct answers are in parentheses.

Stimulus items:

/d/: mistake, gone, spilled, reach (spilled)

/g/: together, big, pail, earth (big)

/m/: hunted, blueberry, storing, time (time)

/z/: covered, small, noise, mouthful (noise)

/v/: drove, hustling, instead, gasped (drove)

/r/: moving, followed, nowhere, make (nowhere)

/ch/: thought, goodness, next, munch (munch)

/p/: stump, store, putting, partridge (stump)

/t/: entire, kept, followed, paddle (kept)

/s/: crept, across, tell, forest (across)

7. Identifying initial sound in words.

What to say to the student: "I'll say a word two times. Tell me what sound is missing the second time. '______, _______.'" (stimulus words)

EXAMPLE: "What sound do you hear in '_____'" (stimulus word) "that is missing in '_____?'" (stimulus word) (e.g., "What sound do you hear in 'time,' that is missing in 'I'm'?") (/t/)

NOTE: Give letter sound not letter name. Use pictured items and/or manipulatives if necessary. Use any of the following stimulus words and/or others you select from the story. Correct answers are in parentheses.

Stimulus items:

"tin, in. What sound do you hear in tin that is missing in in?" (/t/)

"bear, air. What sound do you hear in bear that is missing in air?" (/b/)

"lick, -ick. What sound do you hear in lick that is missing in -ick?" (/l/)

"Sal, Al. What sound do you hear in Sal that is missing in Al?" (/s/)

"thought, ought. What sound do you hear in thought that is missing in ought?" (/voiceless th/)

"hill, ill. What sound do you hear in hill that is missing in ill?" (/h/)

"sit, it. What sound do you hear in sit that is missing in it?" (/s/)

"clump, lump. What sound do you hear in clump that is missing in lump?" (/k/)

"many, any. What sound do you hear in many that is missing in any?" (/m/)

"around, round. What sound do you hear in around that is missing in round?" (/a/)

8. Identifying final sound in words.

What to say to the student: "I'll say a word two times. Tell me what sound is missing the second time. '_______, _______.'" (stimulus words)

EXAMPLE: "What sound do you hear in '_____'" (stimulus word) "that is missing in '_____'?" (stimulus word) (e.g., "What sound do you hear in 'time' that is missing in 'tie'?") (/m/)

> *NOTE: Give letter sound not letter name. Use pictured items and/or manipulatives if necessary. Use any of the following stimulus words and/or others you select from the story. Correct answers are in parentheses.*

Stimulus items:

"turned, turn. What sound do you hear in turned that is missing in turn?" (/d/)

"follow, fall. What sound do you hear in follow that is missing in fall?" (/long O/)

"berry, bear. What sound do you hear in berry that is missing in bear?" (/long E/)

"drop, draw. What sound do you hear in drop that is missing in draw?" (/p/)

"tired, tire. What sound do you hear in tired that is missing in tire?" (/d/)

"gulp, gull. What sound do you hear in gulp that is missing in gull?" (/p/)

"side, sigh. What sound do you hear in side that is missing in sigh?" (/d/)

"feet, fee. What sound do you hear in feet that is missing in fee?" (/t/)

"lips, lip. What sound do you hear in lips that is missing in lip?" (/s/)

"gasp, gas. What sound do you hear in gasp that is missing in gas?" (/p/)

9. Segmenting initial sound in words.

What to say to the student: "Listen to the word I say and tell me the first sound you hear."

EXAMPLE: "What's the first sound in '_____'?" (stimulus word) (e.g., "What's the first sound in 'berry'?") (/b/)

> *NOTE:* *Give letter sound not letter name. Use pictured items and/or manipulatives if necessary. Use any of the following stimulus words and/or others you select from the story. Use any group of 10 stimulus items you select per teaching set.*

Stimulus items:

/p/: padded, pail, partridge, peek, people, person, pick, picking, possibly, pulled, put

/b/: back, bear, because, behind, berries, berry, besides, big, blueberry, bottom, brought, bushes, but

/t/: take, taste, time, tin, tired, to, together, took, tramped, tramping, turned

/d/: day, didn't, down, dropped, drove

/k/: came, can, canning, catch, caw, close, clump, cold, could, covered, crow, kept, kind, kuplank, kuplink, kuplunk, quickly

/g/: garumpf, gasped, get, go, gone, goodness, grow, gulp

/ch/: child, children, choking

/dz/: (as in jelly): just

/m/: make, many, mean, middle, mistake, mixed, more, mother, mouthful, moving, munch, must, my

/n/: knew, next, noise, not, now, nowhere

/s/: said, Sal, sat, saying, seen, side, single, sitting, slow, small, so, sound, spilled, standing, started, stopped, store, stored, storing, struggled, stump, swallow

/f/: far, fast, feet, few, find, flew, followed, food, for, four, from, full

/v/: very

/h/: had, hadn't, handful, he, heard, her, hill, hold, home, hunt, hunted, hurried, hustle, hustled, hustling,whole

/r/: earth, reach, reached, really, rest, right, rock, run

/l/: large, licking, like, lips, little, long, look, lots

/w/, /wh/: one, walked, walking, wanted, wants, was, way, we, went, were, what, where, will, winter, with, without

/sh/: she, shy, surely

/voiceless th/: thinking, thought, three, through

/voiced th/: that, the, them, they, there, though

/y/ (as in yellow): you, yours

vowels: ahead, all, along, already, among, and, as, ate, away, eat, eaten, eating, enough, entire, even, every, I, in, inside, instead, is, off, old, on, other, out, over, own, up

10. Segmenting final sound in words.

What to say to the student: "Listen to the word I say and tell me the last sound you hear."

EXAMPLE: "What's the last sound in the word '_____'?" (stimulus word) (e.g., "What's the last sound in the word 'took'?") (/k/)

> ***NOTE:*** *Give letter sound not letter name. Use pictured items and/or manipulatives if necessary. Use any of the following stimulus words and/or others you select from the story. Use any group of 10 stimulus items you select per teaching set.*

Stimulus items:

/p/: clump, gasp, gulp, stump, up

/t/: ate, brought, but, didn't, dropped, eat, fast, feet, get, hadn't, hunt, just, kept, mixed, must, next, not, out, put, rest, right, sat, stopped, taste, that, thought, walked, went, what, without

/d/: ahead, and, around, behind, child, cold, could, covered, find, followed, food, had, heard, hold, hunted, hustled, inside, kind, old, padded, pulled, said, side, sound, spilled, started, stored, struggled, tired, turned, wanted

/k/: back, kuplank, kuplink, kuplunk, like, look, make, mistake, peek, rock, take, took

/g/: big

/ch/: catch, munch, reach

/dz/: (as in jelly): partridge, large

/m/: bottom, came, from, home, them, time

/n/: can, children, down, eaten, even, gone, in, mean, on, one, own, run, seen, tin

/ng/: along, among, canning, choking, eating, hustling, licking, long, moving, picking, putting, saying, sitting, standing, thinking, tramping

/s/: close, goodness, lips, lots, tremendous, wants

/z/: as, because, berries, besides, bushes, is, noise, was

/f/: enough, garumpf, off

/v/: drove

/r/: another, bear, entire, fear, for, four, her, more, mother, nowhere, other, store, there, together, were, where, winter

/l/: all, full, handful, hill, hustle, little, pail, people, middle, mouthful, Sal, single, small, single, whole, will

/voiceless th/: earth, with

/long A/: away, day, they, way

/long E/: already, berry, blueberry, he, many, quickly, really, three, very, we

/long I/: my, shy

/long O/: crow, go, grow, so, swallow, though

/oo/: flew, knew, through, too, you

/ah/: caw

/ow/: now

11. Generating words from the story beginning with a particular sound.

What to say to the student: "Let's think of words **from the story** that start with certain sounds."

EXAMPLE: "Tell me a word **from the story** that starts with / /." (stimulus sound) (e.g., "the sound /p/") (partridge)

> ***NOTE:*** *Give letter sound not letter name. Use pictured items if necessary. Use any of the following stimulus words and/or others you select from the story. You say the sound (e.g., a voiceless /p/ sound) and the student is to say a word from the story that begins with that sound. Use any group of 10 stimulus items you select per teaching set.*

Stimulus items:

/p/: padded, pail, partridge, peek, people, person, pick, picking, possibly, pulled, put

/b/: back, bear, because, behind, berries, berry, besides, big, blueberry, bottom, brought, bushes, but

/t/: take, taste, time, tin, tired, to, together, took, tramped, tramping, turned

/d/: day, didn't, down, dropped, drove

/k/: came, can, canning, catch, caw, close, clump, cold, could, covered, crow, kept, kind, kuplank, kuplink, kuplunk, quickly

/g/: garumpf, gasped, get, go, gone, goodness, grow, gulp

/ch/: child, children, choking

/dz/: (as 1st sound in jelly): just

/m/: make, many, mean, middle, mistake, mixed, more, mother, mouthful, moving, munch, must, my

/n/: knew, next, noise, not, now, nowhere

/s/: said, Sal, sat, saying, seen, side, single, sitting, slow, small, so, sound, spilled, standing, started, stopped, store, stored, storing, struggled, stump, swallow

/f/: far, fast, feet, few, find, flew, followed, food, for, four, from, full

/v/: very

/h/: had, hadn't, handful, he, heard, her, hill, hold, home, hunt, hunted, hurried, hustle, hustled, hustling, whole

/r/: earth, reach, reached, really, rest, right, rock, run

/l/: large, licking, like, lips, little, long, look, lots

/w/, /wh/: one, walked, walking, wanted, wants, was, way, we, went, were, what, where, will, winter, with, without

/sh/: she, shy, surely

/voiceless th/: thinking, thought, three, through

/voiced th/: that, the, them, they, there, though

/y/ (as 1st sound in yellow): you, yours

vowels: ahead, all, along, already, among, and, as, ate, away, eat, eaten, eating, enough, entire, even, every, I, in, inside, instead, is, off, old, on, other, out, over, own, up

12. Blending sounds in monosyllabic words divided into onset-rime beginning with two consonant cluster + rime.

What to say to the student: "Now we'll put sounds together to make words."
EXAMPLE: "Put these sounds together to make a word (/ / + / /)." (stimulus sounds) "What's the word?" (e.g., "gr + ow: What's the word?") (grow)

> *NOTE: Give letter sound not letter name. Use pictured items and/or manipulatives if necessary. Use any of the following stimulus words and/or others you select from the story. Correct answers are in parentheses.*

Stimulus items:

st + ore (store)	cr + oh (crow)
dr + op (drop)	sp + ill (spill)
cl + ump (clump)	st + ump (stump)
br + ought (brought)	pl + ank (plank)
dr + ove (drove)	st + and (stand)

13. Blending sounds in monosyllabic words divided into onset-rime beginning with single consonant + rime.

What to say to the student: "Let's put sounds together to make words."
EXAMPLE: "Put these sounds together to make a word (/ / + / /)." (stimulus sounds) "What's the word?" (e.g., "/d/ + ay: what's the word?") (day)

> *NOTE: Give letter sound not letter name. Use pictured items and/or manipulatives if necessary. Use any of the following stimulus words and/or others you select from the story. Correct answers are in parentheses.*

Stimulus items:

/k/ + old (cold)	/m/ + unch (munch)
/t/ + ake (take)	/p/ + ick (pick)
/g/ + ulp (gulp)	/b/ + air (bear)
/s/ + ound (sound)	/n/ + oise (noise)
/p/ + ail (pail)	/s/ + al (Sal)

14. Blending sounds to form a monosyllabic word beginning with a continuant sound.

What to say to the student: "We'll put sounds together to make words."
EXAMPLE: "Put these sounds together to make a word (/ / + / / + / /)." (stimulus sounds) (e.g., "/m/ /long A/ /k/.") (make)

> **NOTE:** *Give letter sound not letter name. Use pictured items and/or manipulatives if necessary. Use any of the following stimulus words and/or others you select from the story. Correct answers are in parentheses.*

Stimulus items:

/f/ /long I/ /n/ /d/ (find)
/S/ /short A/ /l/ (Sal)
/th/ /ah/ /t/ (thought)
/m/ /long E/ /n/ (mean)
/s/ /long E/ /n/ (seen)
/sh/ /long I/ (shy)
/m/ /short U/ /s/ /t/ (must)
/w/ /ah/ /n/ /t/ (want)
/f/ /l/ /oo/ (flew)
/r/ /short U/ /n/ (run)

15. Blending sounds to form a monosyllabic word beginning with a noncontinuant sound.

What to say to the student: "We'll put sounds together to make words."
EXAMPLE: "Put these sounds together to make a word (/ / + / / + / /)." (stimulus sounds) (e.g., "/p/ /long A/ /l/.") (pail)

> **NOTE:** *Give letter sound not letter name. Use pictured items and/or manipulatives if necessary. Use any of the following stimulus words and/or others you select from the story. Correct answers are in parentheses.*

Stimulus items:

/g/ /short A/ /s/ /p/ (gasp)
/k/ /short A/ /n/ (can)
/ch/ /long I/ /l/ /d/ (child)
/g/ /short U/ /l/ /p/ (gulp)
/k/ /r/ /long O/ (crow)
/k/ /ah/ (caw)
/b/ /short A/ /k/ (back)
/ch/ /long O/ /k/ (choke)
/p/ /short I/ /k/ (pick)
/k/ /w/ /short I/ /k/ (quick)

16. Substituting initial sound in words.

What to say to the student: "We're going to change beginning/first sounds in words."
EXAMPLE: "Say '_____.'" (stimulus word) "Instead of / /" (stimulus sound) "say / /." (stimulus sound) (e.g., Say 'bear.' Instead of /b/ say /ch/. What's your new word?") (chair)

> ***NOTE:*** *Give letter sound not letter name. Use pictured items and/or manipulatives if necessary. Use any of the following stimulus words and/or others you select from the story. Correct answers are in parentheses.*

Stimulus items:

"Say child. Instead of /ch/ say /m/." (mild)

"Say berry. Instead of /b/ say /m/." (marry)

"Say hill. Instead of /h/ say /b/." (bill)

"Say lips. Instead of /l/ say /sh/." (ships)

"Say Sal. Instead of /s/ say /p/." (pal)

"Say three. Instead of /voiceless th/ say /f/." (free)

"Say caw. Instead of /k/ say /p/." (paw)

"Say take. Instead of /t/ say /b/." (bake)

"Say mixed. Instead of /m/ say /f/." (fixed)

"Say pail. Instead of /p/ say /w/." (whale)

17. Substituting final sound in words.

What to say to the student: "We're going to change ending/last sounds in words."
EXAMPLE: "Say '_____.'" (stimulus word) "Instead of / /" (stimulus sound) "say / /." (stimulus sound) (e.g., "Say 'ate.' Instead of /t/ say /m/. What's your new word?") (aim)

> ***NOTE:*** *Give letter sound not letter name. Use pictured items and/or manipulatives if necessary. Use any of the following stimulus words and/or others you select from the story. Correct answers are in parentheses.*

Stimulus items:

"Say hunt. Instead of /t/ say /long E/." (honey)

"Say tin. Instead of /n/ say /p/." (tip)

"Say heard. Instead of /d/ say /z/."(hers)

"Say off. Instead of /f/ say /n/." (on)

"Say hunt. Instead of /t/, say /k/." (hunk)

"Say up. Instead of /p/ say /s/." (us)

"Say sat. Instead of /t/ say /k/." (sack)

"Say that. Instead of /t/ say /n/." (than)

"Say had. Instead of /d/ say /z/." (has)

"Say lick. Instead of /k/ say /p/." (lip)

18. Segmenting middle sound in monosyllabic words.

What to say to the student: "Tell me the middle sound in the word I say."
EXAMPLE: "What's the middle sound in the word '_____'?" (stimulus word) (e.g., "What's the middle sound in the word 'feet'?") (/long E/)

> ***NOTE:** Give letter sound not letter name. Use pictured items and/or manipulatives if necessary. Use any of the following stimulus words and/or others you select from the story. Correct answers are in parentheses.*

Stimulus items:

sat (/short A/)	old (/l/)
side (/long I/)	tin (/short I/)
back (/short A/)	take (/long A/)
peek (/long E/)	lip (/short I/)
not (/ah/)	pail (/long A/)

19. Substituting middle sound in words.

What to say to the student: "We're going to change the middle sound in words."
EXAMPLE: "Say '_____.'" (stimulus word) "Instead of / /" (stimulus sound) "say / /." (stimulus sound) (e.g., "Say 'Sal.' Instead of /short A/ say /long E/. What's your new word?") (seal)

> *NOTE: Give letter sound not letter name. Use pictured items and/or manipulatives if necessary. Use any of the following stimulus words and/or others you select from the story. Correct answers are in parentheses.*

Stimulus items:

"Say ate. Instead of /t/ say /p/." (ape)

"Say pail. Instead of /long A/ say /short I/." (pill)

"Say like. Instead of /long I/ say /long A/."(lake)

"Say moon. Instead of /oo/ say /short A/." (man)

"Say hill. Instead of /short I/, say /long O/." (hole)

"Say rock. Instead of /ah/ say /long A/." (rake)

"Say sat. Instead of /short A/ say /short I/." (sit)

"Say tin. Instead of /short I/ say /long E/." (teen)

"Say bear. Instead of /long A/ say /long O/." (bore)

"Say pick. Instead of /short I/, say /short A/." (pack)

20. Identifying all sounds in monosyllabic words.

What to say to the student: "Now tell me all the sounds you hear in the word I say."
EXAMPLE: "What sounds do you hear in the word '_____'?" (stimulus word) (e.g., "What sounds do you hear in the word 'Sal'?") (/s/ /short A/ /l/)

> *NOTE: Give letter sound not letter name. Use pictured items and/or manipulatives if necessary. Use any of the following stimulus words and/or others you select from the story. Correct answers are in parentheses.*

Stimulus items:

pail (/p/ /long A/ /l/)

ate (/long A/ /t/)

mean (/m/ /long E/ /n/)

home (/h/ /long O/ /m/)

gone (/g/ /ah/ /n/)

taste (/t/ /long A/ /s/ /t/)

gasp (/g/ /short A/ /s/ /p/)

choke (/ch/ /long O/ /k/)

munch (/m/ /short U/ /n/ /ch/)

spill (/s/ /p/ /short I/ /l/)

21. Deleting sounds within words.

What to say to the student: "We're going to leave out sounds in words."
EXAMPLE: "Say '_____'" (stimulus word) "without / /." (stimulus sound) (e.g., "Say 'blue' without /l/." (boo) Say: "The word that was left, 'boo,' is a real word. Sometimes the word won't be a real word.")

> ***NOTE:*** *Give letter sound not letter name. Use pictured items and/or manipulatives if necessary. Use any of the following stimulus words and/or others you select from the story. Correct answers are in parentheses.*

Stimulus items:

"Say store without /t/." (sore)

"Say stand without /t/." (sand)

"Say and without /n/." (ad)

"Say drove without /r/." (dove)

"Say brought without /r/." (bought)

"Say spill without /p/." (sill)

"Say grow without /r/." (go)

"Say slow without /l/." (so)

"Say stump without /t/." (sump)

"Say quick without /w/." (kick)

22. Substituting consonant in words having a two-sound cluster.

What to say to the student: "We're going to substitute sounds in words."
EXAMPLE: "Say '_____'" (stimulus word). "Instead of / /" (stimulus sound) "say / /" (stimulus sound) (e.g., "Say 'climb.' Instead of /l/ say /r/.") (crime). Say: "Sometimes the new word will be a made-up word."

NOTE: Give letter sound not letter name. Use pictured items and/or manipulatives if necessary. Use any of the following stimulus words and/or others you select from the story. Correct answers are in parentheses.

Stimulus items:

"Say store. Instead of /t/ say /n/." (snore)

"Say clump. Instead of /l/ say /r/." (crump)

"Say plank. Instead of /l/ say /r/." (prank)

"Say blue. Instead of /l/ say /r/." (brew)

"Say stop. Instead of /t/ say /l/."(slop)

"Say spill. Instead of /p/ say /k/." (skill)

"Say grow. Instead of /r/ say /l/." (glow)

"Say stump. Instead of /t/ say /l/." (slump)

"Say kuplink. Instead of /l/ say /r/" (kuprink)

"Say instead. Instead of /t/ say /p/." (insped)

23. Phoneme reversing.

What to say to the student: "We're going to say words backward."
EXAMPLE: "Say the word '_____'" (stimulus word) "backward." (e.g., "If we say 'gulp' backward, the word is 'plug.'")

NOTE: This is a difficult phoneme-level task and should only be done with older students. Give letter sound, not letter name. Use pictured items and/or manipulatives if necessary. Use any of the following stimulus words and/or others you select from the story. Correct answers are in parentheses.

Stimulus items:

my	(I'm)	back	(cab)
tin	(nit)	take	(Kate)
can	(knack)	but	(tub)
gone	(nog)	choke	(coach)
seen	(niece)	lick	(kill)

24. Phoneme switching.

What to say to the student: "We're going to switch the first sounds in two words."
EXAMPLE: "Switch the first sounds in '_____' and '_____.'" (stimulus words) (e.g., "Switch the first sounds in 'sat down.'") (dat sown)

> *NOTE: This is a difficult phoneme-level task and should only be done with older students. Give letter sound not letter name. Use pictured items and/or manipulatives if necessary. Use any of the following stimulus words and/or others you select from the story. Correct answers are in parentheses.*

Stimulus items:

her pail	(per hail)
my child	(chy mild)
sat munching	(mat sunching)
tin pail	(pin tail)
little Sal	(sittle lal)
for winter	(wore finter)
heard noise	(nerd hoise)
bear ate	(air bate)
hunt berries	(bunt herries)
my birthday	(by mirthday)

25. Pig latin.

What to say to the student: "We're going to talk in a secret language using words from the story. In pig latin, you take off the first sound of a word, put it at the end of the word, and add a long A sound."
EXAMPLE: "Say Sal in pig latin." (alsay)

> *NOTE: This is a difficult phoneme-level task and should only be done with older students. Use pictured items and/or manipulatives if necessary. Use any of the following stimulus words and/or others you select from the story. Correct answers are in parentheses.*

Stimulus items:

far	(arfay)
big	(igbay)
time	(imetay)
bush	(ooshbay)
bear	(airbay)
peek	(eekpay)
many	(anymay)
hill	(illhay)
berries	(airiesbay)
rock	(ockray)

CHAPTER

PHONOLOGICAL AWARENESS ACTIVITIES TO USE WITH *CORDUROY*

Text version used for selection of stimulus items:

Freeman, D. (1976). *Corduroy*. New York: Puffin Books.

PHONOLOGICAL AWARENESS ACTIVITIES AT THE WORD LEVEL

1. Counting words.

What to say to the student: "We're going to count words."

EXAMPLE: "How many words do you hear in this sentence (or phrase)? 'Big store.'" (2)

> *NOTE: Use pictured items and/or manipulatives if necessary. Use any of the following stimulus phrases or sentences and/or others you select from the story. Correct answers are in parentheses.*

Stimulus items:

look new (2)

big hug (2)

the right size (3)

on her lap (3)

in a box (3)

I can find it (4)

this must be home (4)

rows and rows of beds (5)

it fell with a crash (5)

you must be a friend (5)

2. Identifying missing word from list.

What to say to the student: "Listen to the words I say. I'll say them again. You tell me which word I leave out."

EXAMPLE: "Listen to the words I say: 'sofa, friend, green.' I'll say them again. Tell me which one I leave out: 'sofa, friend.'" (green)

> ***NOTE:*** *Use pictured items and/or manipulatives if necessary. Use any of the following stimulus words and/or others you select from the story. Correct answers are in parentheses.*

Stimulus set #1	Stimulus set #2
button, floor	floor (button)
pop, bright	pop (bright)
crash, mother, rounds	crash, rounds (mother)
dolls, fuzzy, yanked	dolls, fuzzy (yanked)
brown, crawled, world	crawled, world (brown)
paws, hiding, locked, home	paws, locked, home (hiding)
flashed, waited, shelf, home	flashed, shelf, home (waited)
sleep, little, bear, mattress	sleep, little, bear (mattress)
Corduroy, mommy, chair, room	Corduroy, mommy, chair (room)
around, chest, bright, crash	around, bright, crash (chest)

3. Identifying missing word in phrase or sentence.

What to say to the student: "Listen to the sentence I read. Tell me which word is missing the second time I read the sentence.

EXAMPLE: "' shoulder strap.' Listen again and tell me which word I leave out. 'shoulder ____.'" (strap)

> ***NOTE:*** *Use pictured items and/or manipulatives if necessary. Use any of the following stimulus sentences and/or others you select from the story. Correct answers are in parentheses.*

Stimulus items:

I've lost a button. I've lost a _____. (button)

Dashing down the escalator. Dashing _____ the escalator. (down)

He tucked him under his arm. He tucked him under his _____. (arm)

I saved money in my piggy bank. I saved _____ in my piggy bank. (money)

The room was small. The room was _____. (small)

Shall I put him in a box? Shall I put him _____ a box? (in)

Over it fell with a crash. Over it _____ with a crash. (fell)

I've always wanted to sleep in a bed. I've always wanted to _____ in a bed. (sleep)

He climbed down from his shelf. He climbed down from his _____. (shelf)

Sew a button on his overalls. Sew a _____ on his overalls. (button)

4. Supplying missing word as adult reads.

What to say to the student: "I want you to help me read the story. You fill in the words I leave out."

EXAMPLE: "I've always wanted to climb a _____." (mountain)

> ***NOTE:*** *Use pictured items and/or manipulatives if necessary. Use any of the following stimulus sentences and/or others you select from the story. Correct answers are in parentheses.*

Stimulus items:

Corduroy lived in a toy _____. (department or store)

The lamp fell with a _____. (crash)

The store was filled with _____. (shoppers)

A small _____ in green overalls. (bear)

He lost the button to his shoulder _____. (strap)

Lisa sat down with _____. (Corduroy)

I've always wanted a _____. (friend)

Why, here's my_____. (button)

He crawled up onto the _____. (shelf or mattress)

My mother said I could bring you _____. (home)

5. Rearranging words.

What to say to the student: "I'll say some words out of order. You put them in the right order so they make sense."

EXAMPLE: "'bank piggy.' Put those words in the right order." (piggy bank)

NOTE: *Use pictured items and/or manipulatives if necessary. Use any of the following stimulus words and/or others you select from the story. Correct answers are in parentheses. This word-level activity can be more difficult than some of the syllable- or phoneme-level activities because of the memory load. If your students are only able to deal with two or three words to be rearranged, add more two- and three-word samples from the story and omit the four-word level items.*

Stimulus items:

size right (right size)

room own her (her own room)

a floor tall lamp (a tall floor lamp)

button a sew (sew a button)

today not dear (not today dear)

mountain a climb (climb a mountain)

accident by quite (quite by accident)

hug a him gave (gave him a hug)

bear own very my (my very own bear)

here's why button my (why here's my button)

PHONOLOGICAL AWARENESS ACTIVITIES AT THE SYLLABLE LEVEL

1. Syllable counting.

What to say to the student: "We're going to count syllables (or parts) of words."
EXAMPLE: "How many syllables do you hear in '_____'?" (stimulus word) (e.g., "How many syllables in 'bear'?") (1)

> ***NOTE:*** *Use pictured items and/or manipulatives if necessary. Use any of the following stimulus words and/or others you select from the story. Use any group of 10 stimulus items you select per teaching set.*

Stimulus items:

One-syllable words: paws, pick, pop, pulled, put, bang, bank, be, bear, bed, big, both, box, bright, bring, brown, but, by, day, dear, did, dolls, doors, down, came, can, climb, come, could, crash, cried, quite, gave, get, girl, go, gone, green, guess, chair, chairs, chest, just, me, more, most, much, must, my, know, new, next, night, no, not, now, said, same, sat, save, saw, see, seen, set, sew, sight, size, sleep, small, spent, stairs, stood, store, straight, strap, right, room, round, rows, fell, felt, find, first, flights, floor, for, friend, from, had, he, he'd, her, here, him, his, home, how, hug, who, right, room, rounds, rows, lamp, lap, large, last, late, light, like, live, look, lost, once, one, want, warm, way, went, were, what, when, why, wide, with, shall, she, shelf, shut, thank, thick, things, think, that, the, them, then, there, they, this, you, your, all, an, and, are, arm, as, ears, else, eyes, I'd, I'm, I've, in, is, it, of, off, oh, on, own, up

Two-syllable words: palace, piggy, before, began, besides, biggest, button, buying, dashing, didn't, doesn't, drawers, carried, counted, cover, going, mattress, mommy, morning, mother, mountain, moving, nothing, sadly, searching, someone, something, sticking, fastened, fuzzy, very, hiding, himself, Lisa, little, looking, waited, waking, wander, wanted, watchman, wondered, shoppers, shoulder, above, after, along, always, around, awake, away, ever, into, only, onto, other, over, under, until, upstairs

Three-syllable words: department, carefully, customer, saleslady, somebody, suddenly, family, furniture, accident, alongside, already, amazing, animals, apartment, enormous, evening, overalls

Four-syllable words: comfortable, escalator

2. Initial syllable deleting.

What to say to the student: "We're going to leave out syllables (or parts of words)."
EXAMPLE: "Say '_____.'" (stimulus word) "Say it again without '_____.'" (stimulus syllable) (e.g., "Say 'besides.' Say it again without 'be.'") (sides)

> **NOTE:** *Use pictured items and/or manipulatives if necessary. Use any of the following stimulus words and/or others you select from the story. Correct answers are in parentheses.*

Stimulus items:

"Say watchman without watch." (man)

"Say saleslady without sales." (lady)

"Say somebody without some." (body)

"Say piggy without pig." (-ee)

"Say biggest without big." (-est)

"Say himself without him." (self)

"Say always without all." (ways)

"Say dashing without dash." (-ing)

"Say only without own" (lee)

"Say something without some." (thing)

3. Final syllable deleting.

What to say to the student: "We're going to leave out syllables (or parts of words)."
EXAMPLE: "Say '_____.'" (stimulus word) "Say it again without '_____.'" (stimulus syllable) (e.g., "Say 'amazing' without '-ing.'") (amaze)

> **NOTE:** *Use pictured items and/or manipulatives if necessary. Use any of the following stimulus words and/or others you select from the story. Correct answers are in parentheses.*

Stimulus items:

"Say apartment without -ment." (apart)

"Say alongside without side." (along)

"Say everywhere without where." (every)

"Say onto without to." (on)

"Say overalls without alls." (over)

"Say upstairs without stairs." (up)

"Say enormous without us." (enorm-)

"Say mummy without -ee." (mum)

"Say only without lee." (own)

"Say department without ment." (depart)

4. Initial syllable adding.

What to say to the student: "Now let's add syllables (or parts) to words."
EXAMPLE: "Add '_____'" (stimulus syllable) "to the beginning of '_____.'" (stimulus syllable) (e.g., "Add 'on' to the beginning of 'to.'") (onto)

> ***NOTE:*** *Use pictured items and/or manipulatives if necessary. Use any of the following stimulus words and/or others you select from the story. Correct answers are in parentheses.*

Stimulus items:

"Add him to the beginning of self." (himself)

"Add shop to the beginning of -ers." (shoppers)

"Add sud- to the beginning of -enly." (suddenly)

"Add search to the beginning of -ing." (searching)

"Add sales to the beginning of lady." (saleslady)

"Add big to the beginning of -est." (biggest)

"Add buy to the beginning of –ing." (buying)

"Add ex- to the beginning of claimed." (excalimed)

"Add a to the beginning of wake." (awake)

"Add fuzz to the beginning of -ee." (fuzzy)

5. Final syllable adding.

What to say to the student: "Now let's add syllables (or parts) to words."
EXAMPLE: "Add '_____'" (stimulus syllable) "to the end of '_____.'" (stimulus syllable) (e.g., "Add 'ment' to the end of 'depart.'") (department)

NOTE: *Use pictured items and/or manipulatives if necessary. Use any of the following stimulus words and/or others you select from the story. Correct answers are in parentheses.*

Stimulus items:

"Add roy to the end of Courdu-." (Corduroy)

"Add one to the end of some." (someone)

"Add -ers the end of shop." (shoppers)

"Add -ment to the end of apart." (apartment)

"Add stairs to the end of up." (upstairs)

"Add alls to the end of over." (overalls)

"Add -mus to the end of enor-." (enormous)

"Add where to the end of every." (everywhere)

"Add sides to the end of be." (besides)

"Add lee to the end of sudden." (suddenly)

6. Syllable substituting.

What to say to the student: "Let's make up some new words."

EXAMPLE: "Say '_____.'" (stimulus word) "Instead of '_____'" (stimulus syllable) "say '_____.'" (stimulus syllable) (e.g., "Say 'buying.' Instead of '-ing' say '-er.' The new word is 'buyer'").

NOTE: *Use pictured items and/or manipulatives if necessary. Use any of the following stimulus words and/or others you select from the story. Correct answers are in parentheses.*

Stimulus items:

"Say department. Instead of ment say -ing." (departing)

"Say carefully. Instead of care say wake." (wakefully)

"Say overalls. Instead of alls say cook." (overcook)

"Say watchman. Instead of man say dog." (watchdog)

"Say himself. Instead of him say her." (herself)

"Say waking. Instead of -ing say -ful." (wakeful)

"Say alongside. Instead of side say shore." (alongshore)

"Say upstairs. Instead of up say down." (downstairs)

"Say biggest. Instead of big say small." (smallest)

"Say until. Instead of til say tie." (untie)

PHONOLOGICAL AWARENESS ACTIVITIES AT THE PHONEME LEVEL

1. Counting sounds.

What to say to the student: "We're going to count sounds in words."
EXAMPLE: "How many sounds do you hear in this word? 'pop.'" (3)

> *NOTE: Use pictured items and/or manipulatives if necessary. Use any of the following stimulus words and/or others you select from the story. Be sure to give the letter sound and not the letter name. Use any group of 10 stimulus items you select per teaching set.*

Stimulus words with two sounds: be, by, day, go, me, my, know, saw, sew, he, she, they, you, as, I'd, I'll, I'm, I've, in, is, it, of, off, on, own, up

Stimulus words with three sounds: paws, pick, pop, put, bang, bear, bed, big, both, but, dear, did, came, can, come, could, gave, get, gone, guess, chair, more, much, night, not, said, same, sat, seen, set, sighed, sight, size, fell, for, had, he'd, here, him, his, home, hug, right, room, rows, lap, late, light, like, live, look, one, what, when, wide, with, shall, shut, thick, that, them, then, this, you'll, you're, and, arm, asked, away, ears, else, other, over

Stimulus words with four sounds: piggy, bank, beds, box, bright, bring, brown, button, dolls, doors, climb, cover, crash, cried, quite, girls, green, chairs, chest, just, mommy, most, mother, must, saved, seemed, sleep, small, smile, stood, store, felt, filled, find, first, floor, from, fuzzy, hello, here's, round, lamp, last, Lisa, little, lived, locked, looked, lost, once, waited, walked, want, warm, watched, went, world, shelf, thank, things, think, above, after, along, arms, awake, into, only, onto, under

Stimulus words with five sounds: palace, before, began, buttons, didn't, doesn't, climbed, gasped, next, sadly, sofas, spent, stairs, stepped, stopped, straight, strap, fastened, flashed, flights, friend, rounds, lamps, wanted, shoppers, shoulder, yanked, always, until

2. Sound categorization or identifying rhyme oddity.

What to say to the student: "Guess which word I say does not rhyme with the other three words."

EXAMPLE: "Tell me which word does not rhyme with the other three. '_____, _____, _____, _____.'" (stimulus words) (e.g., "brown, down, both, crown. Which word doesn't rhyme?") (both)

> ***NOTE:*** *Use pictured items if necessary. Use any of the following stimulus words and/or others you select from the story. Correct answers are in parentheses.*

Stimulus items:

bear, shopper, air, care (shopper)

ears, shelf, elf, self (ears)

cried, dyed, blinked, fried (blinked)

button, mutton, drawers, glutton (drawers)

dashing, lamp, crashing, flashing (lamp)

customer, bright, light, right (customer)

bank, sank, yank, Lisa (Lisa)

fuzzy, thick, stick, tick (fuzzy)

shut, cut, rut, doors (doors)

blink, overalls, sink, wink (overalls)

3. Matching rhyme.

What to say to the student: "We're going to think of rhyming words."

EXAMPLE: "Which word rhymes with '_____'?" (stimulus word) (e.g., "Which word rhymes with 'button:' 'bed, mutton, quite, bang'?") (mutton)

> ***NOTE:*** *Use pictured items if necessary. Use any of the following stimulus words and/or others you select from the story. Correct answers are in parentheses.*

Stimulus items:

bear: department, wear, shoppers, bright (wear)

flights: brown, Corduroy, tights, sofas (tights)

round: seemed, bang, ground, crawled (ground)

blinked: things, shoulder, winked, yanked (winked)

climb: slime, wondered, you'll, amazing (slime)

friend: admiring, green, trend, escalator (trend)

box: enormous, onto, fox, animals (fox)

shoulder: watchman, things, when, bolder (bolder)

locked: shocked, gasped, reached, evening (shocked)

ears: already, overalls, fears, exclaimed (fears)

4. Producing rhyme.

What to say to the student: "Now we'll say rhyming words."

EXAMPLE: "Tell me a word that rhymes with '_____.'" (stimulus word) (e.g., "Tell me a word that rhymes with 'saved.' You can make up a word if you want.") (paved)

> ***NOTE:*** *Use pictured items if necessary. Use any of the following stimulus words and/or others you select from the story (i.e., you say a word from the list below and the student is to think of a rhyming word). Use any group of 10 stimulus items you select per teaching set.*

Stimulus items:

/p/: palace, paws, pick, piggy, pop, pulled, put

/b/: bang, bank, be, bear, bed, bear, before, began, besides, big, biggest, blinked, both, box, bright, bring, brown, but, button, buying, by

/d/: dashing, day, dear, department, did, didn't, doesn't, dolls, doors, down, drawers

/k/: came, can, carefully, carried, climb, come, Corduroy, could, counted, cover, crash, crawled, cried, customer, quite

/g/: gasped, gave, get, girl, go, going, gone, green

/ch/: chair, chest

/dz/: (as 1st sound in jelly): just

/m/: mattress, me, mommy, more, morning, most, mother, mountain, moving, much, must, my

/n/: know, new, next, night, no, not, nothing, now

/s/: sad, said, same, sat, saved, saw, searching, see, seemed, seen, set, sew, sighed, sight, size, sleep, small, smile, sofa, somebody, someone, something, spent, stairs, stepped, sticking, stood, stopped, store, straight, strap, spots, stairs, started, still, stopped, strange, street

/f/: family, fastened, fell, felt, filled, find, first, flashed, flight, floor, for, friend, from, fuzzy

/v/: very

/h/: had, he, he'd, heard, hello, her, here, here's, hiding, him, himself, his, home, how, hug, who

/r/: reached, right, room, round, rows

/l/: lamp, lap, large, last, late, light, like, Lisa, little, live, lock, look, looking, lost

/w/, /wh/: once, one, wag, waited, walked, wandered, want, wanted, warm, watched, way, when, why, wide, with, wondered, world

/sh/: shall, she, shelf, shoppers, shoulder, shut

/voiceless th/: thank, thick, things, think

/voiced th/: that, the, them, then, there, they, this

/y/ (as 1st sound in yellow): yanked, you, you'll, you're, your

vowels: a, after, all, along, an, and, are, arm, around, as, asked, awake, away, ears, else, ever, eyes, I'd, I'll, I'm, I've, in, into, is, it, of, off, oh, on, only, onto, other, over, own, under, up

5. Sound matching (initial).

What to say to the student: "Now we'll listen for the first sound in words."
EXAMPLE: "Listen to this sound: / /." (stimulus sound). "Guess which word I say begins with that sound. '_____, _____, _____, _____.'" (stimulus words) (e.g., "Listen to this sound /w/. Guess which word I say begins with that sound: 'heard, button, cried, wondered.'") (wondered)

> ***NOTE:*** *Give letter sound, not letter name. Use pictured items if necessary. Use any of the following stimulus words and/or others you select from the story. Correct answers are in parentheses.*

Stimulus items:

/b/: dashing, customer, brown, nothing (brown)

/m/: night, something, going, moving (moving)

/long E/: enormous, just, mountain, sofas (enormous)

/s/: wandered, mattress, suddenly, biggest (suddenly)

/sh/: comfortable, both, shoppers, watchman (shoppers)

/k/: Corduroy, before, waking, accident (Corduroy)

/long O/: upstairs, overalls, carefully, paws (overalls)

/p/: drawers, customer, palace, exclaimed (palace)

/f/: comfortable, furniture, mommy, admiring (furniture)

/h/: hug, awake, carried, buying (hug)

6. Sound matching (final).

What to say to the student: "Now we'll listen for the last sound in words."

EXAMPLE: "Listen to this sound: / /." (stimulus sound) "Guess which word I say ends with that sound '_____, _____, _____, _____.'" (stimulus words) (e.g., "Listen to this sound /r/. Guess which word I say ends with that sound: 'counted, friend, customer, Lisa.'") (customer)

> ***NOTE:*** *Give letter sound, not letter name. Use pictured items if necessary. Use any of the following stimulus words and/or others you select from the story. Correct answers are in parentheses.*

Stimulus items:

/t/: heard, looking, department, fastened (department)

/f/: locked, himself, sofas, mountain (himself)

/long E/: blinked, comfortable, already, bear (already)

/z/: family's, shall, Corduroy, apartment (family's)

/s/: alongside, evening, enormous, button (enormous)

/k/: counted, large, escalator, thank (thank)

/n/: home, mountain, answered, mattress (mountain)

/d/: watchman, flights, exclaimed, awake (exclaimed)

/g/: big, pulled, furniture, already (big)

/sh/: customer, crash, drawers, saleslady (crash)

7. Identifying initial sound in words.

What to say to the student: "I'll say a word two times. Tell me what sound is missing the second time. '______, ______.'" (stimulus words)

EXAMPLE: "What sound do you hear in '_____'" (stimulus word) "that is missing in '_____'?" (stimulus word) (e.g., "What sound do you hear in 'bed,' that is missing in '-ed'?") (/b/)

> ***NOTE:*** *Give letter sound not letter name. Use pictured items and/or manipulatives if necessary. Use any of the following stimulus words and/or others you select from the story. Correct answers are in parentheses.*

Stimulus items:

"think, ink. What sound do you hear in think that is missing in ink?" (/th/)

"waking, aching. What sound do you hear in waking that is missing in aching?" (/w/)

"smile, mile. What sound do you hear in smile that is missing in mile?" (/s/)

"bright, right. What sound do you hear in bright that is missing in right?" (/b/)

"crash, rash. What sound do you hear in crash that is missing in rash?" (/k/)

"very, airy. What sound do you hear in very that is missing in airy?" (/v/)

"flashed, lashed. What sound do you hear in flashed that is missing in lashed?" (/f/)

"how, ow. What sound do you hear in how that is missing in ow?" (/h/)

"shoulder, older. What sound do you hear in shoulder that is missing in older?" (/sh/)

"mother, other. What sound do you hear in mother that is missing in other?" (/m/)

8. Identifying final sound in words.

What to say to the student: "I'll say a word two times. Tell me what sound is missing the second time. '______, ______.'" (stimulus words)

EXAMPLE: "What sound do you hear in '_____' (stimulus word) "that is missing in '_____'?" (stimulus word) (e.g., "What sound do you hear in 'brown' that is missing in 'brow'?") (/n/)

NOTE: *Give letter sound, not letter name. Use pictured items and/or manipulatives if necessary. Use any of the following stimulus words and/or others you select from the story. Correct answers are in parentheses.*

Stimulus items:

"lamp, lamb. What sound do you hear in lamp that is missing in lamb?" (/p/)

"gasped, gasp. What sound do you hear in gasped that is missing in gasp?" (/t/)

"chest, chess. What sound do you hear in chest that is missing in chess?" (/t/)

"wide, why. What sound do you hear in wide that is missing in why?" (/d/)

"same, say. What sound do you hear in same that is missing in say?" (/m/)

"exclaimed, exclaim. What sound do you hear in exclaimed that is missing in exclaim?" (/d/)

"like, lie. What sound do you hear in like that is missing in lie?" (/k/)

"heard, her. What sound do you hear in heard that is missing in her?" (/d/)

"home, hoe. What sound do you hear in home that is missing in hoe?" (/m/)

"world, whirl. What sound do you hear in world that is missing in whirl?" (/d/)

9. Segmenting initial sound in words.

What to say to the student: "Listen to the word I say and tell me the first sound you hear."

EXAMPLE: "What's the first sound in '_____'?" (stimulus word) (e.g., "What's the first sound in 'button'?") (/b/)

NOTE: *Give letter sound, not letter name. Use pictured items and/or manipulatives if necessary. Use any of the following stimulus words and/or others you select from the story. Use any group of 10 stimulus items you select per teaching set.*

Stimulus items:

/p/: palace, paws, pick, piggy, pop, pulled, put

/b/: bang, bank, be, bear, bed, bear, before, began, besides, big, biggest, blinked, both, box, bright, bring, brown, but, button, buying, by

/d/: dashing, day, dear, department, did, didn't, doesn't, dolls, doors, down, drawers

/k/: came, can, carefully, carried, climb, come, Corduroy, could, counted, cover, crash, crawled, cried, customer, quite

/g/: gasped, gave, get, girl, go, going, gone, green

/ch/: chair, chest

/dz/: (as 1st sound in jelly): just

/m/: mattress, me, mommy, more, morning, most, mother, mountain, moving, much, must, my

/n/: know, new, next, night, no, not, nothing, now

/s/: sad, said, same, sat, saved, saw, searching, see, seemed, seen, set, sew, sighed, sight, size, sleep, small, smile, sofa, somebody, someone, something, spent, stairs, stepped, sticking, stood, stopped, store, straight, strap, spots, stairs, started, still, stopped, strange, street

/f/: family, fastened, fell, felt, filled, find, first, flashed, flight, floor, for, friend, from, furniture, fuzzy

/v/: very

/h/: had, he, he'd, heard, hello, her, here, here's, hiding, him, himself, his, home, how, hug, who

/r/: reached, right, room, round, rows

/l/: lamp, lap, large, last, late, light, like, Lisa, little, live, lock, look, looking, lost

/w/, /wh/: once, one, wag, waited, walked, wandered, want, wanted, warm, watched, watchman, way, when, why, wide, with, wondered, world

/sh/: shall, she, shelf, shoppers, shoulder, shut

/voiceless th/: thank, thick, things, think

/voiced th/: that, the, them, then, there, they, this

/y/ (as 1st sound in yellow): yanked, you, you'll, your

vowels: a, above, accident, admiring, after, all, along, alongside, already, always, amazing, an, and, animals, answered, apartment, are, arm, around, as, asked, awake, away, ears, else, escalator, evening, ever, everywhere, exclaimed, eyes, I'd, I'll, I'm, I've, in, into, is, it, of, off, oh, on, only, onto, other, over, overalls, own, under, until, up, upstairs

10. Segmenting final sound in words.

What to say to the student: "Listen to the word I say and tell me the last sound you hear. **EXAMPLE:** "What's the last sound in the word '_____'?" (stimulus word) (e.g., "What's the last sound in the word 'lamp'?") (/p/)

***NOTE:** Give letter sound not letter name. Use pictured items and/or manipulatives if necessary. Use any of the following stimulus words and/or others you select from the story. Use any group of 10 stimulus items you select per teaching set.*

Stimulus items:

/p/: lamp, lap, pop, sleep, strap, up

/t/: accident, apartment, asked, biggest, blinked, bright, but, chest, department, didn't, doesn't, felt, first, flashed, gasped, get, it, just, last, late, light, locked, looked, lost, most, must, next, night, not, put, quite, reached, right, sat, set, shut, sight, spent, stepped, stopped, straight, that, walked, want, watched, went, what, yanked

/d/: alongside, and, answered, around, bed, carried, climbed, could, counted, crawled, cried, did, exclaimed, fastened, filled, find, friend, had, he'd, heard, I'd, lived, pulled, round, said, saved, seemed, sighed, stood, wandered, waited, wanted, wide, wondered, world

/k/: pick, bank, like, look, thank, thick, think, awake

/g/: big, hug

/ch/: much

/dz/: (as 1st sound in jelly): large

/m/: arm, came, climb, come, from, him, home, I'm, room, same, them, warm

/n/: an, began, brown, button, can, down, gone, green, in, mountain, on, one, own, seen, someone, then, watchman, when

/ng/: admiring, bring, buying, dashing, evening, going, hiding, looking, morning, moving, nothing, searching, something, sticking, waking, along, bang

/s/: box, else, enormous, guess, lamps, mattress, once, palace, straps, this

/z/: always, animals, arms, as, beds, besides, buttons, chairs, dolls, doors, drawers, ears, eyes, family's, girls, here's, his, is, overalls, paws, rounds, rows, shoppers, size, sofas, stairs, things, upstairs

/f/: himself, shelf, off

/v/: above, gave, I've, live, of

/r/: furniture, after, are, bear, before, chair, cover, customer, dear, escalator, ever, everywhere, floor, for, four, her, here, more, mother, other, over, shoulder, store, there, under, were, you're your, never, other

/l/: all, comfortable, fell, girl, I'll, little, shall, smile, until, you'll

/sh/: crash

/voiceless th/: both, with

/long A/: away, day, they, way

/long E/: already, be, carefully, Corduroy, fuzzy, he, me, mommy, only, piggy, sadly, saleslady, see, she, somebody, suddenly, very

/long I/: my, why

/long O/: go, hello, know, no, oh, sew

/oo/: into, new, onto, who, you

/ow/: how, now

/uh/: a, Lisa

/ah/: saw

11. Generating words from the story beginning with a particular sound.

What to say to the student: "Let's think of words **from the story** that start with certain sounds."

EXAMPLE: "Tell me a word **from the story** that starts with / /." (stimulus sound) (e.g., "the sound /k/.") (Corduroy)

> ***NOTE:*** *Give letter sound not letter name. Use pictured items if necessary. Use any of the following stimulus words and/or others you select from the story. You say the sound (e.g., a voiceless /p/ sound) and the student is to say a word from the story that begins with that sound. Use any group of 10 stimulus items you select per teaching set.*

Stimulus items:

/p/: palace, paws, pick, piggy, pop, pulled, put

/b/: bang, bank, be, bear, bed, bear, before, began, besides, big, biggest, blinked, both, box, bright, bring, brown, but, button, buying, by

/d/: dashing, day, dear, department, did, didn't, doesn't, dolls, doors, down, drawers

/k/: came, can, carefully, carried, climb, come, Corduroy, could, counted, cover, crash, crawled, cried, customer, quite

/g/: gasped, gave, get, girl, go, going, gone, green

/ch/: chair, chest

/dz/: (as 1st sound in jelly): just

/m/: mattress, me, mommy, more, morning, most, mother, mountain, moving, much, must, my

/n/: know, new, next, night, no, not, nothing, now

/s/: sad, said, same, sat, saved, saw, searching, see, seemed, seen, set, sew, sighed, sight, size, sleep, small, smile, sofa, somebody, someone, something, spent, stairs, stepped, sticking, stood, stopped, store, straight, strap, spots, stairs, started, still, stopped, strange, street

/f/: family, fastened, fell, felt, filled, find, first, flashed, flight, floor, for, friend, from, furniture, fuzzy

/v/: very

/h/: had, he, he'd, heard, hello, her, here, here's, hiding, him, himself, his, home, how, hug, who

/r/: reached, right, room, round, rows

/l/: lamp, lap, large, last, late, light, like, Lisa, little, live, lock, look, looking, lost

/w/, /wh/: once, one, wag, waited, walked, wandered, want, wanted, warm, watched, watchman, way, when, why, wide, with, wondered, world

/sh/: shall, she, shelf, shoppers, shoulder, shut

/voiceless th/: thank, thick, things, think

/voiced th/: that, the, them, then, there, they, this

/y/ (as 1st sound in yellow): yanked, you, you'll you're, your

vowels: a, above, accident, admiring, after, all, along, alongside, already, always, amazing, an, and, animals, answered, apartment, are, arm, around, as, asked, awake, away, ears, else, escalator, evening, ever, everywhere, exclaimed, eyes, I'd, I'll, I'm, I've, in, into, is, it, of, off, oh, on, only, onto, other, over, overalls, own, under, until, up, upstairs

12. Blending sounds in monosyllabic words divided into onset-rime beginning with two consonant cluster + rime.

What to say to the student: "Now we'll put sounds together to make words."
EXAMPLE: "Put these sounds together to make a word (/ / + / /)." (stimulus sounds) "What's the word?" (e.g., "bl + ink: What's the word?") (blink)

NOTE: *Give letter sound not letter name. Use pictured items and/or manipulatives if necessary. Use any of the following stimulus words and/or others you select from the story. Correct answers are in parentheses.*

Stimulus items:

cl + ime (climb)	st + ore (store)
st + raps (straps)	cr + ied (cried)
br + ing (bring)	sp + ent (spent)
gr + een (green)	br + ite (bright)
fl + ash (flash)	st + airs (stairs)

13. Blending sounds in monosyllabic words divided into onset-rime beginning with single consonant + rime.

What to say to the student: "Let's put sounds together to make words."
EXAMPLE: "Put these sounds together to make a word (/ / + / /)." (stimulus sounds) "What's the word?" (e.g., "/h/ + ug: what's the word?") (hug)

> **NOTE:** *Give letter sound not letter name. Use pictured items and/or manipulatives if necessary. Use any of the following stimulus words and/or others you select from the story. Correct answers are in parentheses.*

Stimulus items:

/s/ + ize (size)	/l/ + amp (lamp)
/r/ + ound (round)	/d/ + oors (doors)
/m/ + ore (more)	/n/ + ite (night)
/l/ + arge (large)	/f/ + ell (fell)
/w/ + ide (wide)	/l/ + ate (late)

14. Blending sounds to form a monosyllabic word beginning with a continuant sound.

What to say to the student: "We'll put sounds together to make words."
EXAMPLE: "Put these sounds together to make a word (/ / + / / + / /)." (stimulus sounds) (e.g., "/n /long I/ /t/.") (night)

> **NOTE:** *Give letter sound not letter name. Use pictured items and/or manipulatives if necessary. Use any of the following stimulus words and/or others you select from the story. Correct answers are in parentheses.*

Stimulus items:

/m/ /ah/ /m/ (mom)
/s/ /l/ /long E/ /p/ (sleep)
/r/ /oo/ /m/ (room)
/l/ /short A/ /m/ /p/ (lamp)
/f/ /l/ /long I/ /t/ (flight)
/sh/ /short E/ /l/ /f/ (shelf)
/y/ /long A/ /ng/ /k/ (yank)
/n/ /short E/ /k/ /s/ /t/ (next)
/s/ /long A/ /m/ (same)
/f/ /r/ /short E/ /n/ /d/ (friend)

15. Blending sounds to form a monosyllabic word beginning with a noncontinuant sound.

What to say to the student: "We'll put sounds together to make words."
EXAMPLE: "Put these sounds together to make a word (/ / + / / + / /)." (stimulus sounds) (e.g., "/p/ /short I/ /k/.") (pick)

> *NOTE: Give letter sound not letter name. Use pictured items and/or manipulatives if necessary. Use any of the following stimulus words and/or others you select from the story. Correct answers are in parentheses.*

Stimulus items:

/b/ /short O /k/ /s/ (box)
/k/ /w/ /long I/ /t/ (quite)
/g/ /short A/ /s/ /p/ /t/ (gasped)
/k/ /r/ /short A/ /sh/ (crash)
/b/ /r/ /ow/ /n/ (brown)
/d/ /ah/ /l/ /z/ (dolls)
/ch/ /short E /s/ /t/ (chest)
/k/ /r/ /short A/ /sh/ (crash)
/p/ /ah/ /z/ (paws)
/b/ /short E/ /d/ /z/ (beds)

16. Substituting initial sound in words.

What to say to the student: "We're going to change beginning/first sounds in words."
EXAMPLE: "Say '_____.'" (stimulus word) "Instead of / /" (stimulus sound) "say / /." (stimulus sound) (e.g., Say 'box.' Instead of /b/ say /f/. What's your new word?") (fox)

> *NOTE: Give letter sound not letter name. Use pictured items and/or manipulatives if necessary. Use any of the following stimulus words and/or others you select from the story. Correct answers are in parentheses.*

Stimulus items:

"Say cried. Instead of /k/ say /t/." (tried)

"Say button. Instead of /b/ say /m/." (mutton)

"Say mountain. Instead of /m/ say /f/." (fountain)

"Say friend. Instead of /f/ say /t/." (trend)

"Say locked. Instead of /l/ say /sh/." (shocked)

"Say flashed. Instead of /f/ say /k/." (clashed)

"Say bank. Instead of /b/ say /voiceless th/." (thank)

"Say chair. Instead of /ch/ say /h/." (hair)

"Say home. Instead of /h/ say /k/." (comb)

"Say walked. Instead of /w/ say /t/." (talked)

17. Substituting final sound in words.

What to say to the student: "We're going to change ending/last sounds in words. **EXAMPLE:** "Say '_____.'" (stimulus word) "Instead of / /" (stimulus sound) "say / /." (stimulus sound) (e.g., "Say 'night.' Instead of /t/ say /n/. What's your new word?") (nine)

> ***NOTE:*** *Give letter sound not letter name. Use pictured items and/or manipulatives if necessary. Use any of the following stimulus words and/or others you select from the story. Correct answers are in parentheses.*

Stimulus items:

"Say spent. Instead of /t/ say /d/." (spend)

"Say straight. Instead of t/ say /n/." (strain)

"Say fills. Instead of /z/ say /d/." (filled)

"Say he'd. Instead of /d/ say /p/." (heap)

"Say like. Instead of /k/ say /m/." (lime)

"Say saved. Instead of /d/ say /m/." (same)

"Say green. Instead of /n/ say /d/." (greed)

"Say home. Instead of /m/ say /p/." (hope)

"Say arm. Instead of /m/ say /t/." (art)

"Say wide. Instead of /d/ say /z/." (wise)

18. Segmenting middle sound in monosyllabic words.

What to say to the student: "Tell me the middle sound in the word I say."
EXAMPLE: "What's the middle sound in the word '_____'?" (stimulus word) (e.g., "What's the middle sound in the word 'hug'?") (/short U/)

> ***NOTE:*** *Give letter sound not letter name. Use pictured items and/or manipulatives if necessary. Use any of the following stimulus words and/or others you select from the story. Correct answers are in parentheses.*

Stimulus items:

pop (/ah/)	thick (/short I/)
bed (/short E/)	much (/short U/)
arm (/r/)	guess (/short E/)
shut (/short U/)	size (/long I/)
hug (short /U/)	gone (/ah/)

19. Substituting middle sound in words.

What to say to the student: "We're going to change the middle sound in words."
EXAMPLE: "Say '_____.'" (stimulus word) "Instead of / /" (stimulus sound) "say / /." (stimulus sound) (e.g., "Say 'brown.' Instead of /ow/ say /long A/. What's your new word?") (brain)

> ***NOTE:*** *Give letter sound not letter name. Use pictured items and/or manipulatives if necessary. Use any of the following stimulus words and/or others you select from the story. Correct answers are in parentheses.*

Stimulus items:

"Say strap. Instead of /short A/ say /short I/." (strip)

"Say bright. Instead of /long I/ say /ah/." (brought)

"Say crash. Instead of /short A/ say /short U/."(crush)

"Say sleep. Instead of /long E/ say /short A/." (slap)

"Say home. Instead of /long O/ say /short A/." (ham)

"Say chair. Instead of /long A/ say /long E/." (cheer)

"Say lap. Instead of /short A/ say /short I/." (lip)

"Say fill. Instead of /short I/ say /ah/." (fall)

"Say quite. Instead of /long I/ say /short I/." (quit)

"Say shut. Instead of /short U/, say /long E/." (sheet)

20. Identifying all sounds in monosyllabic words.

What to say to the student: "Now tell me all the sounds you hear in the word I say."
EXAMPLE: "What sounds do you hear in the word '_____'?" (stimulus word) (e.g., "What sounds do you hear in the word 'gave'?") (/g/ /long A/ /v/)

> ***NOTE:*** *Give letter sound not letter name. Use pictured items and/or manipulatives if necessary. Use any of the following stimulus words and/or others you select from the story. Correct answers are in parentheses.*

Stimulus items:

green (/g/ /r/ /long E/ /n/)

straps (/s/ /t/ /short A/ /p/ /s/)

next (/n/ /short E/ /k/ /s/ /t/)

saved (/s/ /long A/ /v/ /d/)

climb (/k/ /l/ /long I/ /m/)

straight (/s/ /t/ /r/ /long A/ /t/)

cried (/k/ /r/ /long I/ /d/)

brown (/b/ /r/ /ow/ /n/)

lived (/l/ /short I/ /v/ /d/)

search (/s/ /long E/ /r/ /ch/)

21. Deleting sounds within words.

What to say to the student: "We're going to leave out sounds in words."
EXAMPLE: "Say '_____'" (stimulus word) "without / /." (stimulus sound) (e.g., "Say 'crash' without /r/." (cash) "The word that was left, 'cash,' is a real word. Sometimes the word won't be a real word.")

> ***NOTE:*** *Give letter sound not letter name. Use pictured items and/or manipulatives if necessary. Use any of the following stimulus words and/or others you select from the story. Correct answers are in parentheses.*

Stimulus items:

"Say floor without /l/." (for)

"Say quite without /w/." (kite)

"Say store without /t/." (sore)

"Say flights without /l/." (fights)

"Say bring without /r/." (bing)

"Say friend without /r/." (fend)

"Say bright without /r/." (bite)

"Say climb without /l/." (kime)

"Say sticking without /t/." (sicking)

"Say spent without /p/." (sent)

22. Substituting consonant in words having a two-sound cluster.

What to say to the student: "We're going to substitute sounds in words."
EXAMPLE: "Say '_____'" (stimulus word). "Instead of /_/" (stimulus sound) "say /_/" (stimulus sound) (e.g., "Say 'store.' Instead of /t/ say /n/.") (snore). Say: "Sometimes the new word will be a made-up word."

> ***NOTE:*** *Give letter sound not letter name. Use pictured items and/or manipulatives if necessary. Use any of the following stimulus words and/or others you select from the story. Correct answers are in parentheses.*

Stimulus items:

"Say green. Instead of /r/ say /l/." (glean)

"Say climb. Instead of /l/ say /r/." (crime)

"Say straps. Instead of /t/ say /k/." (scraps)

"Say stairs. Instead of /t/ say /p/." (spares)

"Say stop. Instead of /t/ say /l/."(slop)

"Say blink. Instead of /l/ say /r/." (brink)

"Say stick. Instead of /t/ say /l/." (slick)

"Say spots. Instead of /p/ say /l/." (slots)

"Say crash. Instead of /r/ say /l/" (clash)

"Say stairs. Instead of /t/ say /k/." (scares)

23. Phoneme reversing.

What to say to the student: "We're going to say words backward."
EXAMPLE: "Say the word '_____'" (stimulus word) "backward." (e.g., "Say 'bed' backward.") (deb)

> ***NOTE:*** *This is a difficult phoneme-level task and should only be done with older students. Give letter sound not letter name. Use pictured items and/or manipulatives if necessary. Use any of the following stimulus words and/or others you select from the story. Correct answers are in parentheses.*

Stimulus items:

came	(make)	shelf	(flesh)
reach	(cheer)	lap	(pal)
seen	(niece)	step	(pets)
can	(knack)	stick	(kits)
gave	(vague)	much	(chum)

24. Phoneme switching.

What to say to the student: "We're going to switch the first sounds in two words."
EXAMPLE: "Switch the first sounds in '_____' and '_____.'" (stimulus words) (e.g., "Switch the first sounds in 'her family.'") (fur hamily)

> ***NOTE:*** *This is a difficult phoneme-level task and should only be done with older students. Give letter sound not letter name. Use pictured items and/or manipulatives if necessary. Use any of the following stimulus words and/or others you select from the story. Correct answers are in parentheses.*

Stimulus items:

tied down	(died town)
right size	(sight rise)
lost button	(bost lutton)
little bed	(bittle led)

big hug	(hig bug)
fuzzy brown	(buzzy frown)
thick mattress	(mick thatress)
both paws	(poth baws)
more comfortable	(core mumfortable)
Corduroy home	(horduroy comb)

25. Pig latin.

What to say to the student: "We're going to talk in a secret language using words from the story. In pig latin, you take off the first sound of a word, put it at the end of the word, and add a long A sound."

EXAMPLE: "Say chest in pig latin." (estchay)

> ***NOTE:*** *This is a difficult phoneme-level task and should only be done with older students. Use pictured items and/or manipulatives if necessary. Use any of the following stimulus words and/or others you select from the story. Correct answers are in parentheses.*

Stimulus items:

doll	(allday)
button	(uttonbay)
sadly	(adlysay)
guess	(essgay)
went	(entway)
thick	(ickthay)
shut	(utshay)
wandered	(anderedway)
dashing	(ashingday)
mountain	(ountainmay)

CHAPTER

PHONOLOGICAL AWARENESS ACTIVITIES TO USE WITH *HAPPY BIRTHDAY, MOON*

Text version used for selection of stimulus items:

Asch, F. (1982). *Happy birthday, moon*. Englewood Cliffs, NJ: Scholastic Inc.

PHONOLOGICAL AWARENESS ACTIVITIES AT THE WORD LEVEL

1. Counting words.

What to say to the student: "We're going to count words."
EXAMPLE: "How many words do you hear in this sentence (or phrase)? 'his voice.'" (2)

> *NOTE: Use pictured items and/or manipulatives if necessary. Use any of the following stimulus phrases or sentences and/or others you select from the story. Correct answers are in parentheses.*

Stimulus items:

he thought (2)

the bank (2)

with the moon (3)

at the sky (3)

found the hat (3)

it fits just right (4)

I still love you (4)

oh boy he thought (4)

bear climbed a tall tree (5)

I would like a hat (5)

2. Identifying missing word from list.

What to say to the student: "Listen to the words I say. I'll say them again. You tell me which word I leave out."

EXAMPLE: "Listen to the words I say: 'did, money, hat.' I'll say them again. Tell me which one I leave out: 'did, hat.'" (money)

> *NOTE: Use pictured items and/or manipulatives if necessary. Use any of the following stimulus words and/or others you select from the story. Correct answers are in parentheses.*

Stimulus set #1	Stimulus set #2
voice, tree	voice (tree)
river, chat	chat (river)
find, yell, moon	find, moon (yell)
tomorrow, bank, blue	tomorrow, blue (bank)
you, branches, hello	branches, hello (you)
crept, top, beautiful	crept, beautiful (top)
okay, moon, voice, top	okay, voice, top (moon)
chased, bought, I'm, shout	bought, I'm, shout (chased)
after, night, through, talk	after, through, talk (night)
fell, reply, love, hat	fell, reply, love (hat)

3. Identifying missing word in phrase or sentence.

What to say to the student: "Listen to the sentence I read. Tell me which word is missing the second time I read the sentence."

EXAMPLE: "'Happy Birthday, Moon.' Listen again and tell me which word I leave out. 'Happy____, Moon.'" (birthday)

> ***NOTE:*** *Use pictured items and/or manipulatives if necessary. Use any of the following stimulus sentences and/or others you select from the story. Correct answers are in parentheses.*

Stimulus items:

Birthday present. Birthday_____. (present)

Hello moon. _____ moon. (Hello)

Into the mountains. Into the ______. (mountains)

His voice echoed. His _____ echoed. (voice)

A beautiful hat. A ____ hat. (beautiful)

My birthday is tomorrow. My birthday is _____. (tomorrow)

He chased after it. He _____ after it. (chased)

When is your birthday? When is _____ birthday? (your)

Bear paddled across the river. Bear _____ across the river. (paddled)

I'm talking to the moon. I'm _____ to the moon. (talking)

4. Supplying missing word as adult reads.

What to say to the student: "I want you to help me read the story. You fill in the words I leave out."

EXAMPLE: "Happy Birthday ____." (moon or bear)

> ***NOTE:*** *Use pictured items and/or manipulatives if necessary. Use any of the following stimulus sentences and/or others you select from the story. Correct answers are in parentheses.*

Stimulus items:

He climbed a tall _____. (tree)

Bear dumped the_____ out of his piggy bank. (money)

Goodbye said the _____. (bear or moon)

My _____ is tomorrow. (birthday)

He hiked through the _____. (forest)

But the _____ did not reply. (moon)

His voice echoed off the _____. (mountains)

He bought the moon a beautiful _____ . (hat)

"Hooray!" Yelled the Bear. "It fits just _____." (right)

He found the hat on his _____. (doorstep)

5. Rearranging words.

What to say to the student: "I'll say some words out of order. You put them in the right order so they make sense."

EXAMPLE: "'home got.' Put those words in the right order." (got home)

> *NOTE: Use pictured items and/or manipulatives if necessary. Use any of the following stimulus words and/or others you select from the story. Correct answers are in parentheses. This word-level activity can be more difficult than some of the syllable- or phoneme-level activities because of the memory load. If your students are only able to deal with two or three words to be rearranged, add more two- and three-word stimulus items from the story and omit the four-word level items.*

Stimulus items:

night one (one night)

mountains other (other mountains)

present birthday (birthday present)

the fell hat (the hat fell)

moon the give (give the moon)

the mountains into (into the mountains)

piggy his bank (his piggy bank)

goodbye the said moon (goodbye said the moon)

right it fits just (it fits just right)

hat blew wind Bear's (wind blew Bear's hat)

PHONOLOGICAL AWARENESS ACTIVITIES AT THE SYLLABLE LEVEL

1. Syllable counting.

What to say to the student: "We're going to count syllables (or parts) of words."

EXAMPLE: "How many syllables do you hear in '_____'?" (stimulus word) (e.g., "How many syllables in 'piggy'?") (2)

NOTE: Use pictured items and/or manipulatives if necessary. Use any of the following stimulus words and/or others you select from the story. Use any group of 10 stimulus items you select per teaching set.

Stimulus items:

One-syllable words: put, bank, bear, blew, bought, boy, but, talk, tall, tell, time, tool, top, tree, try, did, do, climb, could, crept, gave, get, give, got, chat, chase, just, me, moon, much, know, nice, night, not, now, said, sky, slept, so, speak, spoke still, far, fell, find, first, fit, for, found, voice, hat, he, hear, hike, him, his, home, right, like, look, love, one, want, watch, well, went, what, when, where, while, wind, would, thought, through, that, the, then, this, yell, you, yours, all, am, and, ask, I'm, is, it, of, off, oh, on, out, own, up

Two-syllable words: paddle, piggy, present, birthday, branches, talking, doorstep, downtown, during, cannot, closer, goody, goodbye, maybe, moment, money, morning, mountain, slowly, forest, very, happen, hello, hooray, reply, river, little, waited, shouted, across, after, away, exclaim, into, okay, other

Three-syllable words: perfectly, beautiful, tomorrow, excited

2. Initial syllable deleting.

What to say to the student: "We're going to leave out syllables (or parts of words)." ***EXAMPLE:*** "Say '_____.'" (stimulus word) "Say it again without '_____.'" (stimulus syllable) (e.g., "Say 'doorstep.' Say it again without 'door.'") (step)

NOTE: Use pictured items and/or manipulatives if necessary. Use any of the following stimulus words and/or others you select from the story. Correct answers are in parentheses.

Stimulus items:

"Say okay without oh." (kay)

"Say morning without morn." (-ing)

"Say into without in." (to)

"Say goodbye without good." (bye)

"Say birthday without birth." (day)

"Say forest without for." (-est)

"Say happen without hap." (pen or -en)

"Say away without a-." (way)

"Say slowly without slow." (lee)

"Say cannot without can." (not)

3. Final syllable deleting.

What to say to the student: "We're going to leave out syllables (or parts of words)."
EXAMPLE: "Say '_____.'" (stimulus word) "Say it again without '_____.'" (stimulus syllable) (e.g., "Say 'doorstep' without 'step.'") (door)

> **NOTE:** *Use pictured items and/or manipulatives if necessary. Use any of the following stimulus words and/or others you select from the story. Correct answers are in parentheses.*

Stimulus items:

"Say downtown without town." (down)

"Say goody without -ee." (good)

"Say doorstep without step." (door)

"Say birthday without day." (birth)

"Say morning without -ing." (morn)

"Say perfectly without lee." (perfect)

"Say hurray without -ay." (her)

"Say mountain without -en." (mount)

"Say after without er-." (aft)

"Say forest without -est." (for)

4. Initial syllable adding.

What to say to the student: "Now let's add syllables (or parts) to words."
EXAMPLE: " Add '_____'" (stimulus syllable) "to the beginning of '_____.'" (stimulus syllable) (e.g., "Add 'to' to the beginning of 'morrow.'") (tomorrow)

> **NOTE:** *Use pictured items and/or manipulatives if necessary. Use any of the following stimulus words and/or others you select from the story. Correct answers are in parentheses.*

Stimulus items:

"Add down to the beginning of town." (downtown)

"Add re- to the beginning of -ply." (reply)

"Add birth to the beginning of day." (birthday)

"Add good to the beginning of bye." (goodbye)

"Add slow to the beginning of lee." (slowly)

"Add shout to the beginning of -ed." (shouted)

"Add mo- to the beginning of –ment." (moment)

"Add can to the beginning of not." (cannot)

"Add oh to the beginning of kay." (okay)

"Add good to the beginning of -ee." (goody)

5. Final syllable adding.

What to say to the student: "Now let's add syllables (or parts) to words."

EXAMPLE: "Add '_____'" (stimulus syllable) "to the end of '_____.'" (stimulus syllable) (e.g., "Add 'ing' to the end of 'morn.'") (morning)

> ***NOTE:*** *Use pictured items and/or manipulatives if necessary. Use any of the following stimulus words and/or others you select from the story. Correct answers are in parentheses.*

Stimulus items:

"Add day to the end of birth." (birthday)

"Add lee to the end of perfect." (perfectly)

"Add be to the end of may." (maybe)

"Add ray to the end of her." (hurray)

"Add -er to the end of riv-." (river)

"Add step to the end of door." (doorstep)

"Add -ing to the end of dur-." (during)

"Add way to the end of a-." (away)

"Add bye to the end of good." (goodbye)

"Add claim to the end of ex-." (exclaim)

6. Syllable substituting.

What to say to the student: "Let's make up some new words."

EXAMPLE: "Say '_____.'" (stimulus word) "Instead of '_____'" (stimulus syllable) "say '_____.'" (stimulus syllable) (e.g., "Say 'slowly.' Instead of 'lee' say 'ing.' The new word is 'slowing.'")

NOTE: Use pictured items and/or manipulatives if necessary. Use any of the following stimulus words and/or others you select from the story. Correct answers are in parentheses.

Stimulus items:

"Say doorstep. Instead of step say knob." (doorknob)

"Say cannot. Instead of can say will." (will not)

"Say goodbye. Instead of good say near." (nearby)

"Say morning. Instead of morn- say run." (running)

"Say beautiful. Instead of beauti- say cup." (cupful)

"Say after. Instead of af- say laugh." (laughter)

"Say okay. Instead of oh say bow." (pronounced with long /O/) (bouquet)

"Say tomorrow. Instead of morrow say day." (today)

"Say exclaim. Instead of claim say it." (exit)

"Say hurray. Instead of ray say self." (herself)

PHONOLOGICAL AWARENESS ACTIVITIES AT THE PHONEME LEVEL

1. Counting sounds.

What to say to the student: "We're going to count sounds in words."
EXAMPLE: "How many sounds do you hear in this word? 'moon.'" (3)

NOTE: Use pictured items and/or manipulatives if necessary. Use any of the following stimulus words and/or others you select from the story. Be sure to give the letter sound and not the letter name. Use any group of 10 stimulus items you select per teaching set.

Stimulus words with two sounds: to, do, me, so, he, up, am, off, is, in, it, on

Stimulus words with three sounds: put, bear, bought, but, tree, time, top, talk, did, could, give, got, get, gave, chat, moon, much, night, nice, not, sky, right, fit, him, hike, hat, home, look, like, love, thought, through, this, then, that

Stimulus words with four sounds: piggy, bank, goody, chased, just, money, speak, spoke, still, find, fits, found, first, hiked

Stimulus words with five sounds: paddled, branch, dumped, cannot, closer, crept, chased, slowly, slept, reply, happens, across

2. Sound categorization or identifying rhyme oddity.

What to say to the student: "Guess which word I say does not rhyme with the other three words."

EXAMPLE: "Tell me which word does not rhyme with the other three. '_____, _____, _____, _____.'" (stimulus words) (e.g., " 'night, hat, light, sight.' Which word doesn't rhyme?") (hat)

> *NOTE: Use pictured items if necessary. Use any of the following stimulus words and/or others you select from the story. Correct answers are in parentheses.*

Stimulus items:

moon, loon, spoon, hello (hello)

hear, paddled, saddled, faddled (hear)

love, dove, across, shove (across)

right, light, doorstep, fight (doorstep)

first, thought, bought, sought (first)

boy, mountain, toy, soy (mountain)

where, bear, goody, fair (goody)

climb, away, I'm, rhyme (away)

shout, out, branches, doubt (branches)

top, mop, cop, birthday (birthday)

3. Matching rhyme.

What to say to the student: "We're going to think of rhyming words."

EXAMPLE: "Which word rhymes with '_____'?" (stimulus word) (e.g., "Which word rhymes with 'chat:' 'hat, all, and, then'?") (hat)

> *NOTE: Use pictured items if necessary. Use any of the following stimulus words and/or others you select from the story. Correct answers are in parentheses.*

Stimulus items:

all: bear, should, climbed, fall (fall)

crept: slept, tree, while, is (slept)

hike: very, talk, bike, exclaimed (bike)

voice: blew, choice, goody, birthday (choice)

thought: goodbye, tomorrow, said, sought (sought)

fell: forest, tell, across, dumped (tell)

present: reply, chased, pheasant, during (pheasant)

sky: fly, little, shouted, branches (fly)

bank: slowly, just, sank, tried (sank)

nice: beautiful, get, hear, ice (ice)

4. Producing rhyme.

What to say to the student: "Now we'll say rhyming words."
EXAMPLE: "Tell me a word that rhymes with '_____.'" (stimulus word) (e.g., "Tell me a word that rhymes with 'top.' You can make up a word if you want.") (hop)

> ***NOTE:*** *Use pictured items if necessary. Use any of the following stimulus words and/or others you select from the story, i.e., you say a word from the list below and the student is to think of a rhyming word. Use any group of 10 stimulus items you select per teaching set.*

Stimulus items:

/p/: paddle, piggy, present (emphasis on first syllable), put

/b/: bank, bear, blew, bought, boy, branch, but

/t/: talk, talking, tall, tell, time, too, top, tree, tried

/d/: did, do, dumped

/k/: climb, close, could, crept

/g/: gave, get, give, goody, got

/ch/: chat, chase

/dz/: (as 1st sound in jelly): just

/m/: me, money, moon, mountain, much

/n/: know, nice, night, now

/s/: said, sky, slept, slow, so, speak, spoke, still

/f/: far, fell, find, first, fit, for, found

/v/: very, voice

/h/: hat, he, hear, hello, hike, him, his, home, hooray

/r/: right, river

/l/: like, little, look, love

/w/, /wh/: one, wait, want, watch, well, went, what, when, where, while, wind (with a short /I/), would

/sh/: shouted

/voiceless th/: thought, through

/voiced th/: that, the, then, this

/y/ (as 1st sound in yellow): yell, you, your

vowels: a, after, all, am, and, ask, I, I'm, in, is, it, of, off, oh, on, other, out, own, up

5. Sound matching (initial).

What to say to the student: "Now we'll listen for the first sound in words."
EXAMPLE: "Listen to this sound: / /." (stimulus sound). "Guess which word I say begins with that sound. '_____, _____, _____, _____.'" (stimulus words) (e.g., "Listen to this sound /n/. Guess which word I say begins with that sound: 'very, night, shouted, river.'") (night)

Stimulus items:

> ***NOTE:*** *Give letter sound not letter name. Use pictured items if necessary. Use any of the following stimulus words and/or others you select from the story. Correct answers are in parentheses.*

/r/: this, river, am, voice (river)

/m/: got, after, nice, moon (moon)

/b/: birthday, shouted, know, tree (birthday)

/p/: tall, very, piggy, happens (piggy)

/g/: mountains, looked, first, gave (gave)

/l/: present, little, speak, whole (little)

/w/: chat, cannot, watch, found (watch)

/y/: yelled, tried, love, okay (yelled)

/t/: wind, chased, paddled, tomorrow (tomorrow)

/d/: spoke, time, downtown, beautiful (downtown)

6. Sound matching (final).

What to say to the student: "Now we'll listen for the last sound in words."

EXAMPLE: "Listen to this sound: / /" (stimulus sound). "Guess which word I say ends with that sound? '_____, _____, _____, _____.'" (stimulus words) (e.g., "Listen to this sound /p/. Guess which word I say ends with that sound: chat, top, home, fits.") (top)

> *NOTE: Give letter sound not letter name. Use pictured items if necessary. Use any of the following stimulus words and/or others you select from the story. Correct answers are in parentheses.*

Stimulus items:

/v/: morning, cannot, gave, money (gave)

/t/: hurray, night, moon, excited (night)

/k/: replied, hello, goodbye, talk (talk)

/z/: tried, downtown, branches, just (branches)

/p/: doorstep, after, chased, talking (doorstep)

/k/: moment, while, spoke, river (spoke)

/n/: thought, moon, yelled, bank (moon)

/l/: cannot, happens, found, beautiful (beautiful)

/d/: replied, hear, then, paddle (replied)

/s/: crept, across, tell, forest (across)

7. Identifying initial sound in words.

What to say to the student: "I'll say a word two times. Tell me what sound is missing the second time. '______, _______.'" (stimulus words)

EXAMPLE: "What sound do you hear in '_____'" (stimulus word) "that is missing in '_____'?" (stimulus word) (e.g., "What sound do you hear in 'slept,' that is missing in '-lept'?") (/s/)

> *NOTE: Give letter sound not letter name. Use pictured items and/or manipulatives if necessary. Use any of the following stimulus words and/or others you select from the story. Correct answers are in parentheses.*

Stimulus items:

"shout, -out. What sound do you hear in shout that is missing in out?" (/sh/)

"branch, -ranch. What sound do you hear in branch that is missing in ranch?" (/b/)

"thought, -ought. What sound do you hear in thought that is missing in -ought?" (/th/)

"while, -aisle. What sound do you hear in while that is missing in aisle?" (/w/)

"climb, -lime. What sound do you hear in climb that is missing in -lime?" (/k/)

"door, -or. What sound do you hear in door that is missing in or?" (/d/)

"paddle, -addle. What sound do you hear in paddle that is missing in addle?" (/p/)

"time, -I'm. What sound do you hear in time that is missing in I'm?" (/t/)

"blew, -lew. What sound do you hear in blew that is missing in lew?" (/b/)

"chat, -at. What sound do you hear in chat that is missing in at?" (/ch/)

8. Identifying final sound in words.

What to say to the student: "I'll say a word two times. Tell me what sound is missing the second time. '______, _______.'" (stimulus words)

EXAMPLE: "What sound do you hear in '_____'" (stimulus word) "that is missing in '_____'?" (stimulus word) (e.g., "What sound do you hear in 'right' that is missing in 'rye'?") (/t/)

> *NOTE: Give letter sound not letter name. Use pictured items and/or manipulatives if necessary. Use any of the following stimulus words and/or others you select from the story. Correct answers are in parentheses.*

Stimulus items:

"first, firs-. What sound do you hear in first that is missing in firs-?" (/t/)

"paddled, paddle-. What sound do you hear in paddled that is missing in paddle-?" (/d/)

"home, hoe-. What sound do you hear in home that is missing in hoe-?" (/m/)

"piggy, pig-.What sound do you hear in piggy that is missing in pig-?" (/ee/ pronounced long E)

"wind, (pronounced with short /I/), win-. What sound do you hear in wind that is missing in win-?" (/d/)

"thought, thaw-. What sound do you hear in thought that is missing in thaw-?" (/t/)

"closer, close-. What sound do you hear in closer that is missing in close?" (/r/)

"dumped, dump-. What sound do you hear in dumped that is missing in dump-?" (/t/)

"time, tie-. What sound do you hear in time that is missing in tie-?" (/m/)

"moon, moo-. What sound do you hear in moon that is missing in moo-?" (/n/)

9. Segmenting initial sound in words.

What to say to the student: "Listen to the word I say and tell me the first sound you hear."

EXAMPLE: "What's the first sound in '_____'?" (stimulus word) (e.g., "What's the first sound in 'fell'?") (/f/)

> ***NOTE:*** *Give letter sound not letter name. Use pictured items and/or manipulatives if necessary. Use any of the following stimulus words and/or others you select from the story. Use any group of 10 stimulus items you select per teaching set.*

Stimulus items:

/p/: paddled, perfectly, piggy, present, put

/b/: bank, bear, beautiful, birthday, blew, bought, boy, branch, but

/t/: talk, talking, tall, tell, time, tomorrow, too, top, tree, tried

/d/: did, do, doorstep, downtown, dumped, during

/k/: cannot, climbed, closer, could, crept

/g/: gave, get, give, goody, goodbye, got

/ch/: chat, chase

/dz/: (as 1st sound in jelly): just

/m/: maybe, me, moment, money, moon, mountain, much

/n/: know, nice, night, now

/s/: said, sky, slept, slowly, so, speak, spoke, still

/f/: far, fell, find, first, fit, for, forest, found

/v/: very, voice

/h/: happen, hat, he, hear, hello, hike, him, his, home, hooray

/r/: reply, right, river

/l/: like, little, look, love

/w/, /wh/: one, wait, want, watch, well, went, what, when, where, while, wind (with a short /I/), would

/sh/: shouted

/voiceless th/: thought, through

/voiced th/: that, the, then, this

/y/ (as 1st sound in yellow): yell, you, your

vowels: a, across, after, all, am, and, ask, away, excited, exclaim, I, I'm, in, into, is, it, of,

off, oh, okay, on, other, out, own, up

10. Segmenting final sound in words.

What to say to the student: "Listen to the word I say and tell me the last sound you hear." ***EXAMPLE:*** "What's the last sound in the word '_____'?" (stimulus word) (e.g., "What's the last sound in the word 'moon'?") (/n/)

NOTE: *Give letter sound not letter name. Use pictured items and/or manipulatives if necessary. Use any of the following stimulus words and/or others you select from the story. Use any group of 10 stimulus items you select per teaching set.*

Stimulus items:

/p/: doorstep, top, up

/t/: bought, but, cannot, chat, crept, dumped, first, fit, forest, get, got, hat, it, just, moment, night, not, out, present, put, right, slept, that, thought, want, went, what

/d/: and, climbed, could, did, excited, exclaimed, find, found, paddled, replied, said, shouted, waited, wind, would, yelled

/k/: bank, like, look, speak, spoke

/ch/: much, watch

/m/: am, him, home, I'm, time

/n/: downtown, in, moon, mountain, on, one, then, when

/ng/: during, morning, talking

/s/: across, fits, nice, that's, this, voice

/z/: branches, his, is

/f/: off

/v/: gave, give, love, of

/r/: after, bear, closer, far, for, hear, other, river, where, your

/l/: all, beautiful, little, tall, tell, well, while

/long A/: away, birthday, okay

/long E/: goody, he, maybe, me, perfectly, piggy, slowly, tree, very

/long I/: goodbye, reply, sky

/long O/: hello, know, so, tomorrow

/oi/: boy

/oo/: do, to, into

11. Generating words from the story beginning with a particular sound.

What to say to the student: "Let's think of words from the story that start with certain sounds."

EXAMPLE: "Tell me a word from the story that starts with / /." (stimulus sound) (e.g., "the sound /k/") (climbed)

> ***NOTE:*** *Give letter sound not letter name. Use pictured items if necessary. Use any of the following stimulus words and/or others you select from the story. You say the sound (e.g., a voiceless /p/ sound) and the student is to say a word from the story that begins with that sound. Use any group of 10 stimulus items you select per teaching set.*

Stimulus items:

/p/: paddled, perfectly, piggy, present, put

/b/: bank, bear, beautiful, birthday, blew, bought, boy, branch, but

/t/: talk, talking, tall, tell, time, tomorrow, too, top, tree, tried

/d/: did, do, doorstep, downtown, dumped, during

/k/: cannot, climbed, closer, could, crept

/g/: gave, get, give, goody, goodbye, got

/ch/: chat, chase

/dz/: (as 1st sound in jelly): just

/m/: maybe, me, moment, money, moon, mountain, much

/n/: know, nice, night, now

/s/: said, sky, slept, slowly, so, speak, spoke, still

/f/: far, fell, find, first, fit, for, forest, found

/v/: very, voice

/h/: happen, hat, he, hear, hello, hike, him, his, home, hooray

/r/: reply, right, river

/l/: like, little, look, love

/w/, /wh/: one, wait, want, watch, well, went, what, when, where, while, wind (with a short /I/), would

/sh/: shouted

/voiceless th/: thought, through

/voiced th/: that, the, then, this

/y/ (as 1st sound in yellow): yell, you, your

vowels: a, across, after, all, am, and, ask, away, excited, exclaim, I, I'm, in, into, is, it, of, off, oh, okay, on, other, out, own, up

12. Blending sounds in monosyllabic words divided into onset-rime beginning with two consonant cluster + rime.

What to say to the student: "Now we'll put sounds together to make words."
EXAMPLE: "Put these sounds together to make a word (/ / + / /)." (stimulus sounds) "What's the word?" (e.g., "cl + ose: What's the word?") (close)

> ***NOTE:*** *Give letter sound not letter name. Use pictured items and/or manipulatives if necessary. Use any of the following stimulus words and/or others you select from the story. Correct answers are in parentheses.*

Stimulus items:

cl + ime (climb)	sp + eak (speak)
sp + oke (spoke)	tr + ied (tried)
bl + ew (blew)	th + ought (thought)
sl + ept (slept)	br + anch (branch)
st + ill (still)	cr + ept (crept)

13. Blending sounds in monosyllabic words divided into onset-rime beginning with single consonant + rime.

What to say to the student: "Let's put sounds together to make words."
EXAMPLE: "Put these sounds together to make a word (/ / + / /)." (stimulus sounds) "What's the word?" (e.g., "/b/ + ought: what's the word?") (bought)

> **NOTE:** *Give letter sound not letter name. Use pictured items and/or manipulatives if necessary. Use any of the following stimulus words and/or others you select from the story. Correct answers are in parentheses.*

Stimulus items:

/b/ + oy (boy)
/m/ + oon (moon)
/t/ + op (top)
/l/ + ove (love)
/v/ + oice (voice)
/w/ + ent (went)
/b/ + ank (bank)
/f/ + it (fit)
/b/ + air (bear)
/t/ + ok (talk)

14. Blending sounds to form a monosyllabic word beginning with a continuant sound.

What to say to the student: "We'll put sounds together to make words."
EXAMPLE: "Put these sounds together to make a word (/ / + / / + / /)." (stimulus sounds) (e.g., "/m/ /oo/ /n/.") (moon)

> **NOTE:** *Give letter sound not letter name. Use pictured items and/or manipulatives if necessary. Use any of the following stimulus words and/or others you select from the story. Correct answers are in parentheses.*

Stimulus items:

/h/ /short I/ /m/ (him)
/w/ /short E/ /n/ /t/ (went)
/m/ /long E/ /n/ (mean)
/f/ /long I/ /n/ /d/ (find)
/w/ /short I/ /n/ /d/ (wind)
/n/ /oi/ /z/ (noise)
/w/ /short E/ /l/ (well)
/m/ /short U/ /n/ /ch/ (munch)
/r/ /short E/ /s/ /t/ (rest)
/f/ /short E/ /l/ (fell)

15. Blending sounds to form a monosyllabic word beginning with a noncontinuant sound.

What to say to the student: "We'll put sounds together to make words."
EXAMPLE: "Put these sounds together to make a word (/ / + / / + / /)." (stimulus sounds) (e.g., "/g/ /short O/ /t/.") (got)

> *NOTE: Give letter sound not letter name. Use pictured items and/or manipulatives if necessary. Use any of the following stimulus words and/or others you select from the story. Correct answers are in parentheses.*

Stimulus items:

/b/ /ah/ /t/ (bought)
/k/ /l/ /long I/ /m/ (climb)
/k/ /r/ /short E/ /p/ /t/ (crept)
/ch/ /short A/ /t/ (chat)
/t/ /long I/ /m/ (time)
/ch/ /long O/ /k/ (choke)
/t/ /ah/ /k/ (talk)
/p/ /short I/ /k/ (pick)
/k/ /short E/ /p/ /t/ (kept)
/ch/ /long A/ /s/ (chase)

16. Substituting initial sound in words.

What to say to the student. "We're going to change beginning/first sounds in words."
EXAMPLE: "Say '_____.'" (stimulus word) "Instead of / /" (stimulus sound) "say / /." (stimulus sound) (e.g., "Say 'said.' Instead of /s/ say /f/. What's your new word?") (fed)

> *NOTE: Give letter sound not letter name. Use pictured items and/or manipulatives if necessary. Use any of the following stimulus words and/or others you select from the story. Correct answers are in parentheses.*

Stimulus items:

"Say night. Instead of /n/ say /l/." (light)
"Say piggy. Instead of /p/ say /z/." (ziggy)
"Say first. Instead of /f/ say /b/." (burst)
"Say could. Instead of /k/ say /sh/." (should)
"Say blew. Instead of /b/ say /f/." (flew)

"Say moon. Instead of /m/ say /s/." (soon)

"Say bear. Instead of /b/ say /ch/." (chair)

"Say mountains. Instead of /m/ say /f/." (fountains)

"Say found. Instead of /f/ say /b/." (bound)

"Say talking. Instead of /t/ say /w/." (walking)

17. Substituting final sound in words.

What to say to the student: "We're going to change ending/last sounds in words."
EXAMPLE: "Say '_____.'" (stimulus word) "Instead of / /" (stimulus sound) "say / /." (stimulus sound) (e.g., "Say 'like.' Instead of /k/ say /t/. What's your new word?") (light)

> ***NOTE:*** *Give letter sound not letter name. Use pictured items and/or manipulatives if necessary. Use any of the following stimulus words and/or others you select from the story. Correct answers are in parentheses.*

Stimulus items:

"Say yelled. Instead of /d/ say /z/." (yells)

"Say chat. Instead of /t/ say /p/." (chap)

"Say bought. Instead of /t/ say /m/." (bomb)

"Say gave. Instead of /v/ say /t/." (gate)

"Say moon. Instead of /n/, say /z/." (moos)

"Say not. Instead of /t/ say /k/." (knock)

"Say speak. Instead of /k/ say /d/." (speed)

"Say hello. Instead of /o/ say /p/." (help)

"Say love. Instead of /v/ say /k/." (luck)

"Say right. Instead of /t/ say /m/." (rhyme)

18. Segmenting middle sound in monosyllabic words.

What to say to the student: "Tell me the middle sound in the word I say."
EXAMPLE: "What's the middle sound in the word '_____'?" (stimulus word) (e.g., "What's the middle sound in the word 'did'?") (short /I/)

> ***NOTE:*** *Give letter sound not letter name. Use pictured items and/or manipulatives if necessary. Use any of the following stimulus words and/or others you select from the story. Correct answers are in parentheses.*

Stimulus items:

tree (/r/)
chat (/short A/)
gave (/long A/)
shout (/ow/)
hike (/long I/)
much (/short U/)
fit (/short I/)
like (/long I/)
get (/short E/)
sky (/k/)

19. Substituting middle sound in words.

What to say to the student: "We're going to change the middle sound in words."
EXAMPLE: "Say '_____.'" (stimulus word) "Instead of / /" (stimulus sound) "say / /." (stimulus sound) (e.g., "Say 'wait.' Instead of /long A/ say /long I/. What's your new word?") (white)

> ***NOTE:*** *Give letter sound not letter name. Use pictured items and/or manipulatives if necessary. Use any of the following stimulus words and/or others you select from the story. Correct answers are in parentheses.*

Stimulus items:

"Say time. Instead of /long I/ say /long A/." (tame)
"Say chat. Instead of /short A/ say /long E/." (cheat)
"Say love. Instead of /short U/ say /short I/." (live)
"Say night. Instead of /long I/ say /ah/."(not)
"Say bought. Instead of /ah/ say /long I/." (bite)
"Say gave. Instead of /long A/ say /short I/." (give)
"Say hike. Instead of /long I/ say /short A/." (hack)
"Say top. Instead of /ah/ say /short I/." (tip)
"Say hat. Instead of /short A/ say /short I/." (hit)
"Say home. Instead of /long O/ say /short A/." (ham)

20. Identifying all sounds in monosyllabic words.

What to say to the student: "Now tell me all the sounds you hear in the word I say."
EXAMPLE: "What sounds do you hear in the word '_____'?" (stimulus word) (e.g., "What sounds do you hear in the word 'top'?") (/t/ /ah/ /p/)

> *NOTE: Give letter sound not letter name. Use pictured items and/or manipulatives if necessary. Use any of the following stimulus words and/or others you select from the story. Correct answers are in parentheses.*

Stimulus items:

but (/b/ /short U/ /t/)

his (/h/ /short I/ /z/)

ask (/short A/ /s/ /k/)

said (/s/ /short E/ /d/)

right (/r/ /long I/ /t/)

want (/w/ /ah/ /n/ /t/)

home (/h/ /long O/ /m/)

hat (/h/ /short A/ /t/)

love (/l/ /short U/ /v/)

voice (/v/ /oi/ /s/)

21. Deleting sounds within words.

What to say to the student. "We're going to leave out sounds in words."
EXAMPLE: "Say '_____'" (stimulus word) "without / /." (stimulus sound) (e.g., "Say 'blew' without /l/."(boo). "The word that was left, 'boo,' is a real word. Sometimes the word won't be a real word."

> *NOTE: Give letter sound not letter name. Use pictured items and/or manipulatives if necessary. Use any of the following stimulus words and/or others you select from the story. Correct answers are in parentheses.*

Stimulus items:

"Say goodbite without /t/." (goodbye)

"Say present without /r/." (peasant)

"Say branch without /r/." (banch)

"Say crept without /r/." (kept)

"Say speak without /p/." (seek)

"Say sky without /k/." (sigh)

"Say slow without /l/." (so)

"Say and without /n/." (add)

"Say spoke without /p/." (soak)

"Say tree without /r/." (tea)

22. Substituting consonant in words having a two-sound cluster.

What to say to the student: "We're going to substitute sounds in words."
EXAMPLE: "Say '_____'" (stimulus word). "Instead of / /" (stimulus sound) "say / /" (stimulus sound) (e.g., "Say 'sky.' Instead of /k/ say /t/.") (sty). Say: "Sometimes the new word will be a made-up word."

> ***NOTE:*** *Give letter sound not letter name. Use pictured items and/or manipulatives if necessary. Use any of the following stimulus words and/or others you select from the story. Correct answers are in parentheses.*

Stimulus items:

"Say spoke. Instead of /p/ say /m/." (smoke)

"Say present. Instead of /r/ say /l/." (pleasant)

"Say sky. Instead of /k/ say /p/." (spy)

"Say tree. Instead of /t/ say /f/." (free)

"Say still. Instead of /t/ say /k/."(skill)

"Say fits. Instead of /t/ say /n/." (fins)

"Say speak. Instead of /p/ say /l/." (sleek)

"Say sky. Instead of /k/ say /l/." (sly)

"Say still. Instead of /t/ say /p/" (spill)

"Say bank. Instead of /k/ say /g/." (bank)

23. Phoneme reversing.

What to say to the student: "We're going to say words backward."

EXAMPLE: "Say the word '_____'" (stimulus word) "backward."(e.g., "Say 'time' backward.") (might)

> *NOTE: This is a difficult phoneme-level task and should only be done with older students. Give letter sound, not letter name. Use pictured items and/or manipulatives if necessary. Use any of the following stimulus words and/or others you select from the story. Correct answers are in parentheses.*

Stimulus items:

top (pot)	fit (tiff)
tell (let)	talk (cot)
much (chum)	nice (sign)
know (own)	spoke (copes)
got (tog)	but (tub)

24. Phoneme switching.

What to say to the student: "We're going to switch the first sounds in two words."
EXAMPLE: "Switch the first sounds in '_____' and '_____.'" (stimulus words) (e.g., "Switch the first sounds in 'with moon.'") (mith woon)

> *NOTE: This is a difficult phoneme-level task and should only be done with older students. Give letter sound, not letter name. Use pictured items and/or manipulatives if necessary. Use any of the following stimulus words and/or others you select from the story. Correct answers are in parentheses.*

Stimulus items:

bear paddled	(pear baddled)
just right	(rust jight)
my birthday	(by mirthday)
one night	(none white)
piggy bank	(biggy pank)
dumped money	(mumped doney)
got home	(hot gome)

beautiful hat	(heautiful bat)
talk with	(walk tith)
found hat	(hound fat)

25. Pig latin.

What to say to the student: "We're going to talk in a secret language using words from the story. In pig latin, you take off the first sound of a word, put it at the end of the word, and add a long A sound."

EXAMPLE: "Say moon in pig latin." (oonmay)

> ***NOTE:*** *This is a difficult phoneme-level task and should only be done with older students. Use pictured items and/or manipulatives if necessary. Use any of the following stimulus words and/or others you select from the story. Correct answers are in parentheses.*

Stimulus items:

bear	(airbay)
piggy	(iggypay)
boy	(oybay)
tree	(reetay)
night	(ightnay)
voice	(oicevay)
shout	(outshay)
hat	(athay)
bank	(ankbay)
money	(oneymay)

CHAPTER

PHONOLOGICAL AWARENESS ACTIVITIES TO USE WITH *HARRY AND THE TERRIBLE WHATZIT*

Text version used for selection of stimulus items:

Gackenbach, D. (1977). *Harry and the terrible whatzit*. New York: Clarion Books.

PHONOLOGICAL AWARENESS ACTIVITIES AT THE WORD LEVEL

1. Counting words.

What to say to the student: "We're going to count words."

EXAMPLE: "How many words do you hear in this sentence (or phrase)? 'wood bin.'" (2)

> *NOTE: Use pictured items and/or manipulatives if necessary. Use any of the following stimulus phrases or sentences and/or others you select from the story. Correct answers are in parentheses.*

Stimulus items:

some milk (2)

the steps (2)

swung the broom (3)

shrank some more (3)

pulled his tail (3)

came back up (3)

then I saw it (4)

glad to see her (4)

the heads made a face (5)

was down to my size (5)

2. Identifying missing word from list.

What to say to the student: "Listen to the words I say. I'll say them again. You tell me which word I leave out."

EXAMPLE: "Listen to the words I say: 'runt, boy, steps.' I'll say them again. Tell me which one I leave out: 'runt, steps.'" (boy)

> *NOTE: Use pictured items and/or manipulatives if necessary. Use any of the following stimulus words and/or others you select from the story. Correct answers are in parentheses.*

Stimulus set #1	**Stimulus set #2**
face, clues	clues (face)
milk, bin	bin (milk)
swat, broom, yell	swat, yell (broom)
damp, rest, wood	damp, rest (wood)
bright, door, chased	door, chased (bright)
glad, jar, nose	glad, nose (jar)
feel, size, home	feel, size (home)
six, kid, back, time	six, kid, time (back)
tail, dark, mad, down	dark, mad, down (tail)
next, heads, back, wham	next, back, wham (heads)

3. Identifying missing word in phrase or sentence.

What to say to the student: "Listen to the sentence I read. Tell me which word is missing the second time I read the sentence."

EXAMPLE: "'Picking flowers.' Listen again and tell me which word I leave out. 'Picking ____.'" (flowers)

> ***NOTE:*** *Use pictured items and/or manipulatives if necessary. Use any of the following stimulus sentences and/or others you select from the story. Correct answers are in parentheses.*

Stimulus items:

More clues. More ____. (clues)

Cellar steps. ____ steps. (cellar)

Behind some boxes. Behind some ____. (boxes)

House next door. ____ next door. (house)

Looked very sad. Looked ____ sad. (very)

Inside the wood bin. Inside the ____ bin. (wood)

I pulled its tail. I ____ its tail. (pulled)

Was down to my size. Was down to my ____. (size)

Over by the pickle jars. Over by the ____ jars. (pickle)

Gave me some milk and cookies. Gave ____ some milk and cookies. (me)

4. Supplying missing word as adult reads.

What to say to the student: "I want you to help me read the story. You fill in the words I leave out."

EXAMPLE: "Behind some ____." (boxes)

> ***NOTE:*** *Use pictured items and/or manipulatives if necessary. Use any of the following stimulus sentences and/or others you select from the story. Correct answers are in parentheses.*

Stimulus items:

Picking _____. (flowers)

She never believes _____. (me)

The back cellar _____. (door)

It was very black and _____. (gloomy)

Gave me some _____ and cookies. (milk)

I twisted a _____. (nose)

Right where it sits _____. (down)

Found her glasses beside the _____ jars. (pickle)

Went down the cellar _____. (steps)

Hiding behind the _____. (furnace)

5. Rearranging words.

What to say to the student: "I'll say some words out of order. You put them in the right order so they make sense."

EXAMPLE: "'sunlight bright.' Put those words in the right order." (bright sunlight)

> *NOTE: Use pictured items and/or manipulatives if necessary. Use any of the following stimulus words and/or others you select from the story. Correct answers are in parentheses. This word-level activity can be more difficult than some of the syllable- or phoneme-level activities because of the memory load. If your students are only able to deal with two or three words to be rearranged, add more two- and three-word samples from the story and omit the four-word level until a later time.*

Stimulus items:

Whatzit terrible (terrible Whatzit)

door cellar (cellar door)

clues more (more clues)

its pulled tail (pulled its tail)

horned Whatzit long (long horned Whatzit)

Parker's try cellar Sheldon (try Sheldon Parker's cellar)

home at feel (feel at home)

the swung again broom (swung the broom again)

and black gloomy very (very black and gloomy)

found your I glasses (I found your glasses)

PHONOLOGICAL AWARENESS ACTIVITIES AT THE SYLLABLE LEVEL

1. Syllable counting.

What to say to the student: "We're going to count syllables (or parts) of words."

EXAMPLE: "How many syllables do you hear in '_____'?" (stimulus word) (e.g., "How many syllables in 'broom'?") (1)

NOTE: Use pictured items and/or manipulatives if necessary. Use any of the of the following stimulus words and/or others you select from the story. Use any group of 10 stimulus items you select per teaching set.

Stimulus items:

One-syllable words: pulled, back, bet, bin, black, boy, bright, broom, but, by, tail, tell, time, to, toed, told, took, try, damp, dark, did, do, done, door, down, called, came, clawed, clues, could, kid, gave, glad, go, gone, got, chased, jar, jars, just, mad, made, me, milk, more, my, knew, know, need, next, nose, not, now, sad, said, saw, say, see, sits, six, size, so, some, steps, swat, feel, for, found, from, had, have, he's, heads, heard, helped, her, here, his, hit, home, horned, house, rest, right, runt, one, was, we, well, went, wham, what, when, where, why, will, with, wood, she, shrank, sure, thought, three, thanks, that, the, then, there, yell, you, your, a, an, and, are, as, asked, at, else, I, I'm, in, is, it, its, of, on, or, out, up

Two-syllable words: Parker's, peanut, picking, because, before, behind, believe, besides, better, boxes, twisted, double, closet, coming, cookies, crazy, kitchen, getting, glasses, gloomy, maybe, mother, never, noticed, cellar, searching, smaller, someone, something, sunlight, flowers, furnace, very, happened, happens, Harry, headed, hiding, really, later, lying, waited, washer, Whatzit, worried, worry, Sheldon, shouted, about, afraid, after, always, answered, around, away, awful, either, even, inside, into, okay, open, outside, over

Three-syllable words: beginning, terrible, disappeared, discovered, answered, anymore, everything

2. Initial syllable deleting.

What to say to the student: "We're going to leave out syllables (or parts of words)."
EXAMPLE: "Say '_____.'" (stimulus word) "Say it again without '_____'" (stimulus syllable) (e.g., "Say 'peanut' without 'pea.'") (nut)

NOTE: Use pictured items and/or manipulatives if necessary. Use any of the following stimulus words and/or others you select from the story. Correct answers are in parentheses.

Stimulus items:

"Say Whatzit without what." (zit)

"Say Sheldon without shell." (done)

"Say outside without out." (side)

"Say into without in." (to)

"Say behind without be." (hind)

"Say disappeared without dis." (appeared)

"Say maybe without may." (be)

"Say twisted without twist." (ed)

"Say sunlight without sun." (light)

"Say because without be." (cause)

3. Final syllable deleting.

What to say to the student: "We're going to leave out syllables (or parts of words)."
EXAMPLE: "Say '_____.'" (stimulus word) "Say it again without '_____.'" (stimulus syllable) (e.g., "Say 'before' without 'for.'") (be)

> ***NOTE:*** *Use pictured items and/or manipulatives if necessary. Use any of the following stimulus words and/or others you select from the story. Correct answers are in parentheses.*

Stimulus items:

"Say Parker without -er." (park)

"Say sunlight without light." (sun)

"Say Whatzit without zit." (what)

"Say okay without kay." (oh)

"Say everything without thing." (every)

"Say hiding without -ing." (hide)

"Say anymore without more." (any)

"Say cookies without ease." (cook)

"Say maybe without be." (may)

"Say smaller without -er." (small)

4. Initial syllable adding.

What to say to the student: "Now let's add syllables (or parts) to words."
EXAMPLE: " Add '_____'" (stimulus syllable) "to the beginning of '_____.'" (stimulus syllable) (e.g., "Add 'may' to the beginning of 'be.'") (maybe)

NOTE: *Use pictured items and/or manipulatives if necessary. Use any of the following stimulus words and/or others you select from the story. Correct answers are in parentheses.*

Stimulus items:

"Add glass to the beginning of -ez."(or uz) (glasses)

"Add twist to the beginning of -ed." (twisted)

"Add sun to the beginning of light." (sunlight)

"Add search to the beginning of -ing." (searching)

"Add all the beginning of ways." (always)

"Add out to the beginning of side." (outside)

"Add cray to the beginning of zee." (crazy)

"Add be to the beginning of leaves." (believes)

"Add ah to the beginning of full." (awful)

"Add what to the beginning of zit." (Whatzit)

5. Final syllable adding.

What to say to the student: "Now let's add syllables (or parts) to words."
EXAMPLE: "Add '_____'" (stimulus syllable) "to the end of '_____.'" (stimulus syllable) (e.g., "Add 'leaves' to the end of 'be.'") (believes)

NOTE: *Use pictured items and/or manipulatives if necessary. Use any of the following stimulus words and/or others you select from the story. Correct answers are in parentheses.*

Stimulus items:

"Add light to the end of sun." (sunlight)

"Add ease to the end of cook." (cookies)

"Add one to the end of some." (someone)

"Add sides the end of be." (besides)

"Add –ez to the end of box." (boxes)

"Add nut to the end of pea." (peanut)

"Add be to the end of may." (maybe)

"Add -ing to the end of lie." (lying)

"Add side to the end of in." (inside)

"Add -ful to the end of aw." (awful)

6. Syllable substituting.

What to say to the student: "Let's make up some new words."
EXAMPLE: "Say '_____.'" (stimulus word) "Instead of '_____'" (stimulus syllable) "say '_____.'" (stimulus syllable) (e.g., "Say 'inside.' Instead of 'side' say 'stead.' The new word is 'instead.'")

> ***NOTE:*** *Use pictured items and/or manipulatives if necessary. Use any of the following stimulus words and/or others you select from the story. Correct answers are in parentheses.*

Stimulus items:

"Say believe. Instead of leave say cause." (because)

"Say someone. Instead of one say thing." (something)

"Say anymore. Instead of any say some." (some more)

"Say sunlight. Instead of light say shine." (sunshine)

"Say crazy. Instead of kray say lay." (lazy)

"Say outside. Instead of out say be." (beside)

"Say everything. Instead of thing say one." (everyone)

"Say peanut. Instead of nut say pull." (people)

"Say hiding. Instead of hide say search." (searching)

"Say awful. Instead of ah say hand." (handful)

PHONOLOGICAL AWARENESS ACTIVITIES AT THE PHONEME LEVEL

1. Counting sounds.

What to say to the student: "We're going to count sounds in words."
EXAMPLE: "How many sounds do you hear in this word? 'tail.'" (3)

> ***NOTE:*** *Use pictured items and/or manipulatives if necessary. Use any of the following stimulus words and/or others you select from the story. Be sure to give the letter sound and not the letter name. Use any group of 10 stimulus items you select per teaching set.*

Stimulus words with two sounds: boy, by, to, do, go, me, my, knew, know, now, say, see, so, her, we, why, she, sure, the, you, an, as, at, I'll, I'm, in, is, it, of, on, or, out, up

Stimulus words with three sounds: back, bet, bin, but, tail, tell, time, toed, took, try, did, done, door, down, came, could, kid, gave, gone, got, jar, mad, made, more, need, nose, not, sad, said, size, some, face, feel, for, had, have, heard, here, his, hit, home, house, tight, one, was, well, wham, what, will, with, wood, worry, thought, three, that, then, there, yell, your, and, away, awful, either, else, its, okay, over

Stimulus words with four sounds: pulled, better, black, broom, told, damp, dark, double, called, carry, clawed, clues, glad, chased, jars, just, maybe, milk, mother, never, cellar, six, swat, found, from, very, Harry, heads, helped, really, rest, runt, last, later, looked, washer, went, worried, about, after, asked, even, into, open

Stimulus words with five sounds: peanut, pickles, because, before, believe, cookies, crazy, gloomy, next, smaller, smelled, steps, flowers, furnace, happened, happens, headed, horned, waited, Sheldon, shouted, shrank, thanks, afraid, always, answered, around, inside, outside

2. Sound categorization or identifying rhyme oddity.

What to say to the student: "Guess which word I say does not rhyme with the other three words."

EXAMPLE: "Tell me which word does not rhyme with the other three. '_____, _____, _____, _____.'" (stimulus words) (e.g., "'trouble, double, bubble, flowers.' Which word doesn't rhyme?") (flowers)

> ***NOTE:*** *Use pictured items if necessary. Use any of the following stimulus words and/or others you select from the story. Correct answers are in parentheses.*

Stimulus items:

yell, well, tell, damp (damp)

bin, come, from, some (bin)

mad, bet, glad, sad (bet)

bright, light, clawed, tight (clawed)

hit, told, it, sit (told)

your, more, tail, door (tail)

horned, Harry, Mary, Larry (horned)

clues, blues, shoes, face (face)

wood, could, rest, should (rest)

toed, thought, swat, got (toed)

3. Matching rhyme.

What to say to the student: "We're going to think of rhyming words."
EXAMPLE: "Which word rhymes with '_____'?" (stimulus word) (e.g., "Which word rhymes with 'face:' 'some, chase, house, bin'?") (chase)

> ***NOTE:*** *Use pictured items if necessary. Use any of the following stimulus words and/or others you select from the story. Correct answers are in parentheses.*

Stimulus items:

bright: wham, tail, hit, right (right)

dark: bark, found, milk, done (bark)

yell: last, toed, well, feel (well)

clues: damp, shoes, clawed, heads (shoes)

door: more, jars, swat, runt (more)

wood: bet, could, waited, shrank (could)

kid: found, open, steps, slid (slid)

boy: into, toy, hit, took (toy)

mad: heard, rest, up, sad (sad)

time: lime, sure, helped, smelled (lime)

4. Producing rhyme.

What to say to the student: "Now we'll say rhyming words."
EXAMPLE: "Tell me a word that rhymes with '_____.'" (stimulus word) (e.g., "Tell me a word that rhymes with 'hit.' You can make up a word if you want.") (sit)

NOTE: *Use pictured items if necessary. Use any of the following stimulus words and/or others you select from the story, i.e., you say a word from the list below and the student is to think of a rhyming word. Use any group of 10 stimulus items you select per teaching set.*

Stimulus items:

/p/: Parker's, peanut, picking, pickles, pulled

/b/: back, because, before, beginning, behind, believe, besides, bet, better, bin, black, boxes, boy, bright, broom, but, by

/t/: tail, tell, terrible, time, to, toed, told, took, try, twisted

/d/: damp, dark, did, do, done, door, double, down

/k/: called, came, carry, clawed, climbed, closet, clues, coming, cookies, could, crazy, kid, kitchen

/g/: gave, getting, glad, glasses, gloomy, go, gone, got

/ch/: chased

/dz/: (as 1st sound in jelly): jar, jars, just

/m/: mad, made, maybe, me, milk, more, mother, my

/n/: knew, know, need, never, next, nose, not, noticed, now

/s/: cellar, sad, said, saw, say, searching, see, sits, six, size, smaller, smelled, so, some, someone, something, steps, sunlight, swat

/f/: face, feel, flowers, for, found, from, furnace

/v/: very

/h/: had, happened, happens, Harry, have, headed, head, heard, helped, her, here, hiding, his, home, horned, house

/r/: really, rest, right, runt

/l/: last, later, looked, lying

/w/, /wh/: one, waited, was, washer, we, well, went, wham, what, Whatzit, when, where, why, will, with, wood, worried, worry

/sh/: she, Sheldon, shouted, shrank, sure

/voiceless th/: thanks, thought, three

/voiced th/: that, the, then, there

/y/ (as 1st sound in yellow): yell, you, your

vowels: a, about, afraid, after, always, an, and, around, as, asked, at, away, awful, either, else, even, I, I'll, I'm, in, inside, into, is, it, of, okay, on, open, or, out, outside, over, up

5. Sound matching (initial).

What to say to the student: "Now we'll listen for the first sound in words."
EXAMPLE: "Listen to this sound: / /." (stimulus sound). "Guess which word I say begins with that sound. '_____, _____, _____, _____.'" (stimulus words) (e.g., "Listen to this sound /b/. Guess which word I say begins with that sound: 'pulled, time, boxes, just.'") (boxes)

> **NOTE:** *Give letter sound, not letter name. Use pictured items if necessary. Use any of the following stimulus words and/or others you select from the story. Correct answers are in parentheses.*

Stimulus items:

/k/: home, kid, over, glad (kid)

/m/: mother, glasses, noticed, double (mother)

/n/: wham, believe, milk, nose (nose)

/s/: peanut, hiding, really, cellar (cellar)

/f/: shrank, flowers, door, awful (flowers)

/sh/: face, size, thanks, Sheldon (Sheldon)

/d/: damp, clues, terrible, wood (damp)

/b/: dark, pickles, broom, next (broom)

/g/: toed, clawed, gloomy, found (gloomy)

/ch/: chased, mad, crazy, bright (chased)

6. Sound matching (final).

What to say to the student: "Now we'll listen for the last sound in words."
EXAMPLE: "Listen to this sound: / /" (stimulus sound). "Guess which word I say ends with that sound '_____, _____, _____, _____.'" (stimulus words) (e.g., "Listen to this sound /n/. Guess which word I say ends with that sound: 'home, steps, open, last'.") (open)

> **NOTE:** *Give letter sound not letter name. Use pictured items if necessary. Use any of the following stimulus words and/or others you select from the story. Correct answers are in parentheses.*

Stimulus items:

/d/: clawed, chased, took, heads (clawed)

/z/: peanut, toed, house, clues (clues)

/n/: swat, nose, bin, came (bin)

/s/: time, six, Sheldon, bright (six)

/m/: wham, gone, chased, glad (wham)

/r/: black, cellar, awful, rest (cellar)

/p/: out, damp, wood, milk (damp)

/t/: up, kid, runt, sits (runt)

/l/: closet, broom, terrible, furnace (terrible)

/k/: right, twisted, boxes, shrank (shrank)

7. Identifying initial sound in words.

What to say to the student: "I'll say a word two times. Tell me what sound is missing the second time. '______, ______.'" (stimulus words)

EXAMPLE: "What sound do you hear in '_____'" (stimulus word) "that is missing in '_____'?" (stimulus word) (e.g., "What sound do you hear in 'broom,' that is missing in 'room'?'") (/r/)

> **NOTE:** *Give letter sound not letter name. Use pictured items and/or manipulatives if necessary. Use any of the following stimulus words and/or others you select from the story. Correct answers are in parentheses.*

Stimulus items:

"bright, right. What sound do you hear in bright that is missing in right?" (/b/)

"dark, ark. What sound do you hear in dark that is missing in ark?" (/d/)

"glad, lad. What sound do you hear in glad that is missing in lad?"(/g/)

"never, ever. What sound do you hear in never that is missing in ever?" (/n/)

"shrank, rank. What sound do you hear in shrank that is missing in rank?" (/sh/)

"black, lack. What sound do you hear in black that is missing in lack?" (/b/)

"try, rye. What sound do you hear in try that is missing in rye?" (/t/)

"time, I'm. What sound do you hear in time that is missing in I'm?" (/t/)

"door, or. What sound do you hear in door that is missing in or?" (/d/)

"told, old. What sound do you hear in told that is missing in old?" (/t/)

8. Identifying final sound in words.

What to say to the student: "I'll say a word two times. Tell me what sound is missing the second time: '______, _______.'" (stimulus words)

EXAMPLE: "What sound do you hear in '_____'" (stimulus word) "that is missing in '_____'?" (stimulus word) (e.g., "What sound do you hear in 'toed' that is missing in 'toe'?") (/d/)

> *NOTE: Give letter sound, not letter name. Use pictured items and/or manipulatives if necessary. Use any of the following stimulus words and/or others you select from the story. Correct answers are in parentheses.*

Stimulus items:

"worry, were. What sound do you hear in worry that is missing in were?" (/long E/)

"heard, her. What sound do you hear in heard that is missing in her?" (/d/)

"Harry, hair. What sound do you hear in Harry that is missing in hair?" (/long E/)

"horned, horn. What sound do you hear in horned that is missing in horn?" (/d/)

"runt, run. What sound do you hear in runt that is missing in run?" (/t/)

"right, rye. What sound do you hear in right that is missing in rye?" (/t/)

"clawed, claw. What sound do you hear in clawed that is missing in claw?" (/d/)

"made, may. What sound do you hear in made that is missing in may?" (/d/)

"house, how. What sound do you hear in house that is missing in how?" (/s/)

"told, toll. What sound do you hear in told that is missing in toll?" (/d/)

9. Segmenting initial sound in words.

What to say to the student: "Listen to the word I say and tell me the first sound you hear."

EXAMPLE: "What's the first sound in '_____'?" (stimulus word) (e.g., "What's the first sound in 'berry'?") (/b/)

> *NOTE:: Give letter sound not letter name. Use pictured items and/or manipulatives if necessary. Use any of the following stimulus words and/or others you select from the story. Use any group of 10 stimulus items you select per teaching set.*

Stimulus items:

/p/: Parker's, peanut, picking, pickles, pulled

/b/: back, because, before, beginning, behind, believe, besides, bet, better, bin, black, boxes, boy, bright, broom, but, by

/t/: tail, tell, terrible, time, to, toed, told, took, try, twisted

/d/: damp, dark, did, disappeared, discovered, do, done, door, double, down

/k/: called, came, carry, clawed, climbed, closet, clues, coming, cookies, could, crazy, kid, kitchen

/g/: gave, getting, glad, glasses, gloomy, go, gone, got

/ch/: chased

/dz/: (as 1st sound in jelly): jar, jars, just

/m/: mad, made, maybe, me, milk, more, mother, my

/n/: knew, know, need, never, next, nose, not, noticed, now

/s/: cellar, sad, said, saw, say, searching, see, sits, six, size, smaller, smelled, so, some, someone, something, steps, sunlight, swat

/f/: face, feel, flowers, for, found, from, furnace

/v/: very

/h/: had, happened, happens, Harry, have, headed, head, heard, helped, her, here, hiding, his, home, horned, house

/r/: really, rest, right, runt

/l/: last, later, looked, lying

/w/, /wh/: one, waited, was, washer, we, well, went, wham, what, Whatzit, when, where, why, will, with, wood, worried, worry

/sh/: she, Sheldon, shouted, shrank, sure

/voiceless th/: thanks, thought, three

/voiced th/: that, the, then, there

/y/ (as 1st sound in yellow): yell, you, your

vowels: a, about, afraid, after, always, an, and, answered, anymore, around, as, asked, at, away, awful, either, else, even, everything, I, I'll, I'm, in, inside, into, is, it, of, okay, on, open, or, out, outside, over, up

10. Segmenting final sound in words.

What to say to the student: "Listen to the word I say and tell me the last sound you hear."
EXAMPLE: "What's the last sound in the word '_____'?" (stimulus word) (e.g., "What's the last sound in the word 'dark'?") (/k/)

NOTE: *Give letter sound not letter name. Use pictured items and/or manipulatives if necessary. Use any of the following stimulus words and/or others you select from the story. Use any group of 10 stimulus items you select per teaching set*

Stimulus items:

/p/: damp, up

/t/: about, asked, at, bet, bright, but, chased, closet, got, helped, hit, it, just, last, looked, next, not, noticed, out, peanut, rest, right, runt, sunlight, swat, that, thought, went, what, Whatzit

/d/: afraid, and, answered, around, behind, called, clawed, could, did, disappeared, discovered, found, glad, had, happened, headed, heard, horned, inside, kid, mad, made, need, outside, pulled, sad, said, shouted, smelled, toed, told, twisted, waited, wood, worried

/k/: back, black, dark, milk, shrank, took

/m/: broom, came, from, home, I'm, some, time, wham

/n/: an, bin, done, down, even, gone, in, kitchen, on, one, open, Sheldon, someone, then, when

/ng/: beginning, coming, everything, getting, hiding, long, lying, picking, searching, something

/s/: else, face, furnace, glasses, house, its, sits, six, steps, thanks

/z/: always, as, because, believes, besides, boxes, clues, cookies, flowers, happens, he's, heads, his, is, jars, nose, Parker's, pickles, size, was

/r/: after, anymore, are, before, cellar, door, for, her, here, jar, later, more, mother, either, never, or, over, smaller, sure, there, where, your

/l/: awful, double, feel, I'll, tail, tell, terrible, well, will, yell

/voiceless th/: with

/long A/: okay, say

/long E/: carry, crazy, gloomy, Harry, maybe, me, really, see, she, three, very, we, worry

/long I/: by, my, try, why

/long O/: go, know, so

/oo/: do, into, knew, to, you

/ah/: saw

/ow/: now

11. Generating words from the story beginning with a particular sound.

What to say to the student: "Let's think of words **from the story** that start with certain sounds."

EXAMPLE: "Tell me a word **from the story** that starts with / /." (stimulus sound) (e.g., "the sound /p/") (Parker)

> ***NOTE:*** *Give letter sound not letter name. Use pictured items if necessary. Use any of the following stimulus words and/or others you select from the story. You say the sound (e.g., a voiceless /p/ sound) and the student is to say a word from the story that begins with that sound. Use any group of 10 stimulus items you select per teaching set.*

Stimulus items:

/p/: Parker's, peanut, picking, pickles, pulled

/b/: back, because, before, beginning, behind, believe, besides, bet, better, bin, black, boxes, boy, bright, broom, but, by

/t/: tail, tell, terrible, time, to, toed, told, took, try, twisted

/d/: damp, dark, did, disappeared, discovered, do, done, door, double, down

/k/: called, came, carry, clawed, climbed, closet, clues, coming, cookies, could, crazy, kid, kitchen

/g/: gave, getting, glad, glasses, gloomy, go, gone, got

/ch/: chased

/dz/: (as 1st sound in jelly): jar, jars, just

/m/: mad, made, maybe, me, milk, more, mother, my

/n/: knew, know, need, never, next, nose, not, noticed, now

/s/: cellar, sad, said, saw, say, searching, see, sits, six, size, smaller, smelled, so, some, someone, something, steps, sunlight, swat

/f/: face, feel, flowers, for, found, from, furnace

/v/: very

/h/: had, happened, happens, Harry, have, headed, head, heard, helped, her, here, hiding, his, home, horned, house

/r/: really, rest, right, runt

/l/: last, later, looked, lying

/w/, /wh/: one, waited, was, washer, we, well, went, wham, what, Whatzit, when, where, why, will, with, wood, worried, worry

/sh/: she, Sheldon, shouted, shrank, sure

/voiceless th/: thanks, thought, three

/voiced th/: that, the, then, there

/y/ (as 1st sound in yellow): yell, you, your

vowels: a, about, afraid, after, always, an, and, answered, anymore, around, as, asked, at, way, awful, either, else, even, everything, I, I'll, I'm, in, inside, into, is, it, of, okay, on, open, or, out, outside, over, up

12. Blending sounds in monosyllabic words divided into onset-rime beginning with two consonant cluster + rime.

What to say to the student: "Now we'll put sounds together to make words."
EXAMPLE: "Put these sounds together to make a word (/ / + / /)." (stimulus sounds) "What's the word?" (e.g., "gl + ad: What's the word?") (glad)

> **NOTE:** *Give letter sound not letter name. Use pictured items and/or manipulatives if necessary. Use any of the following stimulus words and/or others you select from the story. Correct answers are in parentheses.*

Stimulus items:

bl + ack (black)	tw + ist (twist)
st + eps (steps)	br + ight (bright)
sw + ought (swat)	tr + I (try)
br + oom (broom)	cl + awed (clawed)
cl + imed (climbed)	sm + ell (smell)

13. Blending sounds in monosyllabic words divided into onset-rime beginning with single consonant + rime.

What to say to the student: "Let's put sounds together to make words."
EXAMPLE: "Put these sounds together to make a word (/ / + / /)." (stimulus sounds) "What's the word?" (e.g., "/t/ + ail: what's the word?") (tail)

> **NOTE:** *Give letter sound not letter name. Use pictured items and/or manipulatives if necessary. Use any of the following stimulus words and/or others you select from the story. Correct answers are in parentheses.*

Stimulus items:

/b/ + in (bin)	/f/ + eel (feel)
/t/ + owed (toed)	/k/ + id (kid)
/m/ + ilk (milk)	/s/ + ize (size)
/n/ + ose (nose)	/g/ + on (gone)
/r/ + unt (runt)	/b/ + oy (boy

14. Blending sounds to form a monosyllabic word beginning with a continuant sound.

What to say to the student: "We'll put sounds together to make words."
EXAMPLE: "Put these sounds together to make a word (/ / + / / + / /)." (stimulus sounds) (e.g., "/f/ /long E/ /l/.") (feel)

> ***NOTE:*** *Give letter sound, not letter name. Use pictured items and/or manipulatives if necessary. Use any of the following stimulus words and/or others you select from the story. Correct answers are in parentheses.*

Stimulus items:

/f/ /long A/ /s/ (face)	/s/ /w/ /ah/ /t/ (swat)
/m/ /short A/ /d/ (mad)	/w/ /short E/ /n/ /t/ (went)
/n/ /long O/ /z/ (nose)	/h/ /short I/ /t/ (hit)
/m/ /long E/ /n/ (mean)	/s/ /short A/ /d/ (sad)
/s/ /long I/ /z/ (size)	/r/ /short U/ /n/ /t/ (runt)

15. Blending sounds to form a monosyllabic word beginning with a noncontinuant sound.

What to say to the student: "We'll put sounds together to make words."
EXAMPLE: "Put these sounds together to make a word (/ / + / / + / /)." (stimulus sounds) (e.g., "/b/ /short A/ /k/.") (back)

> ***NOTE:*** *Give letter sound not letter name. Use pictured items and/or manipulatives if necessary. Use any of the following stimulus words and/or others you select from the story. Correct answers are in parentheses.*

Stimulus items:

/b/ /short I/ /n/ (bin)

/k/ /l/ /oo/ /z/ (clues)

/t/ /long O/ /d/ (toed)

/k/ /l/ /ah/ /d/ (clawed)

/b/ /r/ /long I/ /t/ (bright)

/d/ /short A/ /m/ /p/ (damp)

/g/ /l/ /short A/ /d/ (glad)

/ch/ /long A/ /s/ (chase)

/g/ /long A/ /v/ (gave)

/k/ /short I/ /d/ (kid)

16. Substituting initial sound in words.

What to say to the student. "We're going to change beginning/first sounds in words." ***EXAMPLE:*** "Say '_____.'" (stimulus word) "Instead of / /" (stimulus sound) "say / /." (stimulus sound) (e.g., "Say 'boy.' Instead of /b/ say /t/. What's your new word?") (toy)

> ***NOTE:*** *Give letter sound not letter name. Use pictured items and/or manipulatives if necessary. Use any of the following stimulus words and/or others you select from the story. Correct answers are in parentheses.*

Stimulus items:

"Say Harry. Instead of /h/ say /m/." (Mary)

"Say damp. Instead of /d/ say /k/." (camp)

"Say face. Instead of /f/ say /ch/." (chase)

"Say size. Instead of /s/ say /w/." (wise)

"Say right. Instead of /r/ say /t/." (tight)

"Say pickles. Instead of /p/ say /t/." (tickles)

"Say door. Instead of /d/ say /sh/." (shore)

"Say try. Instead of /t/ say /k/." (cry)

"Say later. Instead of /l/ say /w/." (waiter)

"Say nose. Instead of /n/ say /h/." (hose)

17. Substituting final sound in words.

What to say to the student: "We're going to change ending/last sounds in words." ***EXAMPLE:*** "Say '_____.'" (stimulus word) "Instead of / /" (stimulus sound) "say /_/." (stimulus sound) (e.g., "Say 'Harry.' Instead of /long E/ say /z/. What's your new word?") (hairs)

> *NOTE: Give letter sound, not letter name. Use pictured items and/or manipulatives if necessary. Use any of the following stimulus words and/or others you select from the story. Correct answers are in parentheses.*

Stimulus items:

"Say dark. Instead of /k/ say /t/." (dart)

"Say back. Instead of /k/ say /ch/." (batch)

"Say crazy. Instead of /long E/ say /d/."(crazed)

"Say nose. Instead of /z/ say /t/." (note)

"Say sad. Instead of /d/, say /t/." (sat)

"Say wham. Instead of /m/ say /p/." (whap)

"Say inside. Instead of /d/ say /t/." (insight)

"Say will. Instead of /l/ say /sh/." (wish)

"Say some. Instead of /m/ say /ch/." (such)

"Say home. Instead of /m/ say /p/." (hope)

18. Segmenting middle sound in monosyllabic words.

What to say to the student: "Tell me the middle sound in the word I say."
EXAMPLE: "What's the middle sound in the word '_____'?" (stimulus word) (e.g., "What's the middle sound in the word 'right'?") (/long I/)

> *NOTE: Give letter sound not letter name. Use pictured items and/or manipulatives if necessary. Use any of the following stimulus words and/or others you select from the story. Correct answers are in parentheses.*

Stimulus items:

wham (/short A/)

okay (/k/)

jar (/ah/)

head (/short E/)

need (/long E/)

three (/r/)

size (/long I/)

gone (/ah/)

hit (/short I/)

sad (/short A/)

19. Substituting middle sound in words.

What to say to the student: "We're going to change the middle sound in words."
EXAMPLE: "Say '_____.'" (stimulus word) "Instead of / /" (stimulus sound) "say / /." (stimulus sound) (e.g., "Say 'sad.' Instead of /short A/ say /long E/. What's your new word?") (seed)

> *NOTE: Give letter sound not letter name. Use pictured items and/or manipulatives if necessary. Use any of the following stimulus words and/or others you select from the story. Correct answers are in parentheses.*

Stimulus items:

"Say toed. Instead of /long O/ say /long I/." (tied)

"Say shrank. Instead of /long A/ say /short U/." (shrunk)

"Say runt. Instead of /short U/ say /short A/."(rant)

"Say wham. Instead of /short A/ say /short I/." (whim)

"Say nose. Instead of /long O/, say /long E/." (knees)

"Say right. Instead of /long I/ say /long A/." (rate)

"Say clues. Instead of /oo/ say /long O/." (close)

"Say time. Instead of /long I/ say /long A/." (tame)

"Say rest. Instead of /short E/ say /short U/." (rust)

"Say went. Instead of /short E/, say /ah/." (want)

20. Identifying all sounds in monosyllabic words.

What to say to the student. "Now tell me all the sounds you hear in the word I say."
EXAMPLE: "What sounds do you hear in the word '_____'?" (stimulus word) (e.g., "What sounds do you hear in the word 'tail'?") (/t/ /long A/ /l/)

> *NOTE: Give letter sound not letter name. Use pictured items and/or manipulatives if necessary. Use any of the following stimulus words and/or others you select from the story. Correct answers are in parentheses.*

Stimulus items:

last (/l/ /short A/ /s/ /t/)

smelled (/s/ /m/ /short E/ /l/ /d/)

broom (/b/ /r/ /oo/ /m/)

steps (/s/ /t/ /short E/ /p/ /s/)

wham (/w/ short A/ /m/)

runt (/r/ /short U/ /n/ /t/)

search (/s/ /r/ /ch/)

glad (/g/ /l/ short A/ /d/)

house (/h/ /ow /s/)

damp (/d/ /short A/ /m/ /p/)

21. Deleting sounds within words.

What to say to the student. "We're going to leave out sounds in words."
EXAMPLE: "Say '_____'" (stimulus word) "without / /." (stimulus sound) (e.g., "Say 'and' without /n/.") Say: "The word that was left, 'ad,' is a real word. Sometimes the word won't be a real word.")

> ***NOTE:*** *Give letter sound not letter name. Use pictured items and/or manipulatives if necessary. Use any of the following stimulus words and/or others you select from the story. Correct answers are in parentheses.*

Stimulus items:

"Say try without /r/." (tie)

"Say broom without /r/." (boom)

"Say smell without /m/." (sell)

"Say damp without /m/." (dap)

"Say clues without /l/." (coos)

"Say box without /k/." (boss)

"Say shrank without /r/." (shank)

"Say told without /l/." (toad)

"Say next without /k/."(nest)

"Say black without /l/." (back)

22. Substituting consonant in words having a two-sound cluster.

What to say to the student. "We're going to substitute sounds in words."

EXAMPLE: "Say '_____'" (stimulus word). "Instead of / /" (stimulus sound) "say / /" (stimulus sound) (e.g., "Say 'black.' Instead of /l/ say /r/.") (brack). Say: "Sometimes the new word will be a made-up word."

> ***NOTE:*** *Give letter sound, not letter name. Use pictured items and/or manipulatives if necessary. Use any of the following stimulus words and/or others you select from the story. Correct answers are in parentheses.*

Stimulus items:

"Say swat. Instead of /w/ say /k/." (Scott)

"Say glasses. Instead of /l/ say /r/." (grasses)

"Say try. Instead of /t/ say /k/." (cry)

"Say bright. Instead of /r/ say /l/." (blight)

"Say runt. Instead of /n/ say /s/." (rust)

"Say smell. Instead of /m/ say /p/." (spells)

"Say glad. Instead of /l/ say /r/." (grad)

"Say clues. Instead of /l/ say /r/." (cruise)

"Say broom. Instead of /r/ say /l/" (bloom)

"Say milk. Instead of /k/ say /d/." (milled)

23. Phoneme reversing.

What to say to the student: "We're going to say words backward."

EXAMPLE: "Say the word '_____'" (stimulus word) "backward." (e.g., "If we say 'but' backward, the word is 'tub.'")

> ***NOTE:*** *This is a difficult phoneme-level task and should only be done with older students. Give letter sound, not letter name. Use pictured items and/or manipulatives if necessary. Use any of the following stimulus words and/or others you select from the story. Correct answers are in parentheses.*

Stimulus items:

tail	(late)	back	(cab)
door	(road)	face	(safe)
came	(make)	need	(dean)

more	(roam)	my	(I'm)
nose	(zone)	feel	(leaf)

24. Phoneme switching.

What to say to the student: "We're going to switch the first sounds in two words."
EXAMPLE: "Switch the first sounds in '_____' and '_____.'" (stimulus words) (e.g., "Switch the first sounds in 'six toed.'") (tix soed)

> *NOTE:* *This is a difficult phoneme-level task and should only be done with older students. Give letter sound, not letter name. Use pictured items and/or manipulatives if necessary. Use any of the following stimulus words and/or others you select from the story. Correct answers are in parentheses.*

Stimulus items:

pickle jars	(jickle pars)
next door	(dext noor)
long horned	(hong lorned)
some boxes	(bum soxes)
wood bin	(bood win)
terrible Whatzit	(werrible tutzit)
Parker's cellar	(Sarker's pellar)
sits down	(dits sown)
very sad	(serry vad)
came back	(bame cack)

25. Pig latin.

What to say to the student: "We're going to talk in a secret language using words from the story. In pig latin, you take off the first sound of a word, put it at the end of the word, and add a long A sound."
EXAMPLE: "Say nose in pig latin." (osenay)

> *NOTE:* *This is a difficult phoneme-level task and should only be done with older students. Use pictured items and/or manipulatives if necessary. Use any of the following stimulus words and/or others you select from the story. Correct answers are in parentheses.*

Stimulus items:

kitchen	(itchenkay)
door	(orday)
sad	(adsay)
crazy	(razykay)
wham	(amway)
pickles	(icklespay)
Parker	(arkerpay)
harry	(airyhay)
cellar	(ellersay)
runt	(untray)

CHAPTER

PHONOLOGICAL AWARENESS ACTIVITIES TO USE WITH *HARRY THE DIRTY DOG*

Text version used for selection of stimulus items:

Zion, G. (1956). *Harry the dirty dog*. New York: Harper.

PHONOLOGICAL AWARENESS ACTIVITIES AT THE WORD LEVEL

1. Counting words.

What to say to the student: "We're going to count words."

EXAMPLE: "How many words do you hear in this sentence (or phrase)? 'He played tag.'" (3)

> ***NOTE:*** *Use pictured items and/or manipulatives if necessary. Use any of the following stimulus phrases or sentences and/or others you select from the story. Correct answers are in parentheses.*

Stimulus items:

piggy bank (2)

scrub brush (2)

he played dead (3)

a white dog (3)

he slid down (3)

he ran back home (4)

he danced and sang (4)

he took the brush (4)

white dog with black spots (5)

up the stairs he dashed (5)

2. Identifying missing word from list.

What to say to the student: "Listen to the words I say. I'll say them again. You tell me which word I leave out."

EXAMPLE: "Listen to the words I say: 'tub, dirty, house.' I'll say them again. Tell me which one I leave out: 'tub, house.'" (dirty)

> ***NOTE:*** *Use pictured items and/or manipulatives if necessary. Use any of the following stimulus words and/or others you select from the story. Correct answers are in parentheses.*

Stimulus set #1	**Stimulus set #2**
tricks, magic	tricks (magic)
tail, dreaming	tail (dreaming)
scrub, clever, sang	scrub, sang (clever)
soapiest, mouth, bath	soapiest, bath (mouth)
tag, dinner, under	dinner, under (tag)
spots, mummy, garden	spots, garden (mummy)
slowly, Harry, father, look	slowly, father, look (Harry)
hungry, chute, wonder, this	chute, wonder, this (hungry)
asleep, shook, wagged, favorite	asleep, wagged, favorite (shook)
hidden, slept, gate, dirtiest	hidden, slept, gate (dirtiest)

3. Identifying missing word in phrase or sentence.

What to say to the student: "Listen to the sentence I read. Tell me which word is missing the second time I read the sentence."

EXAMPLE: "'He felt tired.' Listen again and tell me which word I leave out. 'He felt ____.'" (tired)

> ***NOTE:*** *Use pictured items and/or manipulatives if necessary. Use any of the following stimulus sentences and/or others you select from the story. Correct answers are in parentheses.*

Stimulus items:

White dog. White _____. (dog)

It's Harry. It's _____. (Harry)

He slept soundly. He _____ soundly. (slept)

Wagged his tail. _____ his tail. (Wagged)

They began shouting. They began _____. (shouting)

Harry ran back home. Harry _____ back home. (ran)

Has anyone seen Harry? Has _____ seen Harry? (anyone)

There's a strange dog. There's a _____ dog. (strange)

He played at the railroad. He played at the _____. (railroad)

He crawled through the fence. He _____ through the fence. (crawled)

3. Supplying missing word as adult reads.

What to say to the student: "I want you to help me read the story. You fill in the words I leave out."

EXAMPLE: "Harry was a white _____." (dog)

> ***NOTE:*** *Use pictured items and/or manipulatives if necessary. Use any of the following stimulus sentences and/or others you select from the story. Correct answers are in parentheses.*

Stimulus items:

He heard the _____. (water)

Harry ran back _____. (home)

The scrubbing _____ was hidden. (brush)

There's a strange _____ in our yard. (dog)

He flip-flopped and flop-_____. (flipped)

A black dog with white _____. (spots)

He played _____ with the other dogs. (tag)

Harry wagged his _____. (tail)

A white dog with _____ spots. (black)

His family combed and _____ him (brushed)

5. Rearranging words.

What to say to the student: "I'll say some words out of order. You put them in the right order so they make sense."

EXAMPLE: "dog dirty." Put those words in the right order." (dirty dog)

> ***NOTE:*** *Use pictured items and/or manipulatives if necessary. Use any of the following stimulus words and/or others you select from the story. Correct answers are in parentheses. This word-level activity can be more difficult than some of the syllable- or phoneme-level activities because of the memory load. If your students are only able to deal with two or three words to be rearranged, add more two- and three-word samples from the story and omit the four-word level items.*

Stimulus items:

dog white (white dog)

tag play (play tag)

barks short (short barks)

fence the through (through the fence)

Harry anyone seen? (anyone seen Harry?)

his under pillow (under his pillow)

place his favorite (his favorite place)

did he tricks these (he did these tricks)

and sang he danced (he sang and danced)

soundly so slept he (he slept so soundly)

PHONOLOGICAL AWARENESS ACTIVITIES AT THE SYLLABLE LEVEL

1. Syllable counting.

What to say to the student: "We're going to count syllables (or parts) of words." *EXAMPLE:* "How many syllables do you hear in '_____'?" (stimulus word) (e.g., "How many syllables in 'brush'?") (1)

> *NOTE: Use pictured items and/or manipulatives if necessary. Use any of the following stimulus words and/or others you select from the story. Use any group of 10 stimulus items you select per teaching set.*

Stimulus items:

One-syllable words: place, play, back, bark, bath, be, brush, but, by, tub, took, tag, to, tricks, tail, day, dead, did, dig, do, dogs, done, door, down, coal, cried, quick, gate, gave, girl, give, got, change, jump, mouth, no, said, sang, sat, scrub, seen, show, slept, slid, so, soon, spots, stairs, still, stop, strange, street, ran, fact, feel, fell, felt, found, from, fun, had, hard, has, he, head, heard, him, his, hole, home, house, how, who, like, look, once, one, walk, wants, was, way, were, when, where, white, why, with, chute, shook, short, things, thought, that, the, them, then, there, these, they, this, yard, you, yours, all, and, as, at, if, in, it, of, oh, old, on, out, up

Two-syllable words: pillow, barking, bathtub, became, before, began, begging, behind, brother, buried, tired, toward, daddy, dinner, dirty, doggy, dreaming, corner, couldn't, garden, getting, children, magic, mummy, never, scrubbing, slowly, sounding, started, stopping, railroad, really, running, father, fixing, flip-flop, flop-flip, happy, Harry, hidden, hungry, little, looking, very, water, without, wonder, shouting, after, again, although, asleep, away, even, ever, except, into, other, over, under

Three-syllable words: anyone, dirtier, dirtiest, carrying, certainly, soapiest, suddenly, family, favorite, following, happily, lovingly wonderful

Four-syllable words: furiously, everyone, everything

2. Initial syllable deleting.

What to say to the student: "We're going to leave out syllables (or parts of words)." *EXAMPLE:* "Say '_____.'" (stimulus word) "Say it again without '_____.'" (stimulus syllable) (e.g., "Say 'railroad.' Say it again without 'rail.'") (road)

> ***NOTE:*** *Use pictured items and/or manipulatives if necessary. Use any of the following stimulus words and/or others you select from the story. Correct answers are in parentheses.*

Stimulus items:

"Say flip-flop without flip." (flop)

"Say shouting without shout." (-ing)

"Say hungry without hung." (-ree)

"Say before without be." (fore)

"Say although without all." (though)

"Say before without be." (fore)

"Say into without in." (to)

"Say dirty without dir-." (tee)

"Say except without ex-" (-cept)

"Say bathtub without bath." (tub)

3. Final syllable deleting.

What to say to the student: "We're going to leave out syllables (or parts of words)." ***EXAMPLE:*** "Say '_____.'" (stimulus word) "Say it again without '_____.'" (stimulus syllable) (e.g., "Say 'became' without 'came.'") (be)

> ***NOTE:*** *Use pictured items and/or manipulatives if necessary. Use any of the following stimulus words and/or others you select from the story. Correct answers are in parentheses.*

Stimulus items:

"Say wonderful without -ful." (wonder)

"Say furiously without -lee." (furious)

"Say anyone without one." (any)

"Say flop-flip without flip." (flop)

"Say bathtub without tub." (bath)

"Say daddy without -ee." (dad)

"Say certainly without -lee." (certain)

"Say mummy without -ee." (mum)

"Say dirtiest without est-." (dirty)

"Say scrubbing without -ing." (scrub)

4. Initial syllable adding.

What to say to the student: "Now let's add syllables (or parts) to words."
EXAMPLE: "Add '_____'" (stimulus syllable) "to the beginning of '_____.'" (stimulus syllable) (e.g., "Add 'dream' to the beginning of '-ing.'") (dreaming)

> *NOTE: Use pictured items and/or manipulatives if necessary. Use any of the following stimulus words and/or others you select from the story. Correct answers are in parentheses*

Stimulus items:

"Add rail to the beginning of road." (railroad)

"Add beg to the beginning of -ing." (begging)

"Add bath to the beginning of tub." (bathtub)

"Add be to the beginning of hind." (behind)

"Add sound to the beginning of -ing." (sounding)

"Add chilled to the beginning of -ren." (children)

"Add hung to the beginning of –ree." (hungry)

"Add corn to the beginning of -er." (corner)

"Add be to the beginning of -gan." (began)

"Add madge to the beginning of -ick." (magic)

5. Final syllable adding.

What to say to the student: "Now let's add syllables (or parts) to words."
EXAMPLE: "Add '_____'" (stimulus syllable) "to the end of '_____.'" (stimulus syllable) (e.g., "Add 'ing' to the end of 'bark.'") (barking)

> *NOTE: Use pictured items and/or manipulatives if necessary. Use any of the following stimulus words and/or others you select from the story. Correct answers are in parentheses.*

Stimulus items:

"Add one to the end of every." (everyone)

"Add -ing to the end of stop." (stopping)

"Add oh to the end of pill." (pillow)

"Add ward to the end of to." (toward)

"Add it to the end of favor." (favorite)

"Add lee to the end of sudden." (suddenly)

"Add -est to the end of soapy." (soapiest)

"Add lee to the end of loving." (lovingly)

"Add den to the end of gar." (garden)

"Add -er to the end of din-." (dinner)

6. Syllable substituting.

What to say to the student: "Let's make up some new words."
EXAMPLE: "Say '_____.'" (stimulus word) "Instead of '_____'" (stimulus syllable) "say '_____.'" (stimulus syllable) (e.g., "Say 'bathtub.' Instead of 'tub' say 'soap.' The new word is 'bathsoap.'")

> *NOTE: Use pictured items and/or manipulatives if necessary. Use any of the following stimulus words and/or others you select from the story. Correct answers are in parentheses.*

Stimulus items:

"Say flip-flop. Instead of flip say flop." (flopflop)

"Say everyone. Instead of one say thing." (everything)

"Say soapiest. Instead of -est say dog." (soapy dog)

"Say mummy. Instead of mum say tum." (tummy)

"Say became. Instead of came say fore." (before)

"Say scrubbing. Instead of scrub say bark." (barking)

"Say railroad. Instead of rail say dirt." (dirt road)

"Say happily. Instead of lee say -est." (happiest)

"Say running. Instead of run say fix." (fixing)

"Say dirtier. Instead of -er say -est." (dirtiest)

PHONOLOGICAL AWARENESS ACTIVITIES AT THE PHONEME LEVEL

1. Counting sounds.

What to say to the student: "We're going to count sounds in words."
EXAMPLE: "How many sounds do you hear in this word? 'dog.'" (3)

> *NOTE: Use pictured items and/or manipulatives if necessary. Use any of the following stimulus words and/or others you select from the story. Be sure to give the letter sound and not the letter name. Use any group of 10 stimulus items you select per teaching set.*

Stimulus words with two sounds: be, by, to, day, do, no, show, so, he, way, shy, they, all, as, at, if, in, it, of, on, up

Stimulus words with three sounds: back, both, beg, but, tub, took, tag, tail, dead, did, dig, dog, done, coal, gate, gave, girl, get, give, got, mouth, said, sat, seen, soon, ran, fact, feel, fell, fun, had, has, head, him, his, hole, home, like, look, once, walk, was, white, with, chute, shook, shout, thought, that, them, then, these, this, even, old

Stimulus words with four sounds: pillow, place, played, black, brush, tired, tried, daddy, dashed, dirty, doggy, dogs, don't dream, combed, cried, quick, change, jump, mummy, never, slid, sound, still, really, rolled, felt, fix, flop, flip, found, from, happy, Harry, hidden, little, looked, very, wagged, water, after, under

Stimulus words with five sounds: became, before, began, brother, tricks, danced, clever, magic, scrub, slept, slowly, spots, stopped, street, wants

2. Sound categorization or identifying rhyme oddity.

What to say to the student: "Guess which word I say does not rhyme with the other three words."
EXAMPLE: "Tell me which word does not rhyme with the other three. '_____, _____, _____, _____.'" (stimulus words) (e.g., "door, bath, four, more. Which word doesn't rhyme?") (bath)

> *NOTE: Use pictured items if necessary. Use any of the following stimulus words and/or others you select from the story. Correct answers are in parentheses.*

Stimulus items:

brush, crush, mush, family (family)

tail, mail, sail, bone (bone)

dead, yard, card, lard (dead)

spot, dot, chute, hot (chute)

dig, pig, dirty, fig (dirty)

dogs, short, court, sort (dogs)

tricks, white, chicks, licks (white)

black, Mac, thought, jack (thought)

scrub, tub, day, rub (day)

mummy, tummy, dashed, rummy (dashed)

3. Matching rhyme.

What to say to the student: "We're going to think of rhyming words."

EXAMPLE: "Which word rhymes with '_____'?" (stimulus word) (e.g., "Which word rhymes with 'tried'? 'dog, cried, spots, buried.'") (cried)

> ***NOTE:*** *Use pictured items if necessary. Use any of the following stimulus words and/or others you select from the story. Correct answers are in parentheses.*

Stimulus items:

spots: scrub, dots, chute, coal (dots)

Harry: family, house, soap, carry (carry)

shook: took, things, yard, father (took)

gate: combed, slept, late, bark (late)

clever: begging, lever, sounding, many (lever)

stairs: dirtiest, tricks, down, cares (cares)

magic: tragic, buried, head, even (tragic)

tag: brush, little, gag, dinner (gag)

coal: goal, tired, began, flopped (goal)

tail: dead, mail, black, under (mail)

4. Producing rhyme.

What to say to the student: "Now we'll say rhyming words."

EXAMPLE: "Tell me a word that rhymes with '_____.'" (stimulus word) (e.g., "Tell me a word that rhymes with 'white.' You can make up a word if you want.") (sight)

> *NOTE: Use pictured items if necessary. Use any of the following stimulus words and/or others you select from the story (i.e., you say a word from the list below and the student is to think of a rhyming word). Use any group of 10 stimulus items you select per teaching set.*

Stimulus items:

/p/: pillow, place, played

/b/: back, barking, barks, bath, bathtub, be, became, before, began, beg, behind, black, brother, brush, buried, but, by

/t/: tub, took, tag, to, tired, tried, tricks, tail

/d/: daddy, danced, dashed, day, dead, did, dig, dinner, dirty, do, doggy, dogs, don't done, door, down, dreaming

/k/: carry, clever, close, coal, combed, corner, cried, quick

/g/: garden, gate, gave, getting, girl, give, got

/ch/: changed, children

/dz/: (as 1st sound in jelly): jumped

/m/: magic, many, mouth, mummy

/n/: never, no

/s/: certainly, said, sang, sat, scrub, seen, show, slept, slid, slow, so, soapy, soon, sound, spots, stairs, started, still, stopped, strange, street

/f/: fact, family, father, favorite, feel, fell, felt, fix, flip, flop, follow, found, from, fun, furious

/v/: very

/h/: had, happy, hard, Harry, has, he, head, heard, hidden, him, his, hole, home, house, how, hungry, who

/r/: rail, road, ran, really, rolled, running

/l/: like, little, look, looking

/w/, /wh/: once, one, wag, walked, wants, was, water, way, were, when, where, white, why, with, wonder, wonderful, worked

/sh/: chute, shook, short, shouting

/voiceless th/: things, thought

/voiced th/: that, the, them, then, there, these, they, this

/y/ (as 1st sound in yellow): yard, you, yours

vowels: a, after, again, all, although, and, anyone, as , asleep, at, away, even, ever, everyone, everything, except, if, in, into, it, of, oh, old, on, other, out, over, under, up

5. Sound matching (initial).

What to say to the student: "Now we'll listen for the first sound in words."
EXAMPLE: "Listen to this sound: / /." (stimulus sound). "Guess which word I say begins with that sound. '_____, _____, _____, _____.'" (stimulus words) (e.g., "Listen to this sound /d/. Guess which word I say begins with that sound: took, spot, daddy, tail.") (daddy)

> ***NOTE:*** *Give letter sound not letter name. Use pictured items if necessary. Use any of the following stimulus words and/or others you select from the story. Correct answers are in parentheses.*

Stimulus items:

/w/: chute, wonderful, thought, again (wonderful)

/s/: worked, brother, spots, dashed (spots)

/t/: tricks, dreaming, flipped, soapiest (tricks)

/f/: day, furiously, doggy, tail (furiously)

/b/: dirtier, without, tried, barking (barking)

/m/: toward, mummy, asleep, thought (mummy)

/sh/: buried, place, shook, lovingly (shook)

/p/: pillow, brush, everything, doggy (pillow)

/b/: although, tag, bathtub, soapiest (bathtub)

/r/: happy, even, running, water (running)

6. Sound matching (final).

What to say to the student: "Now we'll listen for the last sound in words."
EXAMPLE: "Listen to this sound: / /" (stimulus sound). "Guess which word I say ends with that sound '_____, _____, _____, _____.'" (stimulus words) (e.g., "Listen

to this sound /g/. Guess which word I say ends with that sound: dinner, tag, brush, place.") (tag)

> *NOTE:* *Give letter sound not letter name. Use pictured items if necessary. Use any of the following stimulus words and/or others you select from the story. Correct answers are in parentheses.*

Stimulus items:

/b/: girl, quick, bathtub, many (bathtub)

/k/: children, magic, slowly, spots (magic)

/z/: mouth, getting, stairs, combed (stairs)

/ng/: changed, certainly, sounding, coal (sounding)

/t/: soapiest, tag, wonder, brother (soapiest)

/long O/: buried, doggy, dirtier, pillow (pillow)

/s/: became, tricks, except, didn't (tricks)

/d/: dreaming, white, yard, hole (yard)

/p/: asleep, behind, there, bathtub (asleep)

/l/: toward, wonderful, water, began (wonderful)

7. Identifying initial sound in words.

What to say to the student: "I'll say a word two times. Tell me what sound is missing the second time. '______, _______.'" (stimulus words)

EXAMPLE: "What sound do you hear in '_____'" (stimulus word) "that is missing in '_____'?" (stimulus word) (e.g., "What sound do you hear in 'gate,' that is missing in '-ate'?") (/g/)

> *NOTE:* *Give letter sound not letter name. Use pictured items and/or manipulatives if necessary. Use any of the following stimulus words and/or others you select from the story. Correct answers are in parentheses.*

Stimulus items:

"Harry, airy. What sound do you hear in Harry that is missing in airy?" (/h/)

"tricks, ricks. What sound do you hear in tricks that is missing in ricks?" (/t/)

"place, lace. What sound do you hear in place that is missing in lace?" (/p/)

"stopping, topping. What sound do you hear in stopping that is missing in topping? (/s/)

"quick, wick. What sound do you hear in quick that is missing in wick?" (/k/)

"bark, ark. What sound do you hear in bark that is missing in ark?" (/b/)

"shout, out. What sound do you hear in shout that is missing in out?" (/sh/)

"black, lack. What sound do you hear in black that is missing in lack?" (/b/)

"slid, lid. What sound do you hear in slid that is missing in lid?" (/s/)

"slept, lept. What sound do you hear in slept that is missing in lept" (/s/)

8. Identifying final sound in words.

What to say to the student: "I'll say a word two times. Tell me what sound is missing the second time. '______, _______.'" (stimulus words)
EXAMPLE: "What sound do you hear in '_____'" (stimulus word) "that is missing in '_____'?" (stimulus word) (e.g., "What sound do you hear in 'soap' that is missing in 'so'?") (/p/)

> ***NOTE:*** *Give letter sound not letter name. Use pictured items and/or manipulatives if necessary. Use any of the following stimulus words and/or others you select from the story. Correct answers are in parentheses.*

Stimulus items:

"barks, bark. What sound do you hear in barks that is missing in bark?" (/s/)

"Harry, hair. What sound do you hear in Harry that is missing in hair?" (/ee/)

"dirtier, dirty. What sound do you hear in dirtier that is missing in dirty?" (/r/)

"like, lie. What sound do you hear in like that is missing in lie?" (/k/)

"buried, bury. What sound do you hear in buried that is missing in bury?" (/d/

"daddy, dad. What sound do you hear in daddy that is missing in dad?" (/ee/)

"like, lie. What sound do you hear in like that is missing in lie?" (/k/)

"flop, flaw. What sound do you hear in flop that is missing in flaw?" (/p/)

"home, hoe. What sound do you hear in home that is missing in hoe?" (/m/)

"heard, her. What sound do you hear in heard that is missing in her?" (/d/)

9. Segmenting initial sound in words.

What to say to the student: "Listen to the word I say and tell me the first sound you hear."

EXAMPLE: "What's the first sound in '_____'?" (stimulus word) (e.g., "What's the first sound in 'dog'?") (/d/)

> *NOTE: Give letter sound not letter name. Use pictured items and/or manipulatives if necessary. Use any of the following stimulus words and/or others you select from the story. Use any group of 10 stimulus items you select per teaching set.*

Stimulus items:

/p/: pillow, place, played

/b/: back, barking, barks, bath, bathtub, be, became, before, began, beg, behind, black, brother, brush, buried, but, by

/t/: tub, took, tag, to, tired, tried, tricks, tail

/d/: daddy, danced, dashed, day, dead, did, dig, dinner, dirty, do, doggy, dogs, don't done, door, down, dreaming

/k/: carry, clever, close, coal, combed, corner, cried, quick

/g/: garden, gate, gave, getting, girl, give, got

/ch/: changed, children

/dz/: (as 1st sound in jelly): jumped

/m/: magic, many, mouth, mummy

/n/: never, no

/s/: certainly, said, sang, sat, scrub, seen, show, slept, slid, slow, so, soapy, soon, sound, spots, stairs, started, still, stopped, strange, street

/f/: fact, family, father, favorite, feel, fell, felt, fix, flip, flop, follow, found, from, fun, furious

/v/: very

/h/: had, happy, hard, Harry, has, he, head, heard, hidden, him, his, hole, home, house, how, hungry, who

/r/: rail, road, ran, really, rolled, running

/l/: like, little, look, looking

/w/, /wh/: once, one, wag, walked, wants, was, water, way, were, when, where, white, why, with, wonder, wonderful, worked

/sh/: chute, shook, short, shouting

/voiceless th/: things, thought

/voiced th/: that, the, them, then, there, these, they, this

/y/ (as 1st sound in yellow): yard, you, yours

vowels: a, after, again, all, although, and, anyone, as, asleep, at, away, even, ever,everyone, everything, except, if, in, into, it, of, oh, old, on, other, out, over, under, up

10. Segmenting final sound in words.

What to say to the student: "Listen to the word I say and tell me the last sound you hear."

> ***EXAMPLE:*** "What's the last sound in the word '_____'?" (stimulus word) (e.g., "What's the last sound in the word 'gate'?") (/t/)

> ***NOTE:*** *Give letter sound not letter name. Use pictured items and/or manipulatives if necessary. Use any of the following stimulus words and/or others you select from the story. Use any group of 10 stimulus items you select per teaching set.*

Stimulus items:

/p/: asleep, jump, stop, up

/b/: scrub, tub

/t/: at, but, chute, couldn't, didn't, dirtiest, don't, except, fact, favorite, felt, flip-flopped, flop-flipped, gate, got, it, out, sat, short, slept, soapiest, street, that, thought, white without

/d/: and, behind, buried, changed, cried, danced, dashed, dead, did, found, had, hard, head, heard, old, played, railroad, said, slid, started, tired, toward, tried, yard

/k/: back, black, like, look, magic, quick, shook, took, walk, work

/g/: dig, dog, tag, wag

/dz/: (as 1st sound in jelly): strange

/m/: became, comb, come, from, him, home, them

/n/: again, anyone, began, children, done, down, even, everyone, fun, garden, hidden, in, on, one, ran, seen, soon, then, when

/ng/: barking, begging, carrying, dreaming, everything, fixing, following, getting, looking, running, sang, scrubbing, shouting, sounding, stopping, thing

/s/: barks, close, house, once, place, spots, stairs, this, tricks, wants

/z/: has, his

/f/: if

/v/: gave, give

/r/: after, before, brother, clever, corner, dinner, dirtier, door, ever, father, never, other, over, there, under, water, were, where, wonder

/l/: all, coal, feel, fell, girl, hole, little, roll, still, tail, wonderful

/sh/: brush

/voiceless th/: bath, mouth, with

/long A/: away, day, they, way,

/long E/: be, certainly, daddy, dirty, doggy, family, furiously, happily, happy, Harry, he, lovingly, many, mummy, hungry, really, slowly, suddenly, very

/long I/: by, why

/long O/: although, no, pillow, show, so

/oo/: do, into, to, who, you

11. Generating words from the story beginning with a particular sound.

What to say to the student: "Let's think of words **from the story** that start with certain sounds."

EXAMPLE: "Tell me a word **from the story** that starts with / /." (stimulus sound) (e.g., "the sound /h/.") (Harry)

> ***NOTE:*** *Give letter sound, not letter name. Use pictured items if necessary. Use any of the following stimulus words and/or others you select from the story. You say the sound (e.g., a voiceless /p/ sound) and the student is to say a word from the story that begins with that sound. Use any group of 10 stimulus items you select per teaching set.*

Stimulus items:

/p/: pillow, place, played

/b/: back, barking, barks, bath, bathtub, be, became, before, began, beg, behind, black, brother, brush, buried, but, by

/t/: tub, took, tag, to, tired, tried, tricks, tail

/d/: daddy, danced, dashed, day, dead, did, dig, dinner, dirty, do, doggy, dogs, don't, done, door, down, dreaming

/k/: carry, clever, close, coal, combed, corner, cried, quick

/g/: garden, gate, gave, getting, girl, give, got

/ch/: changed, children

/dz/: (as 1st sound in jelly): jumped

/m/: magic, many, mouth, mummy

/n/: never, no

/s/: certainly, said, sang, sat, scrub, seen, show, slept, slid, slow, so, soapy, soon, sound, spots, stairs, started, still, stopped, strange, street

/f/: fact, family, father, favorite, feel, fell, felt, fix, flip, flop, follow, found, from, fun, furious

/v/: very

/h/: had, happy, hard, Harry, has, he, head, heard, hidden, him, his, hole, home, house, how, hungry, who

/r/: rail, road, ran, really, rolled, running

/l/: like, little, look, looking

/w/, /wh/: once, one, wag, walked, wants, was, water, way, were, when, where, white, why, with, wonder, wonderful, worked

/sh/: chute, shook, short, shouting

/voiceless th/: things, thought

/voiced th/: that, the, them, then, there, these, they, this

/y/ (as 1st sound in yellow): yard, you, yours

vowels: a, after, again, all, although, and, anyone, as , asleep, at, away, even, ever, everyone, everything, except, if, in, into, it, of, oh, old, on, other, out, over, under, up

12. Blending sounds in monosyllabic words divided into onset-rime beginning with two consonant cluster + rime.

What to say to the student: "Now we'll put sounds together to make words"

EXAMPLE: "Put these sounds together to make a word (/ / + / /)." (stimulus sounds) "What's the word?" (e.g., "fl + ip: What's the word?") (flip)

> ***NOTE:*** *Give letter sound, not letter name. Use pictured items and/or manipulatives if necessary. Use any of the following stimulus words and/or others you select from the story. Correct answers are in parentheses.*

Stimulus items:

bl + ack (black)	sk + rub (scrub)
tr + ick (trick)	sp + ots (spots)
st + reet (street)	st+ airs (stairs)
br + ush (brush)	st + range (strange)
sl + id (slid)	pl + ace (place)

13. Blending sounds in monosyllabic words divided into onset-rime beginning with single consonant + rime.

What to say to the student: "Let's put sounds together to make words."
EXAMPLE: "Put these sounds together to make a word (/ / + / /)." (stimulus sounds) "What's the word?" (e.g., "/s/ + oap: what's the word?") (soap)

> *NOTE: Give letter sound not letter name. Use pictured items and/or manipulatives if necessary. Use any of the following stimulus words and/or others you select from the story. Correct answers are in parentheses.*

Stimulus items:

/d/ + og (dog)	/w/ + ok (walk)
/h/ + ard (hard)	/f/ + ell (fell)
/d/ + ash (dash)	/s/ + oon (soon)
/b/ + ath (bath)	/h/ + ole (hole)
/t/ + ub (tub)	/g/ + ate (gate)

14. Blending sounds to form a monosyllabic word beginning with a continuant sound.

What to say to the student: "We'll put sounds together to make words."
EXAMPLE: "Put these sounds together to make a word (/ / + / / + / /)." (stimulus sounds) (e.g., "/m/ /ow/ /th/.") (mouth)

> *NOTE: Give letter sound not letter name. Use pictured items and/or manipulatives if necessary. Use any of the following stimulus words and/or others you select from the story. Correct answers are in parentheses.*

Stimulus items:

/s/ /short A/ /t/ (sat)

/s/ /l/ /short E/ /p/ /t/ (slept)

/f/ /r/ /short U/ /m/ (from)

/sh/ /ow/ /t/ (shout)

/f/ /short E/ /l/ /t/ (felt)

/sh/ /oo/ /t/ (chute)

/w/ /short A/ /g/ (wag)

/r/ /short A/ /n/ (ran)

/f/ /l/ /short I/ /p/ (flip)

/s/ /k/ /r/ /short U/ /b/ (scrub)

15. Blending sounds to form a monosyllabic word beginning with a noncontinuant sound.

What to say to the student: "We'll put sounds together to make words."
EXAMPLE: "Put these sounds together to make a word (/ / + / / + / /)." (stimulus sounds) (e.g., "/d/ /ah/ /g/.") (dog)

> **NOTE:** *Give letter sound, not letter name. Use pictured items and/or manipulatives if necessary. Use any of the following stimulus words and/or others you select from the story. Correct answers are in parentheses.*

Stimulus items:

/b/ /short A /k/ (back)

/g/ /long A/ /t/ (gate)

/k/ /r/ /short E/ /p/ /t/ (crept)

/b/ /r/ /short U/ /sh/ (brush)

/b/ /short A/ /th/ (bath)

/t/ /short U/ /b/ (tub)

/b/ /l/ /short A /k/ (black)

/k/ /long O/ /l/ (coal)

/k/ /long O/ /m/ (comb)

/d/ /short I/ /g/ (dig)

16. Substituting initial sound in words.

What to say to the student. "We're going to change beginning/first sounds in words."
EXAMPLE: "Say '_____.'" (stimulus word) "Instead of / /" (stimulus sound) "say / /." (stimulus sound) (e.g., "Say 'tub.' Instead of /t/ say /k/. What's your new word?") (cub)

> **NOTE:** *Give letter sound, not letter name. Use pictured items and/or manipulatives if necessary. Use any of the following stimulus words and/or others you select from the story. Correct answers are in parentheses.*

Stimulus items:

"Say doggy. Instead of /d/ say /f/." (foggy)

"Say bark. Instead of /b/ say /sh/." (shark)

"Say tired. Instead of /t/ say /f/." (fired)

"Say dinner. Instead of /d/ say /voiceless th/." (thinner)

"Say bath. Instead of /b/ say /m/." (math)

"Say jumped. Instead of /j/ say /b/." (bumped)

"Say Harry. Instead of /h/ say /l/." (Larry)

"Say furiously. Instead of /f/ say /k/." (curiously)

"Say yard. Instead of /y/ say /g/." (guard)

"Say wagged. Instead of /w/ say /g/." (gagged)

17. Substituting final sound in words.

What to say to the student: "We're going to change ending/last sounds in words." ***EXAMPLE:*** "Say '_____.'" (stimulus word) "Instead of / /" (stimulus sound) "say / /." (stimulus sound) (e.g., "Say 'wagged.' Instead of /d/ say /z/. What's your new word?") (wags)

> ***NOTE:*** *Give letter sound not letter name. Use pictured items and/or manipulatives if necessary. Use any of the following stimulus words and/or others you select from the story. Correct answers are in parentheses.*

Stimulus items:

"Say down. Instead of /n/ say /t/." (doubt)

"Say done. Instead of /n/ say /k/." (duck)

"Say gate. Instead of /t/ say /v/." (gave)

"Say mouth. Instead of /th/ say /s/." (mouse)

"Say road. Instead of /d/ say /p/." (rope)

"Say coal. Instead of /l/ say /t/." (coat)

"Say doggy. Instead of /ee/ say /z/." (dogs)

"Say seen. Instead of /n/ say /d/." (seed)

"Say flop. Instead of /p/ say /s/." (floss)

"Say home. Instead of /m/ say /p/." (hope)

18. Segmenting middle sound in monosyllabic words.

What to say to the student: "Tell me the middle sound in the word I say."
EXAMPLE: "What's the middle sound in the word '_____'?" (stimulus word) (e.g., "What's the middle sound in the word 'gate'?") (/long A/)

> ***NOTE:*** *Give letter sound not letter name. Use pictured items and/or manipulatives if necessary. Use any of the following stimulus words and/or others you select from the story. Correct answers are in parentheses.*

Stimulus items:

comb (/long O/)
fun (/short U/)
dog (ah)
soap (/long O/)
ran (/short A/)
dash (/short A/)
cry (/r/)
dead (/short E/)
slow (/l/)
walk (/ah/)

19. Substituting middle sound in words.

What to say to the student: "We're going to change the middle sound in words."
EXAMPLE: "Say '_____.'" (stimulus word) "Instead of / /" (stimulus sound) "say / /." (stimulus sound) (e.g., "Say 'flop.' Instead of /ah/ say /short I/. What's your new word?") (flip)

> ***NOTE:*** *Give letter sound not letter name. Use pictured items and/or manipulatives if necessary. Use any of the following stimulus words and/or others you select from the story. Correct answers are in parentheses.*

Stimulus items:

"Say dog. Instead of /ah/ say /short I/." (dig)
"Say mummy. Instead of /short U/ say /ah/." (mommy)
"Say road. Instead of /long O/ say /long I/."(ride)
"Say soap. Instead of /long O/ say /short I/." (sip)
"Say wag. Instead of /short A/, say /short I/." (wig)
"Say mouth. Instead of /ow/ say /short A/." (math)

"Say coal. Instead of /long O/ say /ah/." (call)

"Say dead. Instead of /short E/ say /short A/." (dad)

"Say fun. Instead of /short U/ say /short A/." (fan)

"Say home. Instead of /long O/, say /short I/." (him)

20. Identifying all sounds in monosyllabic words.

What to say to the student: "Now tell me all the sounds you hear in the word I say."
EXAMPLE: "What sounds do you hear in the word '_____'?" (stimulus word) (e.g., "What sounds do you hear in the word 'dog'?") (/d/ /ah/ /g/)

> *NOTE: Give letter sound, not letter name. Use pictured items and/or manipulatives if necessary. Use any of the following stimulus words and/or others you select from the story. Correct answers are in parentheses.*

Stimulus items:

wag (/w/ /short A/ /g/)

black (/b/ /l/ /short A/ /k/)

brush (/b/ /r/ /short U/ /sh/)

white (/w/ /long I/ /t/)

spots (/s/ /p/ /ah/ /t/ /s/)

scrub (/s/ /k/ /r/ /short U/ /b/)

dance (/d/ /short A/ /n/ /s/)

tricks (/t/ /r/ /short I/ /k/ /s/)

chute (/sh/ /oo/ /t/)

home (/h/ /long O/ /m/)

21. Deleting sounds within words.

What to say to the student. "We're going to leave out sounds in words."
EXAMPLE: "Say '_____'" (stimulus word) "without / /." (stimulus sound) (e.g., "Say 'slid' without /l/." (sid) Say: "The word that was left, 'sid,' is a real word. Sometimes the word won't be a real word."

> *NOTE: Give letter sound, not letter name. Use pictured items and/or manipulatives if necessary. Use any of the following stimulus words and/or others you select from the story. Correct answers are in parentheses.*

Stimulus items:

"Say tricks without /r/." (ticks)

"Say place without /l/." (pace)

"Say quick without /w/." (kick)

"Say chrome without /r/." (comb)

"Say played without /l/." (payed)

"Say slow without /l/." (so)

"Say black without /l/." (back)

"Say still without /t/." (sill)

"Say old without /l/." (owed)

"Say sleep without /l/." (seep)

22. Substituting consonant in words having a two-sound cluster.

What to say to the student: "We're going to substitute sounds in words."
EXAMPLE: "Say '_____'" (stimulus word). "Instead of / /" (stimulus sound) "say / /" (stimulus sound) (e.g., "Say 'stop.' Instead of /t/ say /l/.") (slop). Say "Sometimes the new word will be a made-up word."

> *NOTE:* *Give letter sound not letter name. Use pictured items and/or manipulatives if necessary. Use any of the following stimulus words and/or others you select from the story. Correct answers are in parentheses.*

Stimulus items:

"Say cried. Instead of /r/ say /l/." (Clyde)

"Say slid. Instead of /l/ say /k/." (skid)

"Say dream. Instead of /d/ say /k/." (cream)

"Say tricks. Instead of /s/ say /t/." (tricked)

"Say brush. Instead of /r/ say /l/." (blush)

"Say found. Instead of /d/ say /t/." (fount)

"Say hard. Instead of /d/ say /p/." (harp)

"Say tricks. Instead of /k/ say /p/." (trips)

"Say crash. Instead of /r/ say /l/" (clash)

"Say stairs. Instead of /t/ say /k/." (scares)

23. Phoneme reversing.

What to say to the student: "We're going to say words backward."
EXAMPLE: "Say the word '_____'" (stimulus word) "backward." (e.g., "Say 'door' backward.") (rode)

> *NOTE: This is a difficult phoneme-level task and should only be done with older students. Give letter sound, not letter name. Use pictured items and/or manipulatives if necessary. Use any of the following stimulus words and/or others you select from the story. Correct answers are in parentheses.*

Stimulus items:

back	(cab)	tub	(but)
feel	(leaf)	stop	(pots)
seen	(niece)	gave	(vague)
tail	(late)	spots	(stops)
no	(own)	soon	(noose)

24. Phoneme switching.

What to say to the student: "We're going to switch the first sounds in two words."
EXAMPLE: "Switch the first sounds in '_____' and '_____.'" (stimulus words) (e.g., "Switch the first sounds in 'one day.'") (done way)

> *NOTE: This is a difficult phoneme-level task and should only be done with older students. Give letter sound, not letter name. Use pictured items and/or manipulatives if necessary. Use any of the following stimulus words and/or others you select from the story. Correct answers are in parentheses.*

Stimulus items:

very happy	(Harry vappy)
felt tired	(telt fired)
mummy daddy	(dummy maddy)
got dirty	(dot girty)
back yard	(yack bard)

happy barks	(bappy harks)
hungry too	(tungry who)
white dog	(dite wog)
family thought	(thamily fought)
dirty Harry	(hurty dairy)

25. Pig latin.

What to say to the student: "We're going to talk in a secret language using words from the story. In pig latin, you take off the first sound of a word, put it at the end of the word, and add a long A sound."

EXAMPLE: "Say dog in pig latin." (ogday)

> *NOTE: This is a difficult phoneme-level task and should only be done with older students. Use pictured items and/or manipulatives if necessary. Use any of the following stimulus words and/or others you select from the story. Correct answers are in parentheses.*

Stimulus items:

Harry	(airyhay)
bath	(athbay)
dinner	(innerday)
family	(amilyfay)
chute	(uteshay)
mummy	(ummyfay)
girl	(irlgay)
pillow	(illowpay)
tail	(ailtay)
children	(ildrenchay)

CHAPTER

PHONOLOGICAL AWARENESS ACTIVITIES TO USE WITH *STONE SOUP*

Text version used for selection of stimulus items:
Paterson, D. (1984). *Stone soup*. Mahwah, NJ: Troll Communications.

PHONOLOGICAL AWARENESS ACTIVITIES AT THE WORD LEVEL

1. Counting words.

What to say to the student: "We're going to count words."

EXAMPLE: "How many words do you hear in this sentence (or phrase)? 'some salt.'" (2)

> ***NOTE:*** *Use pictured items and/or manipulatives if necessary. Use any of the following stimulus phrases or sentences and/or others you select from the story. Correct answers are in parentheses.*

Stimulus items:

warm bread (2)

stone soup (2)

bit of meat (3)

spare some food (3)

he ran off (3)

in the first place (4)

a place to sleep (4)

a few stale crusts (4)

I might just have one (5)

if we do not ask (5)

2. Identifying missing word from list.

What to say to the student: "Listen to the words I say. I'll say them again. You tell me which word I leave out."

EXAMPLE: "Listen to the words I say: 'make, barley, tired.' I'll say them again. Tell me which one I leave out: 'make, barley.'" (tired)

> *NOTE: Use pictured items and/or manipulatives if necessary. Use any of the following stimulus words and/or others you select from the story. Correct answers are in parentheses.*

Stimulus set #1	Stimulus set #2
bread, third	bread (third)
barrels, little	little (barrels)
meat, king, fire	meat, fire (king)
heard, pot, village	heard, pot (village)
buzzed, chunks, town	chunks, town (buzzed)
cider, lucky, built	cider, lucky (built)
soup, soldier, next, glad	soup, next, glad (soldier)
milk, cut, boil, orange	milk, cut, boil (orange)
flavor, waited, share, house	flavor, waited, house (share)
salt, tables, must, roast	salt, must, roast (tables)

3. Identifying missing word in phrase or sentence.

What to say to the student: "Listen to the sentence I read. Tell me which word is missing the second time I read the sentence."

EXAMPLE: "'Home from war.' Listen again and tell me which word I leave out. 'Home from____.'" (war)

> *NOTE: Use pictured items and/or manipulatives if necessary. Use any of the following stimulus sentences and/or others you select from the story. Correct answers are in parentheses.*

Stimulus items:

Stone soup. Stone_____. (soup)

Great distance. ____ distance. (Great)

Dozen peeled onions. Dozen ______ onions. (peeled)

You have no food. You have ______ food. (no)

They ate and drank and danced. They _____ and drank and danced. (ate)

The stones are cooking nicely. The stones are cooking _____. (nicely)

He returned with some barley. He returned with _____ barley. (some)

You have taught us something. You have _____ us something. (taught)

Goodbye called the soldiers. _____ called the soldiers. (Goodbye)

The soup was fit for a king. The soup was _____ for a king. (fit)

3. Supplying missing word as adult reads.

What to say to the student: "I want you to help me read the story. You fill in the words I leave out."

EXAMPLE: "Perfect stone _____." (soup)

> ***NOTE:*** *Use pictured items and/or manipulatives if necessary. Use any of the following stimulus sentences and/or others you select from the story. Correct answers are in parentheses.*

Stimulus items:

Since you have no _____. (food)

Several stalks of _____. (celery)

Busy hiding their _____. (food)

Came back with big _____ of meat. (chunks)

Brought him a bucket of _____. (milk)

Get a _____ of warm bread. (loaf)

They all sniffed the _____. (soup)

The villagers buzzed with _____. (excitement)

Let us borrow a large cooking _____. (pot)

They could hardly believe it had been made from _____. (stones)

5. Rearranging words.

What to say to the student: "I'll say some words out of order. You put them in the right order so they make sense."

EXAMPLE: "'pieces small.' Put those words in the right order." (small pieces)

NOTE: Use pictured items and/or manipulatives if necessary. Use any of the following stimulus words and/or others you select from the story. Correct answers are in parentheses. This word-level activity can be more difficult than some of the syllable- or phoneme-level activities because of the memory load. If your students are only able to deal with two or three words to be rearranged, add more two- and three-word samples from the story and omit the four-word level until a later time.

Stimulus items:

soup stone (stone soup)

chunks big (big chunks)

month last (last month)

carrots crisp orange (crisp orange carrots)

loaves brought they so out (so they brought out loaves)

and salt pepper (salt and pepper)

beds most comfortable (most comfortable beds)

they potatoes their hid (they hid their potatoes)

smells already better it (it smells better already)

king it for was a fit (it was fit for a king)

PHONOLOGICAL AWARENESS ACTIVITIES AT THE SYLLABLE LEVEL

1. Syllable counting.

What to say to the student: "We're going to count syllables (or parts) of words."
EXAMPLE: "How many syllables do you hear in '_____'?" (stimulus word) (e.g., "How many syllables in 'bed'?") (1)

NOTE: Use pictured items and/or manipulatives if necessary. Use any of the of the following stimulus words and/or others you select from the story. Use any group of 10 stimulus items you select per teaching set.

Stimulus items:

One-syllable words: part, place, pot, put, back, bad, barn, be, bed, been, big, bowl, bread, bring, brought, built, but, taught, to, tossed, town, tucked, turned, danced, dined, don't, door, down, drank, dropped, called, came, can, can't, could, crisp, crusts, cut, king, get, glad, good, great, chased, chunks, just, made, make, may, meat, might, milk, mill, much, must, knew, know, next, nice, none, not, now, said, salt, same, sat, saw, seen, sense, set, since, sleep, slice, small, smells, smooth, sniffed, so, some, soon, soup, spare, square, stale, stalks, still, stirred, stones, such, few, filled, find, first, fit, food, for, found, from, had, half, has, have, he, heard, hid, his, home, house, how, hung, ran, rich, right, road, roasts, land, large, last, let, loaf, long, once, one, walked, want, war, warm, was, we, wells, went, were, what, when, which, who, wife, will, with, would, share, she, shook, should, thick, thin, third, thought, thank, the, their, them then, they, this, yes, you, a, all, an, and, as, ask, at, each, eat, I, if, in, is, it, it's, of, off, on, or, out, us

Two-syllable words: peasant, pepper, perhaps, pieces, pity, barley, barrels, before, believe, beneath, better, boil, borrow, busy, tables, tasted, tired, traveled, distance, dozen, carrots, closets, coming, cooking, quickly, gathered, goodbye, marching, mayor, miller, minutes, missing, never, nicely, nothing, cellars, cider, saying, second, simply, sniffing, soldier, someone, something, strangers, farmer's, faster, finding, flavor, very, village, happy, hardly, hidden, hiding, hoping, houses, hungry, hurried, ready, really, returned, lacking, little, lowered, lucky, waited, water, welcomed, whispered, women, thicken, themselves, about, added, after, again, ago, agreed, alone, also, always, answer, any, armful, arrived, asking, away, even, ever, except, extra, idea, inside, into, onions, orange, under

Three-syllable words: potatoes, townspeople, decided, delicious, disappeared, celery, satisfied, several, faraway, finally, villagers, already, another, entire, excitement, imagine, important, overhead

Four-syllable words: pillowcases, comfortable, everyone, everything, vegetables

2. Initial syllable deleting.

What to say to the student: "We're going to leave out syllables (or parts of words)." ***EXAMPLE:*** "Say '_____.'" (stimulus word) "Say it again without '_____.'" (stimulus syllable) (e.g., "Say 'someone' without 'some.'") (one)

> ***NOTE:*** *Use pictured items and/or manipulatives if necessary. Use any of the following stimulus words and/or others you select from the story. Correct answers are in parentheses.*

Stimulus items:

"Say barley without bar." (lee)

"Say townspeople without towns." (people)

"Say answer without an." (sir)

"Say perhaps without per-." (haps)

"Say inside without in." (side)

"Say bucket without buck." (-et)

"Say returned without re-." (turned)

"Say also without all." (so)

"Say beneath without be." (neath)

"Say goodbye without good." (bye)

3. Final syllable deleting.

What to say to the student: "We're going to leave out syllables (or parts of words)." *EXAMPLE:* "Say '_____.'" (stimulus word) "Say it again without '_____.'" (stimulus syllable) (e.g., "Say 'armful' without 'ful.'") (arm)

> *NOTE: Use pictured items and/or manipulatives if necessary. Use any of the following stimulus words and/or others you select from the story. Correct answers are in parentheses.*

Stimulus items:

"Say excitement without -ment." (excite)

"Say themselves without selves." (them)

"Say overhead without head." (over)

"Say farmer without -er." (farm)

"Say whispered without purred." (whis-)

"Say lacking without -ing." (lack)

"Say hardly without lee." (hard)

"Say pepper without -er." (pep)

"Say several without -al." (sever)

"Say hurried without -eed." (her)

4. Initial syllable adding.

What to say to the student: "Now let's add syllables (or parts) to words." *EXAMPLE:* " Add '_____'" (stimulus syllable) "to the beginning of '_____.'" (stimulus syllable) (e.g., "Add 'be' to the beginning of 'neath.'") (beneath)

NOTE: *Use pictured items and/or manipulatives if necessary. Use any of the following stimulus words and/or others you select from the story. Correct answers are in parentheses.*

Stimulus items:

"Add far to the beginning of away." (faraway)

"Add side to the beginning of -er." (cider)

"Add all to the beginning of ready." (already)

"Add af- to the beginning of -ter." (after)

"Add bee to the beginning of leave." (believe)

"Add nice to the beginning of lee." (nicely)

"Add march to the beginning of -ing." (marching)

"Add good to the beginning of bye." (goodbye)

"Add bar to the beginning of oh." (borrow)

"Add lack to the beginning of -ing." (lacking)

5. Final syllable adding.

What to say to the student: "Now let's add syllables (or parts) to words."
EXAMPLE: "Add '_____'" (stimulus syllable) "to the end of '_____.'" (stimulus syllable) (e.g., "Add 'selves' to the end of 'them.'") (themselves)

NOTE: *Use pictured items and/or manipulatives if necessary. Use any of the following stimulus words and/or others you select from the story. Correct answers are in parentheses.*

Stimulus items:

"Add tire to the end of en-." (entire)

"Add -ment to the end of excite." (excitement)

"Add toes to the end of pota-." (potatoes)

"Add yuns the end of un-." (onions)

"Add lee to the end of ree-." (really)

"Add -uts to the end of care." (carrots)

"Add ways to the end of all." (always)

"Add –unt to the end of import." (important)

"Add lee to the end of quick." (quickly)

"Add -cept to the end of ex-." (except)

6. Syllable substituting.

What to say to the student: "Let's make up some new words."
EXAMPLE: "Say '_____.'" (stimulus word) "Instead of '_____'" (stimulus syllable) "say '_____.'" (stimulus syllable) (e.g., "Say 'under.' Instead of '-der' say 'do.' The new word is 'undo.'")

> ***NOTE:*** *Use pictured items and/or manipulatives if necessary. Use any of the following stimulus words and/or others you select from the story. Correct answers are in parentheses.*

Stimulus items:

"Say excitement. Instead of -ment say -ing." (exciting)

"Say perhaps. Instead of -haps say mit." (permit)

"Say disappeared. Instead of dis- say re-." (reappeared)

"Say barley. Instead of lee say king." (barking)

"Say townspeople. Instead of towns say good." (goodpeople)

"Say goodbye. Instead of bye say -ness." (goodness)

"Say extra. Instead of -tra say -cept." (except)

"Say armful. Instead of arm say care." (careful)

"Say welcome. Instead of well say be." (become)

"Say borrow. Instead of bar say sar-." (sorrow)

PHONOLOGICAL AWARENESS ACTIVITIES AT THE PHONEME LEVEL

1. Counting sounds.

What to say to the student: "We're going to count sounds in words."
EXAMPLE: "How many sounds do you hear in this word? 'glad.'" (4)

> ***NOTE:*** *Use pictured items and/or manipulatives if necessary. Use any of the following stimulus words and/or others you select from the story. Be sure to give the letter sound and not the letter name. Use any group of 10 stimulus items you select per teaching set.*

Stimulus words with two sounds: be, to, may, knew, no, now, saw, so, few, he, how, we, were, who, she, the, they, you, all, an, as, at, each, eat, if, in, is, it, of, off, on, one, or, out, us

Stimulus words with three sounds: pot, put, back, bad, bed, been, big, boil, bowl, but, taught, town, door, down, came, can, could, cut, king, get, good, made, make, meat, might, mill, much, nice, not, said, same, sat, seen, set, some, soon, soup, such, fire, fit, food, for, had, half, has, have, heard, hid, his, home, house, hung, ran, rich, right, road, roasts, let, loaf, long, was, what, when, which, wife, will, with, would, share, shook, should, thick, thin, third, thought, their, them, then, yes, ago, and, any, ask, away, even, ever, it's, once

Stimulus words with four sounds: pails, part, peeled, pepper, pity, place, barn, beds, better, borrow, bread, bring, brought, built, busy, buzzed, tired, tossed, tucked, turned, dined, don't dozen, called, can't, glad, great, chased, just, milk, miller, must, knocked, never, ready, really, cider, salt, sense, served, since, sleep, slice, small, smooth, spare, stale, still, stirred, stone, filled, find, first, foods, found, from, very, happy, hidden, hurried, land, large, last, little, loaves, looked, lowered, lucky, waited, walked, want, water, wells, went, women, thicken, thank, about, added, after, again, alone, also, answer, asked, into, under

Stimulus words with five sounds: pieces, barley, barrels, before, believe, beneath, tables, tasted, danced, drank, dropped, coming, cooking, crisp, gathered, goodbye, chunks, mayor's, next, nicely, nothing, roasts, celery, cellars, several, sliced, smells, sniffed, square, stones, stuffed, flavor, village, hoping, houses, hungry, agreed, always, another, arrived, entire, inside

2. Sound categorization or identifying rhyme oddity.

What to say to the student: "Guess which word I say does not rhyme with the other three words."

EXAMPLE: "Tell me which word does not rhyme with the other three. '_____, _____, _____, _____.'" (stimulus words) (e.g., "right, might, bite, pot. Which word doesn't rhyme?") (pot)

> ***NOTE:*** *Use pictured items if necessary. Use any of the following stimulus words and/or others you select from the story. Correct answers are in parentheses.*

Stimulus items:

bowl, boil, roll, troll (boil)

chunk, drank, thank, spank (chunk)

stones, bones, cider, phones (cider)

there, square, spare, stalks (stalks)

door, war, sniffed, or (sniffed)

thought, sleep, bought, taught (sleep)

found, roast, boast, coast (found)

eat, meat, treat, thought (thought)

taste, tired, mired, fired (taste)

mill, still, will, turned (turned)

3. Matching rhyme.

What to say to the student: "We're going to think of rhyming words."
EXAMPLE: "Which word rhymes with '_____'?" (stimulus word) (e.g., "Which word rhymes with 'roasts'? 'mayor, house, boasts, who.'") (boasts)

> **NOTE:** *Use pictured items if necessary. Use any of the following stimulus words and/or others you select from the story. Correct answers are in parentheses.*

Stimulus items:

salt: shook, thick, fault, happy (fault)

stale: pail, pepper, bowl, celery (pail)

chunks: hidden, welcomed, extra, bunks (bunks)

fire: milk, tire, someone, food (tire)

soup: loop, imagine, onion, walked (loop)

dined: strangers, faster, lined, whispered (lined)

armful: finally, harmful, slice, overhead (harmful)

wife: third, lowered, finding, life (life)

miller: important, thriller, hoping, finding (thriller)

carrots: orange, themselves, parrots, finally (parrots)

4. Producing rhyme.

What to say to the student: "Now we'll say rhyming words."
EXAMPLE: "Tell me a word that rhymes with '_____.'" (stimulus word) (e.g., "Tell me a word that rhymes with 'stone.' You can make up a word if you want." (bone)

> **NOTE:** *Use pictured items if necessary. Use any of the following stimulus words and/or others you select from the story (i.e., you say a word from the list below and the student is to think of a rhyming word). Use any group of 10 stimulus items you select per teaching set.*

Stimulus items:

/p/: pails, part, peasant, peeled, pepper, perhaps, pieces, pillowcases, pity, place, pot, potatoes, put

/b/: back, bad, barley, barn, barrels, be, bed, beds, been, before, believe, beneath, better, big, boil, borrow, bowl, bread, bring, brought, built, busy, but, buzzed

/t/: tables, tasted, taught, tired, to, tossed, town, traveled, tucked, turned

/d/: danced, decided, dined, distance, don't, door, down, dozen, drank, dropped

/k/: called, came, can, can't, carrots, closets, cooking, could, crisp, crusts, cut, king, quickly

/g/: gathered, get, glad, good, goodbye, great

/ch/: chased, chunks

/dz/: (as 1st sound in jelly): just

/m/: made, make, marching, may, mayor, meat, might, milk, mill, miller, minutes, missing, much, must

/n/: knew, knocked, know, never, next, nice, no, none, not, nothing, now

/s/: celery, cellars, cider, said, salt, same, sat, saw, saying, second, seen, sense, served, set, several, simply, since, sleep, slice, small, smells, smooth, sniffed, sniffing, so, soldier, some, soon, soup, spare, square, stale, stalks, still, stirred, stone, stones, strangers, stuffed, such

/f/: farmer, faster, few, filled, find, finding, fire, first, fit, flavor, food, for, found, from

/v/: very, village

/h/: had, half, happy, hardly, has, have, he, heard, hid, hidden, hiding, his, home, hoping, house, houses, how, hung, hungry, hurried

/r/: ran, ready, really, rich, right, road, roasts

/l/: lacking, land, large, last, let, little, loaf, loaves, long, looked, lowered, lucky

/w/, /wh/: once, one, waited, walked, want, war, warm, was, water, we, welcomed, wells, went, were, what, when, which, who, wife, will, with, women, would

/sh/: share, she, shook, should

/voiceless th/: thick, thicken, thin, third, thought, thank

/voiced th/: the, their, them, then, there, they, this

/y/ (as 1st sound in yellow): yes, you

vowels: a, about, added, after, again, ago, agreed, all, alone, already, also, an, and, as, asked, asking, at, away, each, eat, entire, even, ever, except, extra, I, idea, if, in, inside, into, is, it, it's, of, off, on, or, orange, out, under, us

5. Sound matching (initial).

What to say to the student: "Now we'll listen for the first sound in words."

EXAMPLE: "Listen to this sound: / /." (stimulus sound). "Guess which word I say begins with that sound. '_____, _____, _____, _____.'" (stimulus words) (e.g., "Listen to this sound /w/. Guess which word I say begins with that sound: 'house, fire, women, lucky.'") (women)

> ***NOTE:*** *Give letter sound not letter name. Use pictured items if necessary. Use any of the following stimulus words and/or others you select from the story. Correct answers are in parentheses.*

Stimulus items:

/p/: town, boil, potatoes, stones (potatoes)

/f/: share, flavor, war, barn (flavor)

/short I/: important, away, pillowcases, beneath (important)

/t/: buzzed, faraway, townspeople, roasts (townspeople)

/w/: soldiers, whispered, tossed, peasant (whispered)

/s/: soup, onions, hiding, villagers (soup)

/ch/: imagine, hungry, chased, barrels (chased)

/k/: disappeared, marching, walked, quickly (quickly)

/m/: crisp, mill, comfortable, satisfied (mill)

/b/: pieces, danced, vegetables, buzzed (buzzed)

6. Sound matching (final).

What to say to the student: "Now we'll listen for the last sound in words."

EXAMPLE: "Listen to this sound: / /" (stimulus sound). "Guess which word I say ends with that sound '_____, _____, _____, _____.'" (stimulus words) (e.g., "Listen to this sound /l/. Guess which word I say ends with that sound: 'bowl, taught, shook, loaves.'") (bowl)

> ***NOTE:*** *Give letter sound not letter name. Use pictured items if necessary. Use any of the following stimulus words and/or others you select from the story. Correct answers are in parentheses.*

Stimulus items:

/f/: before, bread, half, small (half)

/long E/: peasant, celery, fire, village (celery)

/d/: stirred, pieces, cooking, mayor (stirred)

/z/: stalks, goodbye, soldiers, carrots (soldiers)

/n/: stone, sniffed, hardly, themselves (stone)

/s/: imagine, just, delicious, cooking (delicious)

/ch/: orange, barrels, asking, rich (rich)

/t/: dined, peasant, armful, everyone (peasant)

/r/: pepper, vegetables, borrow, sliced (pepper)

/v/: entire, simply, believe, everything (believe)

7. Identifying initial sound in words.

What to say to the student: "I'll say a word two times. Tell me what sound is missing the second time. '_______, _______.'" (stimulus words)

EXAMPLE: "What sound do you hear in '_____'" (stimulus word) "that is missing in '_____'?" (stimulus word) (e.g., "What sound do you hear in 'small,' that is missing in 'mall'?'") (/s/)

> **NOTE:** *Give letter sound not letter name. Use pictured items and/or manipulatives if necessary. Use any of the following stimulus words and/or others you select from the story. Correct answers are in parentheses.*

Stimulus items:

"traveled, -raveled. What sound do you hear in traveled that is missing in raveled?" (/t/)

"bring, ring. What sound do you hear in bring that is missing in ring?" (/b/)

"share, air. What sound do you hear in share that is missing in air?" (/sh/)

"stone, tone. What sound do you hear in stone that is missing in tone?" (/s/)

"land, and. What sound do you hear in land that is missing in and?" (/l/)

"thought, ought. What sound do you hear in thought that is missing in ought?" (/th/)

"part, art. What sound do you hear in part that is missing in art?" (/p/)

"never, ever. What sound do you hear in never that is missing in ever?" (/n/)

"ready, Eddy. What sound do you hear in ready that is missing in Eddy?" (/r/)

"brought, rot. What sound do you hear in brought that is missing in rot?" (/b/)

8. Identifying final sound in words.

What to say to the student: "I'll say a word two times. Tell me what sound is missing the second time. '_______, _______.'" (stimulus words)

EXAMPLE: "What sound do you hear in '_____'" (stimulus word) "that is missing in '_____'?" (stimulus word) (e.g., "What sound do you hear in 'stone' that is missing in 'stow'?"(/n/)

> *NOTE: Give letter sound not letter name. Use pictured items and/or manipulatives if necessary. Use any of the following stimulus words and/or others you select from the story. Correct answers are in parentheses.*

Stimulus items:

"soup, Sue. What sound do you hear in soup that is missing in Sue?" (/p/)

"knocked, knock. What sound do you hear in knocked that is missing in knock?" (/t/)

"buzzed, buzz. What sound do you hear in buzzed that is missing in buzz?" (/d/)

"made, may. What sound do you hear in made that is missing in may?" (/d/)

"tables, table. What sound do you hear in tables that is missing in table?" (/z/)

"chunks, chunk. What sound do you hear in chunks that is missing in chunk?" (/s/)

"crisp, Kris. What sound do you hear in crisp that is missing in Kris?" (/p/)

"heard, her. What sound do you hear in heard that is missing in her?" (/d/)

"miller, mill. What sound do you hear in miller that is missing in mill?" (/r/)

"finally, final. What sound do you hear in finally that is missing in final?" (/long E/)

9. Segmenting initial sound in words.

What to say to the student: "Listen to the word I say and tell me the first sound you hear."

EXAMPLE: "What's the first sound in '_____'?" (stimulus word) (e.g., "What's the first sound in 'tossed'?") (/t/)

NOTE: Give letter sound not letter name. Use pictured items and/or manipulatives if necessary. Use any of the following stimulus words and/or others you select from the story. Use any group of 10 stimulus items you select per teaching set.

Stimulus items:

/p/: pails, part, peasant, peeled, pepper, perhaps, pieces, pillowcases, pity, place, pot, potatoes, put

/b/: back, bad, barley, barn, barrels, be, bed, beds, been, before, believe, beneath, better, big, boil, borrow, bowl, bread, bring, brought, built, busy, but, buzzed

/t/: tables, tasted, taught, tired, tossed, town, townspeople, traveled, tucked, turned, two

/d/: danced, decided, dined, disappeared, distance, don't, door, down, dozen, drank, dropped

/k/: called, came, can, can't, carrots, closets, comfortable, cooking, could, crisp, crusts, cut, king, quickly

/g/: gathered, get, glad, good, goodbye, great

/ch/: chased, chunks

/dz/: (as 1st sound in jelly): just

/m/: made, make, marching, may, mayor, meat, might, milk, mill, miller, minutes, missing, much, must

/n/: knew, knocked, know, never, next, nice, nicely, no, none, not, nothing, now

/s/: celery, cellars, cider, said, salt, same, sat, satisfied, saw, saying, second, seen, sense, served, set, several, simply, since, sleep, slice, small, smells, smooth, sniffed, sniffing, so, soldier, some, someone, something, soon, soup, spare, square, stale, stalks, still, stirred, stone, strangers, stuffed, such

/f/: faraway, farmer, faster, few, filled, finally, find, finding, fire, first, fit, flavor, food, for, found, from

/v/: vegetables, very, village, villagers

/h/: had, half, happy, hardly, has, have, he, heard, hid, hidden, hiding, his, home, hoping, house, houses, how, hung, hungry, hurried

/r/: ran, ready, really, returned, rich, right, road, roasts

/l/: lacking, land, large, last, let, little, loaf, loaves, long, looked, lowered, lucky

/w/, /wh/: once, one, waited, walked, want, war, warm, was, water, we, welcomed, wells, went, were, what, when, which, whispered, who, wife, will, with, women, would

/sh/: share, she, shook, should

/voiceless th/: thick, thicken, thin, third, thought, thank

/voiced th/: the, their, them, themselves, then, there, they, this

/y/ (as 1st sound in yellow): yes, you

vowels: a, about, added, after, again, ago, agreed, all, alone, already, also, always, an, and, armful, arrived, as, asked, asking, at, away, each, eat, entire, even, ever, everyone, everything, except, excitement, extra, I, idea, if, imagine, important, in, inside, into, is, it, it's, of, off, on, onions, or, orange, overhead, out, under, us

10. Segmenting final sound in words.

What to say to the student: "Listen to the word I say and tell me the last sound you hear."

EXAMPLE: "What's the last sound in the word '_____'?" (stimulus word) (e.g., "What's the last sound in the word 'vegetables'?") (/z/)

> **NOTE:** *Give letter sound not letter name. Use pictured items and/or manipulatives if necessary. Use any of the following stimulus words and/or others you select from the story. Use any group of 10 stimulus items you select per teaching set.*

Stimulus items:

/p/: crisp, soup

/t/: about, asked, at, brought, built, but, can't, chased, cut, danced, don't, dropped, eat, except, excitement, first, fit, get, great, important, it, just, knocked, last, let, looked, meat, might, must, next, not, out, part, peasant, pot, put, right, salt, sat, set, sliced, sniffed, stuffed, taught, thought, tossed, tucked, walked, want, went, what

/d/: added, agreed, and, arrived, bad, bed, bread, buzzed, called, decided, dined, disappeared, filled, find, food, found, gathered, glad, good, had, heard, hid, hurried, inside, land, lowered, made, overhead, peeled, returned, road, said, satisfied, second, served, should, stirred, tasted, third, tired, traveled, turned, waited, welcomed, whispered, would

/k/: ask, back, drank, make, milk, shook, thank, thick

/g/: big

/ch/: each, much, rich, such, which

/dz/: (as in jelly): large, orange, village

/m/: came, from, home, same, some, them, warm

/n/: again, alone, an, barn, been, can, down, dozen, even, everyone, hidden, imagine, in, none, on, one, ran, seen, someone, soon, stone, then, thicken, thin, town, when, women

/ng/: asking, bring, coming, cooking, everything, finding, hiding, hoping, hung, king, lacking, long, marching, missing, nothing, saying, sniffing, something

/s/: carrots, chunks, closets, crusts, delicious, distance, house, it's, minutes, nice, once, perhaps, place, roasts, sense, since, stalks, this, us, yes

/z/: always, as, barrels, beds, cellars, farmer's, foods, has, his, houses, is, loaves, mayor's, onions, pieces, pillowcases, potatoes, smells, soldiers, stones, strangers, tables, themselves, vegetables, villagers, was, wells

/f/: half, if, loaf, off, wife

/v/: believe, have, of

/r/: after, another, answer, are, before, better, cider, door, entire, ever, faster, fire, flavor, for, mayor, miller, never, or, pepper, share, soldier, spare, square, their, under, war, water, were

/l/: all, armful, boil, bowl, comfortable, little, mill, pails, several, small, stale, still, townspeople, will

/voiceless th/: beneath, with

/voiced th/: smooth

/long A/: away, faraway, may, they

/long E/: already, any, barley, be, busy, celery, finally, happy, hardly, he, hungry, lucky, nicely, pity, quickly, ready, really, she, simply, very, we

/long I/: goodbye, I

/long O/: ago, also, borrow, know, no, so

/short U/: extra

/oo/: into, knew, too, who

/ah/: saw

/ow/: now

11. Generating words from the story beginning with a particular sound.

What to say to the student: "Let's think of words **from the story** that start with certain sounds."

EXAMPLE: "Tell me a word **from the story** that starts with / /." (stimulus sound) (e.g., "the sound /w/") (water)

NOTE: *Give letter sound not letter name. Use pictured items if necessary. Use any of the following stimulus words and/or others you select from the story. You say the sound (e.g., a voiceless /p/ sound) and the student is to say a word from the story that begins with that sound. Use any group of 10 stimulus items you select per teaching set.*

Stimulus items:

/p/: pails, part, peasant, peeled, pepper, perhaps, pieces, pillowcases, pity, place, pot, potatoes, put

/b/: back, bad, barley, barn, barrels, be, bed, beds, been, before, believe, beneath, better, big, boil, borrow, bowl, bread, bring, brought, built, busy, but, buzzed

/t/: tables, tasted, taught, tired, to, tossed, town, townspeople, traveled, tucked, turned, two

/d/: danced, decided, dined, disappeared, distance, don't, door, down, dozen, drank, dropped

/k/: called, came, can, can't, carrots, closets, comfortable, cooking, could, crisp, crusts, cut, king, quickly

/g/: gathered, get, glad, good, goodbye, great

/ch/: chased, chunks

/dz/: (as 1st sound in jelly): just

/m/: made, make, marching, may, mayor, meat, might, milk, mill, miller, minutes, missing, much, must

/n/: knew, knocked, know, never, next, nice, nicely, no, none, not, nothing, now

/s/: celery, cellars, cider, said, salt, same, sat, satisfied, saw, saying, second, seen, sense, served, set, several, simply, since, sleep, slice, small, smells, smooth, sniffed, sniffing, so, soldier, some, someone, something, soon, soup, spare, square, stale, stalks, still, stirred, stone, strangers, stuffed, such

/f/: faraway, farmer, faster, few, filled, finally, find, finding, fire, first, fit, flavor, food, for, found, from

/v/: vegetables, very, village, villagers

/h/: had, half, happy, hardly, has, have, he, heard, hid, hidden, hiding, his, home, hoping, house, houses, how, hung, hungry, hurried

/r/: ran, ready, really, returned, rich, right, road, roasts

/l/: lacking, land, large, last, let, little, loaf, loaves, long, looked, lowered, lucky

/w/, /wh/: once, one, waited, walked, want, war, warm, was, water, we, welcomed, wells, went, were, what, when, which, whispered, who, wife, will, with, women, would

/sh/: share, she, shook, should

/voiceless th/: thick, thicken, thin, third, thought, thank

/voiced th/: the, their, them, themselves, then, there, they, this

/y/ (as 1st sound in yellow): yes, you

vowels: a, about, added, after, again, ago, agreed, all, alone, already, also, always, an, and, armful, arrived, as, asked, asking, at, away, each, eat, entire, even, ever, everyone, everything, except, excitement, extra, I, idea, if, imagine, important, in, inside, into, is, it, it's, of, off, on, onions, or, orange, overhead, out, under, us

12. Blending sounds in monosyllabic words divided into onset-rime beginning with two consonant cluster + rime.

What to say to the student: "Now we'll put sounds together to make words."
EXAMPLE: "Put these sounds together to make a word (/ / + / /)." (stimulus sounds) "What's the word?" (e.g., "gl + ad: What's the word?") (glad)

> **NOTE:** *Give letter sound not letter name. Use pictured items and/or manipulatives if necessary. Use any of the following stimulus words and/or others you select from the story. Correct answers are in parentheses.*

Stimulus items:

st + uft (stuffed)

pl + ace (place)

cr + isp (crisp)

st + ale (stale)

kw + ick (quick)

st + ocks (stalks)

sh + air (share)

th + ick (thick)

cr + ust (crust)

th + ank (thank)

13. Blending sounds in monosyllabic words divided into onset-rime beginning with single consonant + rime.

What to say to the student: "Let's put sounds together to make words."
EXAMPLE: "Put these sounds together to make a word (/ / + / /)." (stimulus sounds) "What's the word?" (e.g., "/b/ + arn: what's the word?") (barn)

> **NOTE:** *Give letter sound not letter name. Use pictured items and/or manipulatives if necessary. Use any of the following stimulus words and/or others you select from the story. Correct answers are in parentheses.*

Stimulus items:

/s/ + oup (soup)
/t/ + own (town)
/m/ + ilk (milk)
/b/ + oil (boil)
/s/ + ense (sense)
/r/ + itch (rich)
/p/ + ails (pails)
/k/ + ing (king)
/n/ + oise (noise)
/m/ + eat (meat)

14. Blending sounds to form a monosyllabic word beginning with a continuant sound.

What to say to the student: "We'll put sounds together to make words."
EXAMPLE: "Put these sounds together to make a word (/ / + / / + / /)." (stimulus sounds) (e.g., "/m/ /short I/ /l/.") (mill)

> *NOTE: Give letter sound not letter name. Use pictured items and/or manipulatives if necessary. Use any of the following stimulus words and/or others you select from the story. Correct answers are in parentheses.*

Stimulus items:

/w/ /long I/ /f/ (wife)
/m/ /long E/ /t/ (meat)
/s/ /l/ /long I/ /s/ (slice)
/r/ /long O/ /d/ (road)
/s/ /oo/ /p/ (soup)
/f/ /short I/ /l/ /d/ (filled)
/l/ /long O/ /v/ /z/ (loaves)
/sh/ /long A/ /r/ (share)
/f/ /long I/ /n/ /d/ (find)
/m/ /long A/ /d/ (made)

15. Blending sounds to form a monosyllabic word beginning with a noncontinuant sound.

What to say to the student: "We'll put sounds together to make words."
EXAMPLE: "Put these sounds together to make a word (/ / + / / + / /)." (stimulus sounds) (e.g., "/k/ /r/ /short I/ /s/ /p/.") (crisp)

> *NOTE: Give letter sound not letter name. Use pictured items and/or manipulatives if necessary. Use any of the following stimulus words and/or others you select from the story. Correct answers are in parentheses.*

Stimulus items:

/c/ /short U/ /t/ (cut)

/p/ /ah/ /t/ (pot)

/t/ /short U/ /k/ /t/ (tucked)

/ch/ /short U/ /ng/ /k/ (chunk)

/g/ /l/ /short A/ /d/ (glad)

/b/ /long O/ /l/ (bowl)

/g/ /r/ /long A/ /t/ (great)

/b/ /short I/ /l/ /t/ (built)

/p/ /long A/ /l/ /z/ (pails)

/p/ /l/ /long A/ /s/ (place)

16. Substituting initial sound in words.

What to say to the student: "We're going to change beginning/first sounds in words." ***EXAMPLE:*** "Say '_____.'" (stimulus word) "Instead of / /" (stimulus sound) "say / /." (stimulus sound) (e.g., Say 'town.' Instead of /t/ say /d/. What's your new word?") (down)

> ***NOTE:*** *Give letter sound not letter name. Use pictured items and/or manipulatives if necessary. Use any of the following stimulus words and/or others you select from the story. Correct answers are in parentheses.*

Stimulus items:

"Say barn. Instead of /b/ say /y/." (yarn)

"Say meat. Instead of /m/ say /n/." (neat)

"Say carrots. Instead of /k/ say /p/." (parrots)

"Say heard. Instead of /h/ say /b/." (bird)

"Say house. Instead of /h/ say /m/." (mouse)

"Say shook. Instead of /sh/ say /l/." (look)

"Say bread. Instead of /b/ say /t/." (tread)

"Say wife. Instead of /w/ say /l/." (life)

"Say thought. Instead of /th/ say /b/." (bought)

"Say better. Instead of /b/ say /l/." (letter)

17. Substituting final sound in words.

What to say to the student: "We're going to change ending/last sounds in words." ***EXAMPLE:*** "Say '_____.'" (stimulus word) "Instead of / /" (stimulus sound) "say / /." (stimulus sound) (e.g., "Say 'built.' Instead of /t/ say /d/. What's your new word?") (build)

NOTE: Give letter sound not letter name. Use pictured items and/or manipulatives if necessary. Use any of the following stimulus words and/or others you select from the story. Correct answers are in parentheses.

Stimulus items:

"Say barn. Instead of /n/ say /k/." (bark)

"Say loaf. Instead of /f/ say /d/." (load)

"Say thick. Instead of /k/ say /n/." (thin)

"Say dined. Instead of /d/ say /z/." (dines)

"Say should. Instead of /d/ say /k/." (shook)

"Say great. Instead of /t/ say /d/." (grade)

"Say meat. Instead of /t/ say /k/." (meek)

"Say fire. Instead of /r/ say /n/." (fine)

"Say dropped. Instead of /t/ say /s/." (drops)

"Say bowl. Instead of /l/ say /t/." (boat)

18. Segmenting middle sound in monosyllabic words.

What to say to the student: "Tell me the middle sound in the word I say."
EXAMPLE: "What's the middle sound in the word '_____'?" (stimulus word (e.g., "What's the middle sound in the word 'bed'?") (/short E/)

NOTE: Give letter sound not letter name. Use pictured items and/or manipulatives if necessary. Use any of the following stimulus words and/or others you select from the story. Correct answers are in parentheses.

Stimulus items:

half (/short A/)

pot (/ah/)

none (/short U/)

hid (/short I/)

taught (/ah/)

chase (/long A/)

soup (/oo/)

road (/long O/)

home (/long O/)

wife (/long I/)

19. Substituting middle sound in words.

What to say to the student: "We're going to change the middle sound in words."
EXAMPLE: "Say '_____.'" (stimulus word) "Instead of / /" (stimulus sound) "say / /." (stimulus sound) (e.g., "Say 'soup.' Instead of /oo/ say /short I/. What's your new word?") (sip)

> ***NOTE:*** *Give letter sound not letter name. Use pictured items and/or manipulatives if necessary. Use any of the following stimulus words and/or others you select from the story. Correct answers are in parentheses.*

Stimulus items:

"Say loaf. Instead of /long O/ say /long E/." (leaf)

"Say small. Instead of /ah/ say /short E/." (smell)

"Say road. Instead of /long O/ say /long I/."(ride)

"Say mill. Instead of /short I/ say /ah/." (mall)

"Say pot. Instead of /ah/ say /short I/." (pit)

"Say boil. Instead of /oi/ say /ah/." (ball)

"Say nice. Instead of /long I/ say /long E/." (niece)

"Say said. Instead of /short E/ say /short A/." (sad)

"Say hid. Instead of /short I/ say /short A/." (had)

"Say made. Instead of /long A/, say /oo/." (mood)

20. Identifying all sounds in monosyllabic words.

What to say to the student: "Now tell me all the sounds you hear in the word I say."
EXAMPLE: "What sounds do you hear in the word '_____'?" (stimulus word) (e.g., "What sounds do you hear in the word 'let'?") (/l/ /short E/ /t/)

> ***NOTE:*** *Give letter sound not letter name. Use pictured items and/or manipulatives if necessary. Use any of the following stimulus words and/or others you select from the story. Correct answers are in parentheses.*

Stimulus items:

bread (/b/ /r/ /short E/ /d/)

house (/h/ /ow/ /s/)

crisp (/k/ /r/ /short I/ /s/ /p/)

third (/voiceless th/ /r/ /d/)

stone (/s/ /t/ /long O/ /n/)

don't (/d/ /long O/ /n/ /t/)

great (/g/ /r/ /long A/ /t/)

crusts (/k/ /r/ /short U/ /s/ /t/ /s/)

milk (/m/ /short I/ /l/ /k/)

sense (/s/ /short E/ /n/ /s/)

21. Deleting sounds within words.

What to say to the student: "We're going to leave out sounds in words."
EXAMPLE: "Say '_____'" (stimulus word) "without / /." (stimulus sound) (e.g., "Say 'quick' without /w/.") (kick) "The word that was left, 'kick,' is a real word. Sometimes the word won't be a real word."

> ***NOTE:*** *Give letter sound not letter name. Use pictured items and/or manipulatives if necessary. Use any of the following stimulus words and/or others you select from the story. Correct answers are in parentheses.*

Stimulus items:

"Say stale without /t/." (sale)

"Say bread without /r/." (bed)

"Say place without /l/." (pace)

"Say great without /r/." (gate)

"Say flavor without /l/." (favor)

"Say bring without /r/." (bing)

"Say stalks without /t/." (socks)

"Say sleep without /l/." (seep)

"Say brought without /r/." (bought)

"Say smells without /m/." (sells)

22. Substituting consonant in words having a two-sound cluster.

What to say to the student: "We're going to change sounds in words."

EXAMPLE: "Say '_____.'" (stimulus word) "Instead of / /" (stimulus sound) "say / /. (stimulus sound) (e.g., "Say 'spare.' Instead of /p/ say /k/.") (scare). Say "Sometimes the new word will be a made-up word."

> *NOTE: Give letter sound not letter name. Use pictured items and/or manipulatives if necessary. Use any of the following stimulus words and/or others you select from the story. Correct answers are in parentheses.*

Stimulus items:

"Say stale. Instead of /t/ say /k/." (scale)

"Say quick. Instead of /w/ say /l/." (click)

"Say bread. Instead of /r/ say /l/." (bled)

"Say small. Instead of /m/ say /t/." (stall)

"Say spare. Instead of /p/ say /t/."(stare)

"Say smells. Instead of /m/ say /p/." (spells)

"Say stones. Instead of /t/ say /k/." (scones)

"Say stir. Instead of /t/ say /p/." (spur)

"Say stuffed. Instead of /t/ say /n/" (snuffed)

"Say snow. Instead of /n/ say /t/." (stow)

23. Phoneme reversing.

What to say to the student: "We're going to say words backward."

EXAMPLE: "Say the word '_____'" (stimulus word) "backward." (e.g., "If we say 'meat' backward, the word is 'team.'")

> *NOTE: This is a difficult phoneme-level task and should only be done with older students. Give letter sound not letter name. Use pictured items and/or manipulatives if necessary. Use any of the following stimulus words and/or others you select from the story. Correct answers are in parentheses.*

Stimulus items:

pot	(top)	bowl	(lobe)
door	(road)	cut	(tuck)
make	(came)	time	(might)
right	(tire)	back	(cab)
let	(tell)	bed	(Deb)

24. Phoneme switching.

What to say to the student: "We're going to switch the first sounds in two words."
EXAMPLE: "Switch the first sounds in '_____' and '_____.'" (stimulus words) (e.g., "Switch the first sounds in 'no sense.'") (so nence)

> *NOTE: This is a difficult phoneme-level task and should only be done with older students. Give letter sound not letter name. Use pictured items and/or manipulatives if necessary. Use any of the following stimulus words and/or others you select from the story. Correct answers are in parentheses.*

Stimulus items:

good soup	(sood goup)
long tables	(tong labels)
town miller	(mown tiller)
very tired	(terry vired)
cooking pot	(pooking cot)
delicious food	(felicious dude)
two carrots	(coo tarrots)
big chunks	(chig bunks)
busy hiding	(hizzy biding)
thick rich	(rick thich)

25. Pig latin.

What to say to the student: "We're going to talk in a secret language using words from the story. In pig latin, you take off the first sound of a word, put it at the end of the word, and add a long A sound."
EXAMPLE: "Say tossed in pig latin." (ossedtay)

NOTE: *This is a difficult phoneme-level task and should only be done with older students. Use pictured items and/or manipulatives if necessary. Use any of the following stimulus words and/or others you select from the story. Correct answers are in parentheses.*

Stimulus items:

town	(owntay)
cider	(idersay)
dozen	(uzenday)
peasants	(easantspay)
barley	(arleybay)
carrots	(airutskay)
pepper	(epperpay)
milk	(ilkmay)
soup	(oupsay)
potatoes	(otatoespay)

CHAPTER

PHONOLOGICAL AWARENESS ACTIVITIES TO USE WITH *THE HUNGRY THING*

Text version used for selection of stimulus items:
Slepian, J., & Seidler, A. (1967). *The hungry thing*. New York, NY: Scholastic, Inc.

PHONOLOGICAL AWARENESS ACTIVITIES AT THE WORD LEVEL

1. Counting words.

What to say to the student: "We're going to count words."

EXAMPLE: "How many words do you hear in this sentence (or phrase)? 'his neck.'" (2)

NOTE: Use pictured items and/or manipulatives if necessary. Use any of the following stimulus phrases or sentences and/or others you select from the story. Correct answers are in parentheses.

Stimulus items:

sounds like (2)

feed me (2)

ate them all (3)

in far lands (3)

came to town (3)

stand on your head (4)

ate them all up (4)

he'd like some tea (4)

how do you eat them? (5)

trade off the box tops (5)

2. Identifying missing word from list.

What to say to the student: "Listen to the words I say. I'll say them again. You tell me which word I leave out."

EXAMPLE: "Listen to the words I say: 'crusts, king, box.' I'll say them again. Tell me which one I leave out: 'crusts, box.'" (king)

> *NOTE: Use pictured items and/or manipulatives if necessary. Use any of the following stimulus words and/or others you select from the story. Correct answers are in parentheses.*

Stimulus set #1	Stimulus set #2
sweet, dish	sweet (dish)
blue, rice	rice (blue)
feet, ice, baby	ice, baby (feet)
hiccup, shoe, tail	hiccup, tail (shoe)
bread, dogs, mouth	bread, mouth (dogs)
curly, three, jello	curly, three (jello)
chicken, party, tree, cracker	chicken, party, tree (cracker)
town, grows, soup, nice	town, grows, nice (soup)
lady, cook, sign, thank	cook, sign, thank (lady)
giggle, box, cousins, laundry	giggle, box, cousins (laundry)

3. Identifying missing word in phrase or sentence.

What to say to the student: "Listen to the sentence I read. Tell me which word is missing the second time I read the sentence."

EXAMPLE: "'Have some noodles.' Listen again and tell me which word I leave out. 'Have____ noodles.'" (some)

NOTE: Use pictured items and/or manipulatives if necessary. Use any of the following stimulus sentences and/or others you select from the story. Correct answers are in parentheses.

Stimulus items:

Tastes sweet. Tastes_____. (sweet)

His sign. ____ sign. (His)

Cried the townspeople. Cried the______. (townspeople)

In big letters. In ____ letters. (big)

Wiped his mouth. _____ his mouth. (Wiped)

Ate them all up. Ate them _____ up. (all)

Soup with a cracker. Soup with a _____. (cracker)

He turned around three times. He_____ around three times. (turned)

Trade off the box tops. Trade off the ____ tops. (box)

They gave him some jello. They _____ him some jello. (gave)

3. Supplying missing word as adult reads.

What to say to the student: "I want you to help me read the story. You fill in the words I leave out."

EXAMPLE: "Pointed to his sign that said 'feed ____.'" (me)

NOTE: Use pictured items and/or manipulatives if necessary. Use any of the following stimulus sentences and/or others you select from the story. Correct answers are in parentheses.

Stimulus items:

You're all very _____. (silly)

They dine in bare _____. (feet)

The Hungry Thing _____ his head. (shook)

What would you like to _____? (eat)

A special spaghetti to eat holding _____. (hands)

You _____ and laugh with ten in your tummy. (giggle)

The boy _____to the wiseman. (whispered)

Sounds like _____ to me. (pancakes, pickles, meatloaf, lollipops, or cookies)

He turned his sign _____ . (around)

Tickles you know, are curly tailed _____dogs. (hot)

5. Rearranging words.

What to say to the student: "I'll say some words out of order. You put them in the right order so they make sense."

EXAMPLE: "'me feed.' Put those words in the right order." (feed me)

> ***NOTE:*** *Use pictured items and/or manipulatives if necessary. Use any of the following stimulus words and/or others you select from the story. Correct answers are in parentheses. This word-level activity can be more difficult than some of the syllable- or phoneme-level activities because of the memory load. If your students are only able to deal with two or three words to be rearranged, add more two- and three-word samples from the story and omit the four-word level until a later time.*

Stimulus items:

you thank (thank you)

again come (come again)

Thing Hungry (Hungry Thing)

very simple all (all very simple)

how you them eat do? (how do you eat them?)

line laundry of (line of laundry)

head his shook (shook his head)

sign his around turned (turned his sign around)

your on stand head (stand on your head)

all ate up them (ate them all up)

PHONOLOGICAL AWARENESS ACTIVITIES AT THE SYLLABLE LEVEL

1. Syllable counting.

What to say to the student: "We're going to count syllables (or parts) of words."
EXAMPLE: "How many syllables do you hear in '_____'?" (stimulus word) (e.g., "How many syllables in 'tail'?") (1)

> *NOTE: Use pictured items and/or manipulatives if necessary. Use any of the of the following stimulus words and/or others you select from the story. Use any group of 10 stimulus items you select per teaching set.*

Stimulus items:

One-syllable words: plain, please, bare, be, big, bit, blue, boop, box, boy, bread, buy, tail, taste, tea, ten, time, too, tops, town, trade, tree, tried, true, try, turned, do, dear, dogs, dressed, dine, dish, came, can, clear, come, cook, course, cried, king, kings, gave, give, got, grows, guest, just, man, me, meant, men, might, more, mouth, know, known, neck, new, nice, said, sat, say, see, seems, serve, sign, some, sound, sounds, soup, stand, sweet, rain, read, red, rice, row, falls, far, feed, feet, fish, for, from, full, hands, hat, have, he, head, hear, his, hot, how, lands, laugh, left, like, line, look, looked, one, way, we, what, when, why, wiped, with, would, shaped, shoe, shook, thing, think, three, through, thread, thought, thank, that, the, them, then, there, they, you, your, a, and, ate, eat, ice, if, in, is, it, of, of, on, ought, up

Two-syllable words: pancakes, party, patted, pickles, pointed, pudding, baby, beetloaf, better, tickles, tummy, dozens, classmates, coated, cookies, cousins, covered, cracker, curly, quicker, gathered, goodbyes, chicken, children, jello, meatloaf, morning, noodles, sickles, silly, simple, smacker, smello, smiled, special, sucking, fancakes, feetloaf, fellow, foodles, hiccup, holding, hookies, hungry, lady, laundry, letters, little, lookies, wanted, wiseman, shmancakes, sugar, yummy, again, answered, around, eaten, excuse

Three-syllable words: cereal, politely, banana, townspeople, dollipops, gollipops, spaghetti, fanana, lollipops, anything, underfed

2. Initial syllable deleting.

What to say to the student: "We're going to leave out syllables (or parts of words)."
EXAMPLE: "Say '_____.'" (stimulus word). "Say it again without '_____.'" (stimulus syllable) (e.g., "Say 'anything' without 'any.'") (thing)

NOTE: Use pictured items and/or manipulatives if necessary. Use any of the following stimulus words and/or others you select from the story. Correct answers are in parentheses.

Stimulus items:

"Say wiseman without wise." (man)

"Say meatloaf without meat." (loaf)

"Say schmancakes without schman." (cakes)

"Say goodbyes without good." (byes)

"Say classmates without class." (mates)

"Say hiccup without hick." (up)

"Say party without par-." (tee)

"Say jello without jell." (oh)

"Say townspeople without town." (people)

"Say baby without bay." (be)

3. Final syllable deleting.

What to say to the student: "We're going to leave out syllables (or parts of words)." *EXAMPLE:* "Say '_____.'" (stimulus word) "Say it again without '_____.'" (stimulus syllable) (e.g., "Say 'goodbyes' without 'byes.'") (good)

NOTE: Use pictured items and/or manipulatives if necessary. Use any of the following stimulus words and/or others you select from the story. Correct answers are in parentheses.

Stimulus items:

"Say morning without -ing." (morn)

"Say dollipops without pops." (dolly)

"Say feetloaf without loaf." (feet)

"Say laundry without -dree." (lawn)

"Say fancakes without cakes." (fan)

"Say cousins without -ins." (cuz)

"Say cracker without -er." (crack)

"Say underfed without fed." (under)

"Say wiseman without man." (wise)

"Say cookies without -eez." (cook)

4. Initial syllable adding.

What to say to the student: "Now let's add syllables (or parts) to words."
EXAMPLE: " Add '_____'" (stimulus syllable) "to the beginning of '_____.'" (stimulus syllable) (e.g., "Add 'chilled' to the beginning of 'ren.'") (children)

> ***NOTE:*** *Use pictured items and/or manipulatives if necessary. Use any of the following stimulus words and/or others you select from the story. Correct answers are in parentheses.*

Stimulus items:

"Add meat to the beginning of loaf." (meatloaf)

"Add schman to the beginning of cakes." (schmancakes)

"Add smack to the beginning of -ers." (smackers)

"Add hook to the beginning of ease." (hookies)

"Add bay to the beginning of bee." (baby)

"Add gol- to the beginning of ipops." (gollipops)

"Add ker- to the beginning of lee." (curly)

"Add hick to the beginning of up." (hiccup)

"Add food to the beginning of -uls." (foodles)

"Add lay to the beginning of -deez." (ladies)

5. Final syllable adding.

What to say to the student: "Now let's add syllables (or parts) to words."
EXAMPLE: "Add '_____'" (stimulus syllable) "to the end of '_____.'" (stimulus syllable) (e.g., "Add '-er' to the end of 'quick.'") (quicker)

> ***NOTE:*** *Use pictured items and/or manipulatives if necessary. Use any of the following stimulus words and/or others you select from the story. Correct answers are in parentheses.*

Stimulus items:

"Add pops to the end of lolly." (lollipops)

"Add cake to the end of pan." (pancake)

"Add -ree to the end of hung." (hungry)

"Add thing to the end of any." (anything)

"Add fed to the end of under." (underfed)

"Add mates to the end of class." (classmates)

"Add loaf to the end of beet." (beetloaf)

"Add ease to the end of cook." (cookies)

"Add byes to the end of good." (goodbyes)

"Add -ite to the end of pole." (polite)

6. Syllable substituting.

What to say to the student: "Let's make up some new words."

EXAMPLE: "Say '_____.'" (stimulus word) "Instead of '_____'" (stimulus syllable) "say '_____.'" (stimulus syllable) (e.g., "Say 'schmancakes.' Instead of 'schman' say 'pan.' The new word is 'pancakes.'")

> ***NOTE:*** *Use pictured items and/or manipulatives if necessary. Use any of the following stimulus words and/or others you select from the story. Correct answers are in parentheses.*

Stimulus items:

"Say pancake. Instead of cake say full." (panful)

"Say meatloaf. Instead of loaf say less." (meatless)

"Say yummy. Instead of yum say tum." (tummy)

"Say anything. Instead of thing say one." (anyone)

"Say wiseman. Instead of man say boy." (wise boy)

"Say hiccup. Instead of hick say back." (backup)

"Say quicker. Instead of -er say lee." (quickly)

"Say noodles. Instead of nood say food." (foodles)

"Say townspeople. Instead of town say nice." (nice people)

"Say cookies. Instead of -eez say -ing." (cooking)

PHONOLOGICAL AWARENESS ACTIVITIES AT THE PHONEME LEVEL

1. Counting sounds.

What to say to the student: "We're going to count sounds in words."
EXAMPLE: "How many sounds do you hear in this word? 'can.'" (3)

> ***NOTE:*** *Use pictured items and/or manipulatives if necessary. Use any of the following stimulus words and/or others you select from the story. Be sure to give the letter sound and not the letter name. Use any group of 10 stimulus items you select per teaching set.*

Stimulus words with two sounds: be, boy, buy, tea, to, do, me, know, say, see, row, he, how, way, we, why, shoe, the, they, you, all, ate, eat, ice, if, in, is, it, of, off, on, ought, up

Stimulus words with three sounds: bare, big, bit, blue, boop, tail, ten, time, town, toys, tree, true, try, dear, dine, dish, came, can, come, cook, gave, man, men, might, more, mouth, known, neck, nice, said, sat, serve, sign, some, soup, rain, read, red, rice, far, feed, feet, fish, for, full, hat, have, head, hear, his, hot, laugh, like, line, look, one, what, when, while, with, would, shook, three, through, thought, that, them, then, there, your, eaten, its

Stimulus words with four sounds: plain, please, baby, better, box, bread, busy, tailed, taste, times, tops, trade, tried, tummy, turned, dogs, clear, course, cried, curly, giggle, grows, guest, chicken, jello, just, meant, seems, silly, sound, sweet, falls, fellow, from, lady, left, little, looked, wiped, shaped, sugar, think, thread, thank, yummy, again, asked

Stimulus words with five sounds: party, pickles, tastes, tickles, dressed, coated, cookies, cracker, quicker, gathered, noodles, cereal, sickles, simple, smacker, smello, smiled, sounds, special, stand, foodles, hiccup, hookies, lands, letters, lookies, around

2. Sound categorization or identifying rhyme oddity.

What to say to the student: "Guess which word I say does not rhyme with the other three words."

EXAMPLE: "Tell me which word does not rhyme with the other three. '_____, _____, _____, _____.'" (stimulus words) (e.g., "blue, shoe, new, silly. Which word doesn't rhyme?") (silly)

> *NOTE: Use pictured items if necessary. Use any of the following stimulus words and/or others you select from the story. Correct answers are in parentheses.*

Stimulus items:

fish, dish, like, wish (like)

eat, cried, sweet, feet (cried)

sickles, pickles, tickles, serve (serve)

jello, smello, tastes, fellow (tastes)

head, dine, red, said (dine)

look, cook, box, shook (box)

gollipops, lollipops, wiseman, dollipops (wiseman)

dear, dogs, clear, hear (dogs)

laugh, blue, you, shoe (laugh)

ice, nice, dine, rice (dine)

3. Matching rhyme.

What to say to the student: "We're going to think of rhyming words."

EXAMPLE: "Which word rhymes with '_____'?" (stimulus word) (e.g., "Which word rhymes with 'tickles'? 'toys, yummy, sugar, pickles.'") (pickles)

> *NOTE: Use pictured items if necessary. Use any of the following stimulus words and/or others you select from the story. Correct answers are in parentheses.*

Stimulus items:

eat: hat, stand, feet, soup (feet)

neck: lady, mouth, times, check (check)

cracker: your, smacker, laugh, course (smacker)

bread: thread, pointed, sweet, hiccup (thread)

hookies: hands, cookies, fancakes, guest (cookies)

hat: bit, kind, sat, plain (sat)

sign: come, box, silly, dine (dine)

nice: new, dogs, rice, cereal (rice)

cried: tried, thought, town, shook (tried)

fish: serve, feed, dish, clear (dish)

4. Producing rhyme.

What to say to the student: "Now we'll say rhyming words."
EXAMPLE: "Tell me a word that rhymes with '_____.'" (stimulus word) (e.g., "Tell me a word that rhymes with 'boy.' You can make up a word if you want.") (toy)

> ***NOTE:*** *Use pictured items if necessary. Use any of the following stimulus words and/or others you select from the story (i.e., you say a word from the list below and the student is to think of a rhyming word). Use any group of 10 stimulus items you select per teaching set.*

Stimulus items:

/p/: pancakes, party, patted, pickles, plain, please, pointed, politely, pudding

/b/: baby, banana, bare, be, beetloaf, better, big, bit, blue, boop, box, boy, bread, busy, by

/t/: tail, tailed, taste, tea, ten, tickles, time, to, tops, town, toys, trade, tree, true, try, tummy, turned

/d/: do, dear, dogs, dressed, dine, dish, dozens, dollipops

/k/: came, can, clear, coated, come, cook, cookies, course, cousins, cracker, cried, curly, kind, quicker

/g/: gathered, gave, giggle, give, gollipops, goodbyes, got, grows, guest

/ch/: chicken, children

/dz/: (as 1st sound in jelly): jello, just

/m/: man, me, meant, meatloaf, men, might, more, morning, mouth

/n/: know, known, neck, new, nice, noodles

/s/: cereal, said, sat, say, see, serve, seems, sickles, sign, silly, simple, smacker, smello, smiled, some, sound, soup, spaghetti, special, stand, sucking, sweet

/f/: falls, fanana, fancakes, far, feed, feetloaf, feet, fellow, fish, foodles, for, from, full

/v/: very

/h/: hands, hat, have, he, head, hear, hiccup, his, holding, hookies, hot, how, hungry

/r/: rain, read, red, rice, row

/l/: lady, lands, laugh, left, letters, like, line, little, lollipops, look, looked, lookies

/w/, /wh/: one, wanted, way, we, what, when, while, whispered, why, wiped, with, would

/sh/: shaped, shmancakes, shoe, shook, sugar

/voiceless th/: thank, thing, think, three, through, thread, thought

/voiced th/: that, the, them, then, there, they

/y/ (as 1st sound in yellow): you, your, yummy

vowels: again, all, anything, are, around, asked, ate, eat, eaten, ice, if, in, is, it, of, off, on, ought, up

5. Sound matching (initial).

What to say to the student: "Now we'll listen for the first sound in words."
EXAMPLE: "Listen to this sound: / /." (stimulus sound). "Guess which word I say begins with that sound '_____, _____, _____, _____.'" (stimulus words) (e.g., "Listen to this sound /l/. Guess which word I say begins with that sound: 'one, laugh, ten, plain.'") (laugh)

> ***NOTE:*** *Give letter sound not letter name. Use pictured items if necessary. Use any of the following stimulus words and/or others you select from the story. Correct answers are in parentheses.*

Stimulus items:

/p/: busy, red, party, simple (party)

/l/: three, laundry, town, please (laundry)

/ch/: sound, jello, curly, chicken (chicken)

/k/: kings, giggle, dogs, mouth (kings)

/s/: coated, silly, fellow, blue (silly)

/sh/: foodles, special, sugar, busy (sugar)

/d/: guest, tails, dozens, excuse (dozens)

/f/: very, fanana, neck, big (fanana)

/m/: dressed, red, nice, might (might)

/b/: bread, whispered, like, head (bread)

6. Sound matching (final).

What to say to the student: "Now we'll listen for the last sound in words."
EXAMPLE: "Listen to this sound / /." (stimulus sound). "Guess which word I say ends with that sound '_____, _____, _____, _____.'" (stimulus words) (e.g., "Listen to this sound /m/. Guess which word I say ends with that sound: feet, time, soup, taste.") (time)

> ***NOTE:*** *Give letter sound not letter name. Use pictured items if necessary. Use any of the following stimulus words and/or others you select from the story. Correct answers are in parentheses.*

Stimulus items:

/d/: boy, guest, trade, men (trade)

/s/: pudding, lollipops, hungry, tummy (lollipops)

/k/: coated, better, shook, time (shook)

/t/: kind, soup, rice, ate (ate)

/v/: serve, toys, cried, laundry (serve)

/g/: tea, yummy, big, ice (big)

/p/: chicken, patted, smiled, boop (boop)

/n/: children, thank, some, cook (children)

/r/: shaped, eaten, quicker, bread (quicker)

/z/: like, noodles, little, box (noodles)

7. Identifying initial sound in words.

What to say to the student: "I'll say a word two times. Tell me what sound is missing the second time. '______, _______.'" (stimulus words)

EXAMPLE: "What sound do you hear in '_____'" (stimulus word) "that is missing in '_____'?" (stimulus word) (e.g., "What sound do you hear in 'red,' that is missing in 'Ed'?") (/r/)

> *NOTE: Give letter sound not letter name. Use pictured items and/or manipulatives if necessary. Use any of the following stimulus words and/or others you select from the story. Correct answers are in parentheses.*

Stimulus items:

"plain, lane. What sound do you hear in plain that is missing in lane?" (/p/)

"tail, ale. What sound do you hear in tail that is missing in ale?" (/t/)

"shmancakes, mancakes. What sound do you hear in shmancakes that is missing in mancakes?" (/sh/)

"dear, ear. What sound do you hear in dear that is missing in ear?" (/d/)

"sweet, wheat. What sound do you hear in sweet that is missing in wheat?" (/s/)

"rice, ice. What sound do you hear in rice that is missing in ice?" (/r/)

"thread, red. What sound do you hear in thread that is missing in red?" (/voiceless th/)

"falls, alls. What sound do you hear in falls that is missing in alls?" (/f/)

"grows, rows. What sound do you hear in grows that is missing in rows?" (/g/)

"bit, it. What sound do you hear in bit that is missing in it?" (/b/)

8. Identifying final sound in words.

What to say to the student: "I'll say a word two times. Tell me what sound is missing the second time. '_______, _______.'" (stimulus words)

EXAMPLE: "What sound do you hear in '_____'" (stimulus word) "that is missing in '_____'?" (stimulus word) (e.g., "What sound do you hear in 'tops' that is missing in 'top'?") (/s/)

> *NOTE: Give letter sound not letter name. Use pictured items and/or manipulatives if necessary. Use any of the following stimulus words and/or others you select from the story. Correct answers are in parentheses.*

Stimulus items:

"eaten, eat. What sound do you hear in eaten that is missing in eat?" (/n/)

"fellow, fell. What sound do you hear in fellow that is missing in fell?" (/long O/)

"silly, sill. What sound do you hear in silly that is missing in sill?" (/long E/)

"course, core. What sound do you hear in course that is missing in core?" (/s/)

"thought, thaw. What sound do you hear in thought that is missing in thaw?" (/t/)

"meant, men. What sound do you hear in meant that is missing in men?" (/t/)

"baby, babe. What sound do you hear in baby that is missing in babe?" (/long E/)

"dressed, dress. What sound do you hear in dressed that is missing in dress?" (/t/)

"time, tie. What sound do you hear in time that is missing in tie?" (/m/)

"cried, cry. What sound do you hear in cried that is missing in cry?" (/d/)

9. Segmenting initial sound in words.

What to say to the student: "Listen to the word I say and tell me the first sound you hear."

EXAMPLE: "What's the first sound in '_____'?" (stimulus word) (e.g., "What's the first sound in 'hungry'?") (/h/)

> ***NOTE:*** *Give letter sound not letter name. Use pictured items and/or manipulatives if necessary. Use any of the following stimulus words and/or others you select from the story. Use any group of 10 stimulus items you select per teaching set.*

Stimulus items:

/p/: pancakes, party, patted, pickles, plain, please, pointed, politely, pudding

/b/: baby, banana, bare, be, beetloaf, better, big, bit, blue, boop, box, boy, bread, busy, by

/t/: tail, tailed, taste, tea, ten, tickles, time, to, tops, town, townspeople, toys, trade, tree, true, try, tummy, turned

/d/: do, dear, dogs, dressed, dine, dish, dozens, dollipops

/k/: came, can, classmates, clear, coated, come, cook, cookies, course, cousins, cracker, cried, curly, kind, quicker

/g/: gathered, gave, giggle, give, gollipops, goodbyes, got, grows, guest

/ch/: chicken, children

/dz/: (as 1st sound in jelly): jello, just

/m/: man, me, meant, meatloaf, men, might, more, morning, mouth

/n/: know, known, neck, new, nice, noodles

/s/: cereal, said, sat, say, see, serve, seems, sickles, sign, silly, simple, smacker, smello, smiled, some, sound, soup, spaghetti, special, stand, sucking, sweet

/f/: falls, fanana, fancakes, far, feed, feetloaf, feet, fellow, fish, foodles, for, from, full

/v/: very

/h/: hands, hat, have, he, head, hear, hiccup, his, holding, hookies, hot, how, hungry

/r/: rain, read, red, rice, row

/l/: lady, lands, laugh, laundry, left, letters, like, line, little, lollipops, look, looked, lookies

/w/, /wh/: one, wanted, way, we, what, when, while, whispered, why, wiped, wiseman, with, would

/sh/: shaped, shmancakes, shoe, shook, sugar

/voiceless th/: thank, thing, think, three, through, thread, thought

/voiced th/: that, the, them, then, there, they

/y/ (as 1st sound in yellow): you, your, yummy

vowels: again, all, answered, anything, are, around, asked, ate, eat, eaten, excuse, ice, if, in, is, it, of, off, on, ought, underfed, up

10. Segmenting final sound in words.

What to say to the student: "Listen to the word I say and tell me the last sound you hear."

EXAMPLE: "What's the last sound in the word '_____'?" (stimulus word) (e.g., "What's the last sound in the word 'smacker'?") (/r/)

> ***NOTE:*** *Give letter sound not letter name. Use pictured items and/or manipulatives if necessary. Use any of the following stimulus words and/or others you select from the story. Use any group of 10 stimulus items you select per teaching set.*

Stimulus items:

/p/: boop, hiccup, soup, up

/t/: asked, ate, bit, dressed, eat, feet, got, guest, hat, hot, it, just, left, looked, meant, might, ought, sat, shaped, sweet, taste, that, thought, what, wiped

/d/: answered, around, bread, coated, covered, cried, feed, gathered, head, kind, patted, pointed, read, red, said, smiled, sound, stand, tailed, thread, tried, turned, underfed, whispered, would

/k/: cook, like, look, neck, shook, thank, think

/g/: big

/m/: came, come, from, some, them, time

/n/: again, can, chicken, children, dine, eaten, in, known, line, man, men, on, one, plain, rain, sign, ten, then, town, when, wiseman

/ng/: anything, holding, morning, pudding, sucking, thing

/s/: box, classmates, course, dollipops, excuse, fancakes, gollipops, ice, lollipops, nice, pancakes, rice, shmancakes, tastes, tops

/z/: cookies, cousins, dogs, dozens, falls, foodles, grows, hands, his, hookies, is, kings, lands, letters, lookies, noodles, pickles, please, seems, sickles, sounds, tickles, times, toys

/f/: beetloaf, feetloaf, if, laugh, meatloaf, off

/v/: gave, give, have, of, serve

/r/: are, bare, better, clear, cracker, dear, far, for, hear, more, quicker, smacker, sugar, there, your

/l/: all cereal, full, giggle, little, simple, special, tail, townspeople, while

/sh/: dish, fish

/voiceless th/: mouth, with

/long A/: say, they, way

/long E/: baby, be, busy, curly, hungry, lady, laundry, me, party, politely, see, silly, spaghetti, tea, three, tree, tummy, very, yummy

/long I/: buy, try, why

/long O/: grow, jello, know, row, smello

/oo/: clue, do, shoe, through, true, you

/ow/: how

11. Generating words from the story beginning with a particular sound.

What to say to the student: "Let's think of words **from the story** that start with certain sounds."

EXAMPLE: "Tell me a word **from the story** that starts with / /." (stimulus sound (e.g., "the sound /p/") (pointed)

> *NOTE: Give letter sound not letter name. Use pictured items if necessary. Use any of the following stimulus words and/or others you select from the story. You say the sound (e.g., a voiceless /p/ sound), and the student is to say a word from the story that begins with that sound. Use any group of 10 stimulus items you select per teaching set.*

Stimulus items:

/p/: pancakes, party, patted, pickles, plain, please, pointed, politely, pudding

/b/: baby, banana, bare, be, beetloaf, better, big, bit, blue, boop, box, boy, bread, busy, by

/t/: tail, tailed, taste, tea, ten, tickles, time, to, tops, town, townspeople, toys, trade, tree, true, try, tummy, turned

/d/: do, dear, dogs, dressed, dine, dish, dozens, dollipops

/k/: came, can, classmates, clear, coated, come, cook, cookies, course, cousins, cracker, cried, curly, kind, quicker

/g/: gathered, gave, giggle, give, gollipops, goodbyes, got, grows, guest

/ch/: chicken, children

/dz/: (as 1st sound in jelly): jello, just

/m/: man, me, meant, meatloaf, men, might, more, morning, mouth

/n/: know, known, neck, new, nice, noodles

/s/: cereal, said, sat, say, see, serve, seems, sickles, sign, silly, simple, smacker, smello, smiled, some, sound, soup, spaghetti, special, stand, sucking, sweet

/f/: falls, fanana, fancakes, far, feed, feetloaf, feet, fellow, fish, foodles, for, from, full

/v/: very

/h/: hands, hat, have, he, head, hear, hiccup, his, holding, hookies, hot, how, hungry

/r/: rain, read, red, rice, row

/l/: lady, lands, laugh, laundry, left, letters, like, line, little, lollipops, look, looked, lookies

/w/, /wh/: one, wanted, way, we, what, when, while, whispered, why, wiped, wiseman, with, would

/sh/: shaped, shmancakes, shoe, shook, sugar

/voiceless th/: thank, thing, think, three, through, thread, thought

/voiced th/: that, the, them, then, there, they

/y/ (as 1st sound in yellow): you, your, yummy

vowels: again, all, answered, anything, are, around, asked, ate, eat, eaten, excuse, ice, if, in, is, it, of, off, on, ought, underfed, up

12. Blending sounds in monosyllabic words divided into onset-rime beginning with two consonant cluster + rime.

What to say to the student: "Now we'll put sounds together to make words."
EXAMPLE: "Put these sounds together to make a word (/ / + / /)." (stimulus sounds) "What's the word?"(e.g., "st + and: What's the word?") (stand)

> ***NOTE:*** *Give letter sound not letter name. Use pictured items and/or manipulatives if necessary. Use any of the following stimulus words and/or others you select from the story. Correct answers are in parentheses.*

Stimulus items:

bl + ue (blue)	cl + ear (clear)
sw + eet (sweet)	cr + ied (cried)
th + ank (thank)	tr + ade (trade)
cr + ack crack)	pl + um (plum)
dr + ess (dress)	br + ead (bread)

13. Blending sounds in monosyllabic words divided into onset-rime beginning with single consonant + rime.

What to say to the student: "Let's put sounds together to make words."
EXAMPLE: "Put these sounds together to make a word (/ / + / /)." (stimulus sounds) "What's the word?" (e.g., "/d/ + ish: what's the word?") (dish)

> ***NOTE:*** *Give letter sound not letter name. Use pictured items and/or manipulatives if necessary. Use any of the following stimulus words and/or others you select from the story. Correct answers are in parentheses.*

Stimulus items:

/t/ + ail (tail)
/h/ + ought (hot)
/g/ + -est (guest)
/m/ + outh (mouth)
/b/ + air (bare)
/s/ + ign (sign)
/n/ + ice (nice)
/b/ + ox (box)
/s/ + oup (soup)
/t/ + aste (taste)

14. Blending sounds to form a monosyllabic word beginning with a continuant sound.

What to say to the student: "We'll put sounds together to make words."
EXAMPLE: "Put these sounds together to make a word (/ / + / / + / /)." (stimulus sounds) (e.g., "/f/ /a/ /l/ /z/.") (falls)

> ***NOTE:*** *Give letter sound not letter name. Use pictured items and/or manipulatives if necessary. Use any of the following stimulus words and/or others you select from the story. Correct answers are in parentheses.*

Stimulus items:

/n/ /long I/ /s/ (nice)
/s/ /oo/ /p/ (soup)
/l/ /short A/ /f/ (laugh)
/m/ /short E/ /n/ /t/ (meant)
/f/ /short I/ /sh/ (fish)
/voiceless th/ /r/ /long E/ (three)
/sh/ /long A/ /p/ /t/ (shaped)
/s/ /w/ /long E/ /t/ (sweet)
/m/ /long I/ /t/ (might)
/r/ /long E/ /d/ (read)

15. Blending sounds to form a monosyllabic word beginning with a noncontinuant sound.

What to say to the student: "We'll put sounds together to make words."
EXAMPLE: "Put these sounds together to make a word (/ / + / / + / /)." (stimulus sounds) (e.g., "/d/ /ah/ /g/ /z/.") (dogs)

> ***NOTE:*** *Give letter sound not letter name. Use pictured items and/or manipulatives if necessary. Use any of the following stimulus words and/or others you select from the story. Correct answers are in parentheses.*

Stimulus items:

/k/ /long I/ /n/ /d/ (kind)

/k/ /short A/ /n/ (can)

/t/ /ah/ /p/ /s/ (tops)

/p/ /l/ /long E/ /z/ (please)

/k/ /r/ /long I/ /d/ (cried)

/t/ /r/ /long A/ /d/ (trade)

/b/ /short I/ /g/ (big)

/g/ /r/ /long O/ /z/ (grows)

/d/ /short I/ /sh/ (dish)

/p/ /l/ /long A/ /n/ (plain)

16. Substituting initial sound in words.

What to say to the student: "We're going to change beginning/first sounds in words." *EXAMPLE:* "Say '_____.'" (stimulus word) "Instead of / /" (stimulus sound) "say / /." (stimulus sound) (e.g., Say 'boy.' Instead of /b/ say /t/. What's your new word?") (toy)

> *NOTE: Give letter sound not letter name. Use pictured items and/or manipulatives if necessary. Use any of the following stimulus words and/or others you select from the story. Correct answers are in parentheses.*

Stimulus items:

"Say dish. Instead of /d/ say /w/." (wish)

"Say meatloaf. Instead of /m/ say /b/." (beetloaf)

"Say banana. Instead of /b/ say /f/." (fanana)

"Say hat. Instead of /h/ say /p/." (pat)

"Say gollipops. Instead of /g/ say /d/." (dollipops)

"Say thread. Instead of /voiceless th/ say /b/." (bread)

"Say tickles. Instead of /t/ say /p/." (pickles)

"Say dine. Instead of /d/ say /l/." (line)

"Say man. Instead of /m/ say /f/." (fan)

"Say noodles. Instead of /n/ say /f/." (foodles)

17. Substituting final sound in words.

What to say to the student: "We're going to change ending/last sounds in words." *EXAMPLE:* "Say '_____.'" (stimulus word) "Instead of / /" (stimulus sound) "say / /." (stimulus sound) (e.g., "Say 'might.' Instead of /t/ say /n/. What's your new word?") (mine)

NOTE: Give letter sound not letter name. Use pictured items and/or manipulatives if necessary. Use any of the following stimulus words and/or others you select from the story. Correct answers are in parentheses.

Stimulus items:

"Say tail. Instead of /l/ say /k/." (take)

"Say off. Instead of /f/ say /n/." (on)

"Say dine. Instead of /n/ say /m/."(dime)

"Say while. Instead of /l/ say /p/." (wipe)

"Say smacker. Instead of /r/, say /s/." (smacks)

"Say like. Instead of /k/ say /t/." (light)

"Say some. Instead of /m/ say /n/." (sun)

"Say tea. Instead of /long E/ say /long I/." (tie)

"Say smello. Instead of /long O/ say /z/." (smells)

"Say plain. Instead of /n/ say /t/." (plate)

18. Segmenting middle sound in monosyllabic words.

What to say to the student: "Tell me the middle sound in the word I say."
EXAMPLE: "What's the middle sound in the word '_____'?" (stimulus word) (e.g., "What's the middle sound in the word 'dine'?") (/long I/)

NOTE: Give letter sound not letter name. Use pictured items and/or manipulatives if necessary. Use any of the following stimulus words and/or others you select from the story. Correct answers are in parentheses.

Stimulus items:

laugh (/short A/)

time (/long I/)

read (/long E/)

ten (/short E/)

boop (/oo/)

tree (/r/)

some (/short U/)

gave (/long A/)

fish (/short I/)

blue (/l/)

19. Substituting middle sound in words.

What to say to the student: "We're going to change the middle sound in words."
EXAMPLE: "Say '_____.'" (stimulus word) "Instead of / /" (stimulus sound) "say / /." (stimulus sound) (e.g., "Say 'rice.' Instead of /long I/ say /long A/. What's your new word?") (race)

> *NOTE: Give letter sound not letter name. Use pictured items and/or manipulatives if necessary. Use any of the following stimulus words and/or others you select from the story. Correct answers are in parentheses.*

Stimulus items:

"Say rain. Instead of /long A/ say /short A/." (ran)

"Say boop. Instead of /oo/ say /ah/." (bop)

"Say mouth. Instead of /ow/ say /short A/."(math)

"Say tail. Instead of /long A/ say /ah/." (tall)

"Say men. Instead of /short E/ say /short A/." (man)

"Say sign. Instead of /long I/ say /long E/." (seen)

"Say feet. Instead of /long E/ say /short I/." (fit)

"Say loaf. Instead of /long O/ say /long E/." (leaf)

"Say feed. Instead of /long E/ say /short E/." (fed)

"Say bread. Instead of /short E/ say /short A/." (brad)

20. Identifying all sounds in monosyllabic words.

What to say to the student: "Now tell me all the sounds you hear in the word I say."
EXAMPLE: "What sounds do you hear in the word '_____'?" (stimulus word) (e.g., "What sounds do you hear in the word 'sat'?") (/s/ /short A/ /t/)

> *NOTE: Give letter sound not letter name. Use pictured items and/or manipulatives if necessary. Use any of the following stimulus words and/or others you select from the story. Correct answers are in parentheses.*

Stimulus items:

blue (/b/ /l/ /oo/)

time (/t/ /long I/ /m/)

like (/l/ /long I/ /k/)

head (/h/ /short E/ /d/)

dish (/d/ /short I/ /sh/)

taste (/t/ /long A/ /s/ /t/)

soup (/s/ /oo/ /p/)

feet (/f/ /long E/ /t/)

neck (/n/ /short E/ /k/)

laugh (/l/ /short A/ /f/)

21. Deleting sounds within words.

What to say to the student: "We're going to leave out sounds in words."
EXAMPLE: "Say '_____'" (stimulus word) "without / /." (stimulus sound) (e.g., "Say 'tried' without /r/.") (tied) "The word that was left, 'tied,' is a real word. Sometimes the word won't be a real word."

> ***NOTE:*** *Give letter sound not letter name. Use pictured items and/or manipulatives if necessary. Use any of the following stimulus words and/or others you select from the story. Correct answers are in parentheses.*

Stimulus items:

"Say plain without /l/." (pain)

"Say stand without /t/." (sand)

"Say sweet without /w/." (seat)

"Say bread without /r/." (bed)

"Say tree without /r/." (tea)

"Say lands without /n/." (lads)

"Say please without /l/." (peas)

"Say grow without /r/." (go)

"Say true without /r/." (to)

"Say blue without /l/." (boo)

22. Substituting consonant in words having a two-sound cluster.

What to say to the student: "We're going to substitute sounds in words."
EXAMPLE: "Say '_____.'" (stimulus word) "Instead of / /" (stimulus sound) "say / /." (stimulus sound) (e.g., "Say 'smack.' Instead of /m/ say /l/.") (slack) Say "Sometimes the new word will be a made up word."

> *NOTE: Give letter sound not letter name. Use pictured items and/or manipulatives if necessary. Use any of the following stimulus words and/or others you select from the story. Correct answers are in parentheses.*

Stimulus items:

"Say sweet. Instead of /w/ say /l/." (sleet)

"Say cried. Instead of /r/ say /l/." (Clyde)

"Say bread. Instead of /r/ say /l/." (bled)

"Say blue. Instead of /l/ say /r/." (brew)

"Say schmancakes. Instead of /m/ say /r/."(shrancakes)

"Say crack. Instead of /r/ say /l/." (clack)

"Say smack. Instead of /m/ say /t/." (stack)

"Say grows. Instead of /r/ say /l/." (glows)

"Say stand. Instead of /t/ say /p/" (spanned)

"Say smello. Instead of /m/ say /t/." (stello)

23. Phoneme reversing.

What to say to the student: "We're going to say words backward."
EXAMPLE: "Say the word '_____'" (stimulus word) "backward." (e.g., "If we say 'came' backward, the word is 'make.'")

> *NOTE: This is a difficult phoneme-level task and should only be done with older students. Give letter sound not letter name. Use pictured items and/or manipulatives if necessary. Use any of the following stimulus words and/or others you select from the story. Correct answers are in parentheses.*

Stimulus items:

tail	(late)	line	(nile)
some	(muss)	ten	(net)
time	(might)	tea	(eat)
can	(knack)	gave	(vague)
more	(roam)	sign	(nice)

24. Phoneme switching.

What to say to the student: "We're going to switch the first sounds in two words."
EXAMPLE: "Switch the first sounds in '_____' and '_____.'" (stimulus words) (e.g., "Switch the first sounds in 'curly tail.'") (turly cail)

> ***NOTE:*** *This is a difficult phoneme-level task and should only be done with older students. Give letter sound not letter name. Use pictured items and/or manipulatives if necessary. Use any of the following stimulus words and/or others you select from the story. Correct answers are in parentheses.*

Stimulus items:

Hungry Thing	(Thungry Hing)
feed me	(meed fee)
little boy	(bittle loy)
sounds like	(lounds sike)
very silly	(sery villy)
big letters	(lig betters)
cook's hat	(hook's cat)
bare feet	(fare beet)
sat down	(dat sown)
thank you	(yank thoo)

25. Pig latin.

What to say to the student: "We're going to talk in a secret language using words from the story. In pig latin, you take off the first sound of a word, put it at the end of the word, and add a long A sound."

EXAMPLE: "Say mouth in pig latin." (outhmay)

NOTE: This is a difficult phoneme-level task and should only be done with older students. Use pictured items and/or manipulatives if necessary. Use any of the following stimulus words and/or others you select from the story. Correct answers are in parentheses.

Stimulus items:

shoe	(oushay)
toys	(oystay)
banana	(ananabay)
party	(artypay)
soup	(oupsay)
tail	(ailtay)
busy	(usybay)
jello	(ellojay)
noodles	(oodlesnay)
lady	(adylay)

CHAPTER

10

PHONOLOGICAL AWARENESS ACTIVITIES TO USE WITH *THE LITTLE RED HEN*

Text version used for selection of stimulus items:
Galdone, P. (1973). *The little red hen*. New York: Clarion Books.

PHONOLOGICAL AWARENESS ACTIVITIES AT THE WORD LEVEL

1. Counting words.

What to say to the student: "We're going to count words."

EXAMPLE: "How many words do you hear in this sentence (or phrase)? 'last crumb.'" (2)

> ***NOTE:*** *Use pictured items and/or manipulatives if necessary. Use any of the following stimulus phrases or sentences and/or others you select from the story. Correct answers are in parentheses.*

Stimulus items:

red hen (2)

back porch (2)

raked the leaves (3)

nap all day (3)

then I will (3)

she cooked the meals (4)

she swept the floor (4)

not I said the mouse (5)

liked to sleep all day (5)

found some grains of wheat (5)

2. Identifying missing word from list.

What to say to the student: "Listen to the words I say. I'll say them again. You tell me which word I leave out."

EXAMPLE: "Listen to the words I say: 'porch, hen, swept.' I'll say them again. Tell me which one I leave out: 'porch, hen.'" (swept)

> ***NOTE:*** *Use pictured items and/or manipulatives if necessary. Use any of the following stimulus words and/or others you select from the story. Correct answers are in parentheses.*

Stimulus set #1	**Stimulus set #2**
bag, mill	bag (mill)
dishes, house	house (dishes)
dog, bowl, warm	bowl, warm (dog)
time, grass, mouse	time, grass (mouse)
milk, crumb, chair	milk, chair (crumb)
nap, leaves, stove, floor	nap, leaves, floor (stove)
flour, little, ripe, plant	flour, ripe, plant (little)
snooze, beds, sticks, eggs	beds, sticks, eggs (snooze)
white, oven, red, time	white, oven, time (red)
grains, washed, shining, three	grains, shining, three (washed)

3. Identifying missing word in phrase or sentence.

What to say to the student: "Listen to the sentence I read. Tell me which word is missing the second time I read the sentence."

EXAMPLE: "'Big bowl.' Listen again and tell me which word I leave out. 'Big____.'" (bowl)

> ***NOTE:*** *Use pictured items and/or manipulatives if necessary. Use any of the following stimulus sentences and/or others you select from the story. Correct answers are in parentheses.*

Stimulus items:

Red hen. Red ____. (hen)

Back porch. ____ porch. (Back)

Cozy little house. Cozy little ____. (house)

Sleep all day. Sleep all ____. (day)

Washed the windows. ____ the windows. (Washed)

A fire in the stove. A fire in the ____. (stove)

She swept the floor. She ____ the floor. (swept)

Bag of fine white flour. Bag of fine white ____. (flour)

The mouse liked to snooze. The ____ liked to snooze. (mouse)

She found some grains of wheat. She found some grains of ____. (wheat)

4. Supplying missing word as adult reads.

What to say to the student: "I want you to help me read the story. You fill in the words I leave out."

EXAMPLE: "Plant the ____." (wheat)

> ***NOTE:*** *Use pictured items and/or manipulatives if necessary. Use any of the following stimulus sentences and/or others you select from the story. Correct answers are in parentheses.*

Stimulus items:

Not _____. (I)

Little Red _____. (hen)

Watered the _____. (wheat)

She swept the _____. (floor)

The cat liked to ____ all day. (sleep)

Three very eager _____. (helpers)

To the very last _____. (crumb)

Washed windows and _____ clothes. (mended)

Found some _____ of wheat. (grains)

A bag of fine white ____. (flour)

5. Rearranging words.

What to say to the student: "I'll say some words out of order. You put them in the right order so they make sense."
EXAMPLE: "'chair warm.' Put those words in the right order." (warm chair)

> *NOTE: Use pictured items and/or manipulatives if necessary. Use any of the following stimulus words and/or others you select from the story. Correct answers are in parentheses. This word-level activity can be more difficult than some of the syllable- or phoneme-level activities because of the memory load. If your students are only able to deal with two or three words to be rearranged, add more two- and three-word samples from the story and omit the four-word level until a later time.*

Stimulus items:

morning each (each morning)

couch soft (soft couch)

hen red little (little red hen)

mouse down jumped (mouse jumped down)

wheat of grains (grains of wheat)

all snooze day (snooze all day)

oven hot was the (the oven was hot)

flour the white fine (the fine white flour)

leaves the raked she (she raked the leaves)

kitchen into the strolled (strolled into the kitchen)

PHONOLOGICAL AWARENESS ACTIVITIES AT THE SYLLABLE LEVEL

1. Syllable counting.

What to say to the student: "We're going to count syllables (or parts) of words."
EXAMPLE: "How many syllables do you hear in '_____'?" (stimulus word) (e.g., "How many syllables in 'porch'?") (1)

NOTE: Use pictured items and/or manipulatives if necessary. Use any of the of the following stimulus words and/or others you select from the story. Use any group of 10 stimulus items you select per teaching set.

Stimulus items:

One-syllable words: pan, plant, porch, poured, pulled, pushed, put, back, bag, be, beds, big, bowl, built, but, by, take, tall, time, to, took, day, did, do, dog, done, down, cake, came, cat, clothes, cooked, couch, cried, crumb, cut, got, grains, grass, ground, grow, chair, jumped, just, made, make, meals, milk, mill, mixed, mouse, mowed, nap, not, now, said, same, sleep, smell, snooze, so, soft, some, soon, sticks, stove, strolled, swept, red, ripe, raked, round, filled, fine, floor, for, found, from, had, hen, his, hoed, hot, house, last, leaves, liked, lived, one, warm, was, washed, weeds, when, wheat, white, work, she, through, three, that, the, them, then, there, this, all, am, and, asked, each, eat, eggs, in, it, of, off, on, out, up

Two-syllable words: planted, batter, began, butter, taking, tended, dishes, cozy, kitchen, garden, gathered, going, mended, morning, myself, scampered, sunny, returned, flour, helpers, hoeing, housework, little, very, watered, windows, shining, sugar, after, eager, into, oven, upon

Three-syllable words: beautiful, together, delicious, carrying, whenever

2. Initial syllable deleting.

What to say to the student: "We're going to leave out syllables (or parts of words)."
EXAMPLE: "Say '_____.'" (stimulus word) "Say it again without '_____.'" (stimulus syllable) (e.g., "Say 'mended' without 'men.'") (did)

NOTE: Use pictured items and/or manipulatives if necessary. Use any of the following stimulus words and/or others you select from the story. Correct answers are in parentheses.

Stimulus items:

"Say myself without my." (self)

"Say garden without gar." (den)

"Say windows without win." (doze)

"Say into without in." (to)

"Say whenever without when." (ever)

"Say housework without house." (work)

"Say returned without re." (turned)

"Say together without to." (gether)

"Say kitchen without kit." (chen)

"Say began without be." (gan)

3. Final syllable deleting.

What to say to the student: "We're going to leave out syllables (or parts of words)."
EXAMPLE: "Say '_____.'" (stimulus word) "Say it again without '_____.'" (stimulus syllable) (e.g., "Say 'into' without 'to.'") (in)

> ***NOTE:*** *Use pictured items and/or manipulatives if necessary. Use any of the following stimulus words and/or others you select from the story. Correct answers are in parentheses.*

Stimulus items:

"Say fireside without side." (fire)

"Say shining without -ing." (shine)

"Say myself without self." (my)

"Say hoeing without -ing." (hoe)

"Say housework without work." (house)

"Say scampered without purred." (scam)

"Say morning without -ing." (morn)

"Say began without -gan." (be)

"Say windows without doze." (win)

"Say returned without turned." (re)

4. Initial syllable adding.

What to say to the student: "Now let's add syllables (or parts) to words."
EXAMPLE: " Add '_____'" (stimulus syllable) "to the beginning of '_____.'" (stimulus syllable) (e.g., "Add 'help' to the beginning of 'erz.'") (helpers)

> ***NOTE:*** *Use pictured items and/or manipulatives if necessary. Use any of the following stimulus words and/or others you select from the story. Correct answers are in parentheses.*

Stimulus items:

"Add my to the beginning of self." (myself)

"Add be to the beginning of -gan." (began)

"Add re- to the beginning of turned." (returned)

"Add when to the beginning of ever." (whenever)

"Add morn to the beginning of -ing." (morning)

"Add in to the beginning of to." (into)

"Add house to the beginning of work." (housework)

"Add dee- to the beginning of –licious." (delicious)

"Add win to the beginning of doze." (windows)

"Add batt to the beginning of -er." (batter)

5. Final syllable adding.

What to say to the student: "Now let's add syllables (or parts) to words."
EXAMPLE: "Add '_____'" (stimulus syllable) "to the end of '_____.'" (stimulus syllable) (e.g., "Add 'side' to the end of 'fire.'") (fireside)

> ***NOTE:*** *Use pictured items and/or manipulatives if necessary. Use any of the following stimulus words and/or others you select from the story. Correct answers are in parentheses.*

Stimulus items:

"Add -ful to the end of beauti-." (beautiful)

"Add -ing to the end of morn." (morning)

"Add on to the end of up." (upon)

"Add den the end of gar." (garden)

"Add -ing to the end of take." (taking)

"Add self to the end of my." (myself)

"Add purred to the end of scam." (scampered)

"Add turned to the end of re-." (returned)

"Add work to the end of house." (housework)

"Add -gan to the end of be." (began)

6. Syllable substituting.

What to say to the student: "Let's make up some new words."
EXAMPLE: "Say '_____.'" (stimulus word) "Instead of '_____'" (stimulus syllable) "say '_____.'" (stimulus syllable) (e.g., "Say 'into.' Instead of 'to' say 'stead.' The new word is 'instead.')

> ***NOTE:*** *Use pictured items and/or manipulatives if necessary. Use any of the following stimulus words and/or others you select from the story. Correct answers are in parentheses.*

Stimulus items:

"Say return. Instead of turn say play." (replay)

"Say housework. Instead of house say home." (homework)

"Say fireside. Instead of side say place." (fireplace)

"Say began. Instead of -gan say for." (before)

"Say myself. Instead of my say her." (herself)

"Say whenever. Instead of when say for." (forever)

"Say windows. Instead of doze say -ter." (winter)

"Say cozy. Instead of co- say cray." (crazy)

"Say mended. Instead of men say ten." (tended)

"Say morning. Instead of morn say shined." (shining)

PHONOLOGICAL AWARENESS ACTIVITIES AT THE PHONEME LEVEL

1. Counting sounds.

What to say to the student: "We're going to count sounds in words."
EXAMPLE: "How many sounds do you hear in this word? 'tail.'" (3)

> ***NOTE:*** *Use pictured items and/or manipulatives if necessary. Use any of the following stimulus words and/or others you select from the story. Be sure to give the letter sound and not the letter name. Use any group of 10 stimulus items you select per teaching set.*

Stimulus words with two sounds: be, by, to, day, do, now, so, who, she, the, all, am, each, eat, in, it, of, off, on, out, up

Stimulus words with three sounds: pan, put, back, bag, big, bowl, but, take, tall, time, took, did, dog, done, down, cake, came, cat, couch, cut, got, grow, chair, made, make, mill, mouse, mowed, nap, not, said, same, some, soon, fine, fire, for, had, hen, his, hoed, hot, house, red, ripe, one, was, when, wheat, white, will, work, through, three, that, them, then, there, this, and, eager, eggs, oven

Stimulus words with four sounds: porch, poured, pulled, pushed, batter, beds, built, butter, clothes, cooked, cozy, cried, crumb, grass, just, meals, milk, sleep, small, smell, snooze, soft, stove, sunny, very, filled, floor, flour, found, from, raked, round, last, leaves, liked, little, lived, warm, washed, weeds, sugar, after, asked, into, upon

Stimulus words with five sounds: plant, began, gathered, grains, ground, jumped, swept, watered

2. Sound categorization or identifying rhyme oddity.

What to say to the student: "Guess which word I say does not rhyme with the other three words."

EXAMPLE: "Tell me which word does not rhyme with the other three. '_____, _____, _____, _____.'" (stimulus words) (e.g., "hot, got, not, did. Which word doesn't rhyme?") (did)

> ***NOTE:*** *Use pictured items if necessary. Use any of the following stimulus words and/or others you select from the story. Correct answers are in parentheses.*

Stimulus items:

when, sticks, hen, then (sticks)

bag, cake, take, make (bag)

come, crumb, one, from (one)

small, tall, all, fire (fire)

red, said, soft, head (soft)

mill, day, will, still (day)

cried, that, cat, mat (cried)

came, soon, same, shame (soon)

time, wheat, feet, meet (time)

ground, round, found, plant (plant)

3. Matching rhyme.

What to say to the student: "We're going to think of rhyming words."

EXAMPLE: "Which word rhymes with '_____'?" (stimulus word) (e.g., "Which word rhymes with 'found'? 'nap, cried, eat, round.'") (round)

> ***NOTE:*** *Use pictured items if necessary. Use any of the following stimulus words and/or others you select from the story. Correct answers are in parentheses.*

Stimulus items:

house: mouse, jumped, last, plant (mouse)

soft: liked, fine, loft, big (loft)

tended: raked, mended, filled, floor (mended)

cake: cat, work, porch, make (make)

seeds: weeds, swept, meals, grass (weeds)

crumb: pan, bowl, from, hen (from)

sunny: funny, cried, garden, time (funny)

snooze: sugar, will, choose, raked (choose)

sleep: white, deep, ripe, ground (deep)

eat: couch, mixed, dog, wheat (wheat)

4. Producing rhyme.

What to say to the student: "Now we'll say rhyming words."

EXAMPLE: "Tell me a word that rhymes with '_____.'" (stimulus word) (e.g., "Tell me a word that rhymes with 'mouse.' You can make up a word if you want.") (house)

> ***NOTE:*** *Use pictured items if necessary. Use any of the following stimulus words and/or others you select from the story (i.e., you say a word from the list below and the student is to think of a rhyming word.) Use any group of 10 stimulus items you select per teaching set.*

Stimulus items:

/p/: pan, plant, planted, porch, poured, pulled, pushed, put

/b/: back, bag, batter, be, beautiful, beds, began, big, bowl, but, butter, by

/t/: take, taking, tall, tended, time, to, together, took

/d/: day, delicious, did, dishes, do, dog, done, down

/k/: cake, came, carrying, cat, clothes, cooked, couch, cozy, cried, crumb, cut, kitchen

/g/: garden, gathered, going, grains, grass, ground, grow

/ch/: chair

/dz/: (as 1st sound in jelly): jumped, just

/m/: made, make, meals, mended, milk, mill, mixed, morning, mouse, mowed, myself

/n/: nap, not, now

/s/: said, same, scampered, sleep, small, smell, snooze, so, soft, some, soon, sticks, stove, strolled, sunny, swept

/f/: filled, fine, fire, fireside, floor, flour, for, found, from

/v/: very

/h/: had, helpers, hen, his, hoed, hoeing, hot, house, housework, who

/r/: red, returned, ripe, raked, round

/l/: last, leaves, liked, little, lived

/w/, /wh/: one, warm, was, washed, watered, weeds, when, wheat, whenever, white, will, windows, work

/sh/: she, shining, sugar

/voiceless th/: through, three

/voiced th/: that, the, them, then, there, this

vowels: after, all, am, and, asked, each, eager, eat, eggs, in, into, it, of, off, on, out, oven, up, upon

5. Sound matching (initial).

What to say to the student: "Now we'll listen for the first sound in words."
EXAMPLE: "Listen to this sound: / /." (stimulus sound). "Guess which word I say begins with that sound. '_____, _____, _____, _____.'" (stimulus words) (e.g., "Listen to this sound /b/. Guess which word I say begins with that sound: 'pushed, bowl, mixed, house.'") (bowl)

> ***NOTE:*** *Give letter sound not letter name. Use pictured items if necessary. Use any of the following stimulus words and/or others you select from the story. Correct answers are in parentheses.*

Stimulus items:

/g/: cozy, grains, fire, eggs (grains)

/p/: three, little, plant, bag (plant)

/s/: flour, leaves, crumb, snooze (snooze)

/m/: nap, couch, mouse, grow (mouse)

/ch/: sugar, meals, chair, jumped (chair)

/d/: beds, dog, porch, white (dog)

/f/: oven, ripe, cake, flour (flour)

/sh/: shining, just, built, last, stove (shining)

/k/: garden, kitchen, small, eager (kitchen)

/t/: tended, raked, filled, hoed (tended)

6. Sound matching (final).

What to say to the student: "Now we'll listen for the last sound in words."

EXAMPLE: "Listen to this sound: / /" (stimulus sound). "Guess which word I say ends with that sound '_____, _____, _____, _____.'" (stimulus words) (e.g., "Listen to this sound /p/. Guess which word I say ends with that sound: 'soft, crumb, ripe, meals.'") (ripe)

> *NOTE:* *Give letter sound not letter name. Use pictured items if necessary. Use any of the following stimulus words and/or others you select from the story. Correct answers are in parentheses.*

Stimulus items:

/z/: pan, smell, eggs, grass (eggs)

/n/: time, made, three, hen (hen)

/m/: crumb, cozy, poured, couch (crumb)

/g/: cake, sleep, swept, bag (bag)

/v/: each, myself, stove, sugar (stove)

/r/: day, beds, found, flour (flour)

/ch/: leaves, porch, mouse, warm (porch)

/d/: snooze, mill, ground, plant (ground)

/k/: milk, big, weeds, down (milk)

/s/: lived, sticks, upon, batter (sticks)

7. Identifying initial sound in words.

What to say to the student: "I'll say a word two times. Tell me what sound is missing the second time. '______, _______.'" (stimulus words)

EXAMPLE: "What sound do you hear in '_____'" (stimulus word) "that is missing in '_____'?" (stimulus word) (e.g., "What sound do you hear in 'time,' that is missing in 'I'm'?") (/t/)

> *NOTE: Give letter sound not letter name. Use pictured items and/or manipulatives if necessary. Use any of the following stimulus words and/or others you select from the story. Correct answers are in parentheses.*

Stimulus items:

"cried, ride. What sound do you hear in cried that is missing in ride?" (/k/)

"small, mall. What sound do you hear in small that is missing in mall?" (/s/)

"grains, rains. What sound do you hear in grains that is missing in rains?" (/g/)

"sticks, ticks. What sound do you hear in sticks that is missing in ticks?" (/s/)

"grow, row. What sound do you hear in grow that is missing in row?" (/g/)

"swept, wept. What sound do you hear in swept that is missing in wept?" (/s/)

"ground, round. What sound do you hear in ground that is missing in round" (/g/)

"sleep, leap. What sound do you hear in sleep that is missing in leap?" (/s/)

"tall, all. What sound do you hear in tall that is missing in all?" (/t/)

"hoeing, owing. What sound do you hear in hoeing that is missing in owing?" (/h/)

8. Identifying final sound in words.

What to say to the student: "I'll say a word two times. Tell me what sound is missing the second time. '______, _______.'" (stimulus words)

EXAMPLE: "What sound do you hear in '_____'" (stimulus word) "that is missing in '_____'?" (stimulus word) (e.g., "What sound do you hear in 'cried' that is missing in 'cry'?") (/d/)

> *NOTE: Give letter sound not letter name. Use pictured items and/or manipulatives if necessary. Use any of the following stimulus words and/or others you select from the story. Correct answers are in parentheses.*

Stimulus items:

"plant, plan. What sound do you hear in plant that is missing in plan?" (/t/)

"ripe, rye. What sound do you hear in ripe that is missing in rye?" (/p/)

"sunny, sun. What sound do you hear in sunny that is missing in sun?" (/long E/)

"house, how. What sound do you hear in house that is missing in how?" (/s/)

"little, lit. What sound do you hear in little that is missing in lit?" (/l/)

"white, why. What sound do you hear in white that is missing in why?" (/t/)

"eggs, egg. What sound do you hear in eggs that is missing in egg?" (/z/)

"time, tie. What sound do you hear in time that is missing in tie?" (/m/)

"built, bill. What sound do you hear in built that is missing in bill?" (/t/)

"poured, pour. What sound do you hear in poured that is missing in pour?" (/d/)

9. Segmenting initial sound in words.

What to say to the student: "Listen to the word I say and tell me the first sound you hear."

EXAMPLE: "What's the first sound in '_____'?" (stimulus word) (e.g., "What's the first sound in 'strolled'?") (/s/)

> ***NOTE:*** *Give letter sound not letter name. Use pictured items and/or manipulatives if necessary. Use any of the following stimulus words and/or others you select from the story. Use any group of 10 stimulus items you select per teaching set.*

Stimulus items:

/p/: pan, plant, planted, porch, poured, pulled, pushed, put

/b/: back, bag, batter, be, beautiful, beds, began, big, bowl, but, butter, by

/t/: take, taking, tall, tended, time, to, together, took

/d/: day, delicious, did, dishes, do, dog, done, down

/k/: cake, came, carrying, cat, clothes, cooked, couch, cozy, cried, crumb, cut, kitchen

/g/: garden, gathered, going, grains, grass, ground, grow

/ch/: chair

/dz/: (as 1st sound in jelly): jumped, just

/m/: made, make, meals, mended, milk, mill, mixed, morning, mouse, mowed, myself

/n/: nap, not, now

/s/: said, same, scampered, sleep, small, smell, snooze, so, soft, some, soon, sticks, stove, strolled, sunny, swept

/f/: filled, fine, fire, fireside, floor, flour, for, found, from

/v/: very

/h/: had, helpers, hen, his, hoed, hoeing, hot, house, housework, who

/r/: red, returned, ripe, raked, round

/l/: last, leaves, liked, little, lived

/w/, /wh/: one, warm, was, washed, watered, weeds, when, wheat, whenever, white, will, windows, work

/sh/: she, shining, sugar

/voiceless th/: through, three

/voiced th/: that, the, them, then, there, this

vowels: after, all, am, and, asked, each, eager, eat, eggs, in, into, it, of, off, on, out, oven, up, upon

10. Segmenting final sound in words.

What to say to the student: "Listen to the word I say and tell me the last sound you hear."

EXAMPLE: "What's the last sound in the word '_____'?" (stimulus word) (e.g., "What's the last sound in the word 'stove'?") (/v/)

NOTE: *Give letter sound not letter name. Use pictured items and/or manipulatives if necessary. Use any of the following stimulus words and/or others you select from the story. Use any group of 10 stimulus items you select per teaching set.*

Stimulus items:

/p/: nap, ripe, sleep, up

/t/: asked, built, but, cat, cooked, cut, eat, got, it, jumped, just, last, not, out, plant, pushed, put, raked, soft, that, washed, wheat, white

/d/: and, cried, did, filled, fireside, found, gathered, ground, had, hoed, liked, lived, made, mended, mixed, mowed, planted, poured, pulled, red, returned, round, said, scampered, strolled, tended, watered

/k/: back, cake, housework, make, milk, take, took, work

/g/: bag, big, dog

/ch/: couch, each, porch

/m/: am, came, crumb, from, same, some, them, time, warm

/n/: began, done, down, fine, garden, hen, in, kitchen, on, one, oven, pan, soon, then, upon, when

/ng/: carrying, going, hoeing, morning, shining, taking

/s/: delicious, grass, house, mouse, sticks, this

/z/: beds, clothes, dishes, eggs, grains, helpers, his, leaves, meals, snooze, was, weeds, windows

/f/: myself, off

/v/: of, stove

/r/: after, batter, butter, chair, eager, fire, floor, flour, for, sugar, there, together, whenever

/l/: all, beautiful, bowl, little, mill, small, smell, tall, will

/voiceless th/: with

/long A/: day

/long E/: be, cozy, she, sunny, three, very

/long I/: by

/long O/: grow, so

/oo/: do, into, through, to, who

/ow/: now

11. Generating words from the story beginning with a particular sound.

What to say to the student: "Let's think of words **from the story** that start with certain sounds."

EXAMPLE: "Tell me a word **from the story** that starts with / /." (stimulus sound) (e.g., "the sound /d/") (dog)

> ***NOTE:*** *Give letter sound not letter name. Use pictured items if necessary. Use any of the following stimulus words and/or others you select from the story. You say the sound (e.g., a voiceless /p/ sound) and the student is to say a word from the story that begins with that sound. Use any group of 10 stimulus items you select per teaching set.*

Stimulus items:

/p/: pan, plant, planted, porch, poured, pulled, pushed, put

/b/: back, bag, batter, be, beautiful, beds, began, big, bowl, but, butter, by

/t/: take, taking, tall, tended, time, to, together, took

/d/: day, delicious, did, dishes, do, dog, done, down

/k/: cake, came, carrying, cat, clothes, cooked, couch, cozy, cried, crumb, cut, kitchen

/g/: garden, gathered, going, grains, grass, ground, grow

/ch/: chair

/dz/: (as 1st sound in jelly): jumped, just

/m/: made, make, meals, mended, milk, mill, mixed, morning, mouse, mowed, myself

/n/: nap, not, now

/s/: said, same, scampered, sleep, small, smell, snooze, so, soft, some, soon, sticks, stove, strolled, sunny, swept

/f/: filled, fine, fire, fireside, floor, flour, for, found, from

/v/: very

/h/: had, helpers, hen, his, hoed, hoeing, hot, house, housework, who

/r/: red, returned, ripe, raked, round

/l/: last, leaves, liked, little, lived

/w/, /wh/: one, warm, was, washed, watered, weeds, when, wheat, whenever, white, will, windows, work

/sh/: she, shining, sugar

/voiceless th/: through, three

/voiced th/: that, the, them, then, there, this

vowels: after, all, am, and, asked, each, eager, eat, eggs, in, into, it, of, off, on, out, oven, up, upon

12. Blending sounds in monosyllabic words divided into onset-rime beginning with two consonant cluster + rime.

What to say to the student: "Now we'll put sounds together to make words."
EXAMPLE: "Put these sounds together to make a word (/ / + / /)." (stimulus sounds) "What's the word?" (e.g., "fl + or: What's the word?") (floor)

NOTE: Give letter sound not letter name. Use pictured items and/or manipulatives if necessary. Use any of the following stimulus words and/or others you select from the story. Correct answers are in parentheses.

Stimulus items:

sm + all (small)
gr + ains (grains)
pl + ant (plant)
st + ove (stove)
sw + ept (swept)
gr + oh (grow)
cr + I'd (cried)
fl + our (flour)
sn + ooze (snooze)
gr + ound (ground)

13. Blending sounds in monosyllabic words divided into onset-rime beginning with single consonant + rime.

What to say to the student: "Let's put sounds together to make words."
EXAMPLE: "Put these sounds together to make a word (/ / + / /)." (stimulus sounds) "What's the word?" (e.g., "/p/ + an: what's the word?") (pan)

NOTE: Give letter sound not letter name. Use pictured items and/or manipulatives if necessary. Use any of the following stimulus words and/or others you select from the story. Correct answers are in parentheses.

Stimulus items:

/k/ + ouch (couch)
/k/ + ake (cake)
/w/ + erk (work)
/f/ + ound (found)
/d/ + og (dog)
/n/ + ap (nap)
/r/ + ipe (ripe)
/b/ + ole (bowl)
/s/ + oft (soft)
/d/ + ay (day)

14. Blending sounds to form a monosyllabic word beginning with a continuant sound.

What to say to the student: "We'll put sounds together to make words."
EXAMPLE: "Put these sounds together to make a word (/ / + / / + / /)." (stimulus sounds) (e.g., "/r/ /long I/ /p/.") (ripe)

NOTE: Give letter sound not letter name. Use pictured items and/or manipulatives if necessary. Use any of the following stimulus words and/or others you select from the story. Correct answers are in parentheses.

Stimulus items:

/s/ /ah/ /f/ /t/ (soft)
/n/ /short A/ /p/ (nap)
/f/ /long I/ /r/ (fire)
/s/ /l/ /long E/ /p/ (sleep)
/m/ /short I/ /l/ /k/ (milk)
/m/ /short I/ /l/ (mill)
/w/ /long I/ /t/ (white)
/s/ /n/ /oo/ /z/ (snooze)
/th/ /r/ /long E/ (three)
/w/ /long E/ /t/ (wheat)

15. Blending sounds to form a monosyllabic word beginning with a noncontinuant sound.

What to say to the student: "We'll put sounds together to make words."
EXAMPLE: "Put these sounds together to make a word (/ / + / / + / /)." (stimulus sounds) (e.g., "/k/ /short A/ /t/.") (cat)

NOTE: Give letter sound not letter name. Use pictured items and/or manipulatives if necessary. Use any of the following stimulus words and/or others you select from the story. Correct answers are in parentheses.

Stimulus items:

/b/ /short A /g/ (bag)
/d/ /short U/ /n/ (done)
/p/ /short A/ /n/ (pan)
/k/ /r/ /short U/ /m/ (crumb)
/g/ /r/ /long O/ (grow)
/d/ /ah/ /g/ (dog)
/b/ /long A/ /k/ (bake)
/g/ /r/ /short A/ /s/ (grass)
/k/ /r/ /long I/ /d/ (cried)
/b/ /short I/ /l/ /t/ (built)

16. Substituting initial sound in words.

What to say to the student: "We're going to change beginning/first sounds in words."
EXAMPLE: "Say '_____.'" (stimulus word) "Instead of / /" (stimulus sound) "say / /." (stimulus sound) (e.g., Say 'take.' Instead of /t/ say /k/. What's your new word?") (cake)

NOTE: Give letter sound not letter name. Use pictured items and/or manipulatives if necessary. Use any of the following stimulus words and/or others you select from the story. Correct answers are in parentheses.

Stimulus items:

"Say chair. Instead of /ch/ say /b/." (bear)

"Say time. Instead of /t/ say /l/." (lime)

"Say mouse. Instead of /m/ say /h/." (house)

"Say weeds. Instead of /w/ say /s/." (seeds)

"Say hen. Instead of /h/ say /t/." (ten)

"Say three. Instead of /voiceless th/ say /f/." (free)

"Say wheat. Instead of /w/ say /sh/." (sheet)

"Say sunny. Instead of /s/ say /f/." (funny)

"Say porch. Instead of /p/ say /t/." (torch)

"Say dishes. Instead of /d/ say /f/." (fishes)

17. Substituting final sound in words.

What to say to the student: "We're going to change ending/last sounds in words." ***EXAMPLE:*** "Say '_____.'" (stimulus word) "Instead of / /" (stimulus sound) "say / /." (stimulus sound) (e.g., "Say 'time.' Instead of /m/ say /p/. What's your new word?") (type)

NOTE: Give letter sound not letter name. Use pictured items and/or manipulatives if necessary. Use any of the following stimulus words and/or others you select from the story. Correct answers are in parentheses.

Stimulus items:

"Say cut. Instead of /t/ say /p/." (cup)

"Say cat. Instead of /t/ say /ch/." (catch)

"Say white. Instead of /t/ say /f/."(wife)

"Say sleep. Instead of /p/ say /t/." (sleet)

"Say eat. Instead of /t/ say /ch/." (each)

"Say back. Instead of /k/ say /t/." (bat)

"Say inside. Instead of /d/ say /t/." (insight)

"Say snooze. Instead of /z/ say /p/." (snoop)

"Say fine. Instead of /n/ say /t/." (fight)

"Say crumb. Instead of /m/ say /sh/." (crush)

18. Segmenting middle sound in monosyllabic words.

What to say to the student: "Tell me the middle sound in the word I say."
EXAMPLE: "What's the middle sound in the word '_____'?" (stimulus word) (e.g., "What's the middle sound in the word 'rake'?") (/long A/)

> *NOTE: Give letter sound not letter name. Use pictured items and/or manipulatives if necessary. Use any of the following stimulus words and/or others you select from the story. Correct answers are in parentheses.*

Stimulus items:

down (/ow/)

meal (/long E/)

dog (/ah/)

mowed (/long O/)

cut (/short U/)

grow (/r/)

fire (/long I/)

wheat (/long E/)

will (/short I/)

ripe (/long I/)

19. Substituting middle sound in words.

What to say to the student: "We're going to change the middle sound in words."
EXAMPLE: "Say '_____.'" (stimulus word) "Instead of / /" (stimulus sound) "say / /." (stimulus sound) (e.g., "Say 'ripe.' Instead of /long I/ say /long O/. What's your new word?") (rope)

> *NOTE: Give letter sound not letter name. Use pictured items and/or manipulatives if necessary. Use any of the following stimulus words and/or others you select from the story. Correct answers are in parentheses.*

Stimulus items:

"Say snooze. Instead of /oo/ say /long E/." (sneeze)

"Say nap. Instead of /short A/ say /short I/." (nip)

"Say mouse. Instead of /ow/ say /long I/" (mice)

"Say sticks. Instead of /short I/ say /short A/." (stacks)

"Say mended. Instead of /short E/ say /long I/." (minded)

"Say butter. Instead of /short U/ say /short A/." (batter)

"Say red. Instead of /short E/ say /ah/." (rod)

"Say pan. Instead of /short A/ say /short U/." (pun)

"Say time. Instead of /long I/ say /long A/." (tame)

"Say crumb. Instead of /short U/ say /short A/." (cram)

20. Identifying all sounds in monosyllabic words.

What to say to the student: "Now tell me all the sounds you hear in the word I say."
EXAMPLE: "What sounds do you hear in the word '_____'?" (stimulus word) (e.g., "What sounds do you hear in the word 'pan'?") (/p/ /short A/ /n/)

> ***NOTE:*** *Give letter sound not letter name. Use pictured items and/or manipulatives if necessary. Use any of the following stimulus words and/or others you select from the story. Correct answers are in parentheses.*

Stimulus items:

beds (/b/ /short E/ /d/ /z/)

time (/t/ /long I/ /m/)

milk (/m/ /short I/ /l/ /k/)

hoed (/h/ /long O/ /d/)

last (/l/ /short A/ /s/ /t/)

couch (/k/ /ow/ /ch/)

stove (/s/ /t/ /long O/ /v/)

crumb (/k/ /r/ /short U/ /m/)

weeds (/w/ /long E/ /d/ /z/)

plant (/p/ /l/ /short A/ /n/ /t/)

21. Deleting sounds within words.

What to say to the student: "We're going to leave out sounds in words."

EXAMPLE: "Say '_____'" (stimulus word) "without / /." (stimulus sound) (e.g., "Say 'grains' without /r/.") (gains) "The word that was left, 'gains,' is a real word. Sometimes the word won't be a real word."

> ***NOTE:*** *Give letter sound not letter name. Use pictured items and/or manipulatives if necessary. Use any of the following stimulus words and/or others you select from the story. Correct answers are in parentheses.*

Stimulus items:

"Say grow without /r/." (go)

"Say sleep without /l/." (seep)

"Say and without /n/." (ad)

"Say grass without /r/." (gas)

"Say floor without /l/." (for)

"Say smell without /m/." (sell)

"Say from without /r/." (fum)

"Say sticks without /t/." (sicks)

"Say plant without /l/." (pant)

"Say mixed without /k/." (missed)

22. Substituting consonant in words having a two-sound cluster.

What to say to the student: "We're going to substitute sounds in words."

EXAMPLE: "Say '_____'" (stimulus word). "Instead of / /" (stimulus sound) "say / /" (stimulus sound) (e.g., "Say 'grow.' Instead of /g/ say /voiceless th/.") (throw). Say: "Sometimes the new word will be a made-up word."

> ***NOTE:*** *Give letter sound not letter name. Use pictured items and/or manipulatives if necessary. Use any of the following stimulus words and/or others you select from the story. Correct answers are in parentheses.*

Stimulus items:

"Say grains. Instead of /g/ say /t/." (trains)

"Say grow. Instead of /r/ say /l/." (glow)

"Say flour. Instead of /f/ say /p/." (plower)
"Say crumb. Instead of /k/ say /f/." (from)
"Say sleep. Instead of /l/ say /t/."(steep)
"Say smell. Instead of /m/ say /p/." (spell)
"Say clothes. Instead of /l/ say /r/." (crows)
"Say swept. Instead of /w/ say /l/." (slept)
"Say grass. Instead of /r/ say /l/" (glass)
"Say small. Instead of /m/ say /t/." (stall)

23. Phoneme reversing.

What to say to the student: "We're going to say words backward."
EXAMPLE: "Say the word '_____'" (stimulus word) "backward." (e.g., "If we say 'back' backward, the word is 'cab.'")

> ***NOTE:*** *This is a difficult phoneme-level task and should only be done with older students. Give letter sound not letter name. Use pictured items and/or manipulatives if necessary. Use any of the following stimulus words and/or others you select from the story. Correct answers are in parentheses.*

Stimulus items:

pan	(nap)	bag	(gab)
cut	(tuck)	tall	(lot)
make	(came)	time	(might)
mill	(limb)	fine	(knife)
eat	(tea)	big	(gib)

24. Phoneme switching.

What to say to the student: "We're going to switch the first sounds in two words."
EXAMPLE: "Switch the first sounds in '_____' and '_____.'" (stimulus words) (e.g., "Switch the first sounds in 'raked leaves.'") (laked reaves)

> ***NOTE:*** *This is a difficult phoneme-level task and should only be done with older students. Give letter sound not letter name. Use pictured items and/or manipulatives if necessary. Use any of the following stimulus words and/or others you select from the story. Correct answers are in parentheses.*

Stimulus items:

soft couch	(coft souch)
red hen	(hed ren)
back porch	(pack borch)
little house	(hittle louse)
beautiful cake	(keautiful bake)
dog got	(gog dot)
cake batter	(bake catter)
fine white	(wine fite)
she cooked	(key shooked)
pulled weeds	(wulled peeds)

25. Pig latin.

What to say to the student: "We're going to talk in a secret language using words from the story. In pig latin, you take off the first sound of a word, put it at the end of the word, and add a long A sound."

EXAMPLE: "Say bowl in pig latin." (olbay)

> *NOTE: This is a difficult phoneme-level task and should only be done with older students. Use pictured items and/or manipulatives if necessary. Use any of the following stimulus words and/or others you select from the story. Correct answers are in parentheses.*

Stimulus items:

dog	(ogday)
nap	(apnay)
mouse	(ousemay)
couch	(ouchkay)
fire	(irefay)
sunny	(unnysay)
ripe	(iperay)
weeds	(eedsway)
raked	(akedray)
cozy	(ozykay)

CHAPTER

PHONOLOGICAL AWARENESS ACTIVITIES TO USE WITH *THE THREE LITTLE PIGS*

Text version used for selection of stimulus items:
Galdone, P. (1970). *The three little pigs.* New York: Clarion Books.

PHONOLOGICAL AWARENESS ACTIVITIES AT THE WORD LEVEL

1. Counting words.

What to say to the student: "We're going to count words."

EXAMPLE: "How many words do you hear in this sentence (or phrase)? 'his house.'" (2)

> *NOTE: Use pictured items and/or manipulatives if necessary. Use any of the following stimulus phrases or sentences and/or others you select from the story. Correct answers are in parentheses.*

Stimulus items:

a house (2)

those bricks (2)

blew the house (3)

load of bricks (3)

the three pigs (3)

give me those sticks (4)

will throw one down (4)

ran to pick it up (5)

first pig met a man (5)

built his house with them (5)

2. Identifying missing word from list.

What to say to the student: "Listen to the words I say. I'll say them again. You tell me which word I leave out."

EXAMPLE: "Listen to the words I say: 'roof, hill, field.' I'll say them again. Tell me which one I leave out: 'roof, hill.'" (field)

> ***NOTE:*** *Use pictured items and/or manipulatives if necessary. Use any of the following stimulus words and/or others you select from the story. Correct answers are in parentheses.*

Stimulus set #1	**Stimulus set #2**
pig, climb	pig (climb)
tree, dinner	dinner (tree)
hair, chin, load	hair, load (chin)
huff, apple, churn	apple, churn (huff)
farm, wolf, rolled	farm, rolled (wolf)
money, time, saw	money, time (saw)
old, tree, garden, pot	old, tree, garden (pot)
straw, told, blew, boiled	straw, blew, boiled (told)
door, fair, house, puffed	door, fair, puffed (house)
cover, build, nice, turnip	build, nice, turnip (cover)

3. Identifying missing word in phrase or sentence.

What to say to the student: "Listen to the sentence I read. Tell me which word is missing the second time I read the sentence."

EXAMPLE: "'Seek their fortune.' Listen again and tell me which word I leave out. 'Seek their____ .'" (fortune)

NOTE: Use pictured items and/or manipulatives if necessary. Use any of the following stimulus sentences and/or others you select from the story. Correct answers are in parentheses.

Stimulus items:

Merry Garden. Merry _____. (Garden)

Butter churn. ____ churn. (butter)

Three little pigs. Three little ______. (pigs)

Clump of bushes. Clump of ______. (bushes)

Bundle of straw. Bundle of _____. (straw)

Came rolling down. Came _____ down. (rolling)

Give me those bricks. Give me _____ bricks. (those)

The churn fell over. The churn fell _____. (over)

I'll blow your house in. I'll blow _____ house in. (your)

He built a blazing fire. He _____ a blazing fire. (built)

3. Supplying missing word as adult reads.

What to say to the student: "I want you to help me read the story. You fill in the words I leave out."

EXAMPLE: "Turnips for ____." (dinner)

NOTE: Use pictured items and/or manipulatives if necessary. Use any of the following stimulus sentences and/or others you select from the story. Correct answers are in parentheses.

Stimulus items:

Bundle of _____. (straw or sticks)

Rolled _____the hill. (down)

Basket full of _____. (apples)

He blew the _____ in. (house)

The little pig _____ his house. (built)

I got a nice potful of _____. (turnips)

Then I'll _____, and I'll puff. (huff)

Sent them off to seek their _____. (fortune)

The _____ was coming down the chimney. (wolf)

Not by the _____of my chinny chin chin. (hair)

5. Rearranging words.

What to say to the student: "I'll say some words out of order. You put them in the right order so they make sense."

EXAMPLE: "'down climb.' Put those words in the right order." (climb down)

> *NOTE: Use pictured items and/or manipulatives if necessary. Use any of the following stimulus words and/or others you select from the story. Correct answers are in parentheses. This word-level activity can be more difficult than some of the syllable- or phoneme-level activities because of the memory load. If your students are only able to deal with two or three words to be rearranged, add more two- and three-word samples from the story and omit the four-word level until a later time.*

Stimulus items:

fire blazing (blazing fire)

around turned (turned around)

home ran (ran home)

pigs three little (three little pigs)

house built his (built his house)

ever happily after (happily ever after)

house your blow in (blow your house in)

that straw me give (give me that straw)

full apples of basket (basket full of apples)

house blow I'll your in (I'll blow your house in)

PHONOLOGICAL AWARENESS ACTIVITIES AT THE SYLLABLE LEVEL

1. Syllable counting.

What to say to the student: "We're going to count syllables (or parts) of words."

EXAMPLE: "How many syllables do you hear in '_____'?" (stimulus word) (e.g., "How many syllables in 'chin'?") (1)

NOTE: *Use pictured items and/or manipulatives if necessary. Use any of the of the following stimulus words and/or others you select from the story. Use any group of 10 stimulus items you select per teaching set.*

Stimulus items:

One-syllable words: pig, pigs, please, pot, puff, put, back, been, blew, blow, bought, bricks, build, built, but, by, time, told, took, tree, turned, two, did, door, down, came, climb, could, keep, get, go, got, great, chin, churn, jumped, just, man, me, met, much, my, knock, know, next, nice, no, not, said, same, seek, sent, six, Smith, so, some, soon, sow, sticks, stopped, straw, ran, right, rolled, roof, round, fair, far, farm, fell, filed, first, five, four, full, had, hair, hard, have, he, hide, hill, him, his, home, house, huff, huffed, hung, last, let, lived, load, once, was, way, we, well, went, what, where, while, will, with, wolf, she, thing, third, thought, three, threw, throw, that, the, their, them, then, this, those, you, yes, your, a, an, and, as, asked, at, ate, eat, I, in, is, it, of, off, oh, old, on, up

Two-syllable words: apple, potful, basket, before, boiled, blazing, bundle, butter, turnips, dinner, climbing, coming, cover, quickly, garden, going, chimney, merry, money, morning, replied, fortune, frightened, happened, later, little, really, second, supper, very, wanted, water, after, again, along, angry, apple, around, ever, indeed, into, o'clock, over, upon

Three-syllable words: afterward, fireplace, together, tomorrow, happily, another

2. Initial syllable deleting.

What to say to the student: "We're going to leave out syllables (or parts of words)."
EXAMPLE: "Say '_____.'" (stimulus word) "Say it again without '_____.'" (stimulus syllable) (e.g., "Say 'quickly' without 'quick.'") (lee)

NOTE: *Use pictured items and/or manipulatives if necessary. Use any of the following stimulus words and/or others you select from the story. Correct answers are in parentheses.*

Stimulus items:

"Say potful without pot." (full)

"Say indeed without in." (deed)

"Say turnips without turn." (ups or ips)

"Say chimney without chim-." (knee)

"Say garden without gar." (den)

"Say fortune without for." (chun or chin)

"Say tomorrow without to." (morrow)

"Say supper without sup." (-er)

"Say before without be." (for)

"Say frighten without fry." (ten)

3. Final syllable deleting.

What to say to the student: "We're going to leave out syllables (or parts of words)."
EXAMPLE: "Say '_____.'" (stimulus word) "Say it again without '_____.'" (stimulus syllable) (e.g., "Say 'around' without 'round.'") (a)

> *NOTE: Use pictured items and/or manipulatives if necessary. Use any of the following stimulus words and/or others you select from the story. Correct answers are in parentheses.*

Stimulus items:

"Say afterward without word." (after)

"Say fireplace without place." (fire)

"Say potful without full." (pot)

"Say blazing without -ing." (blaze)

"Say into without to." (in)

"Say climbing without -ing." (climb)

"Say basket without -ket." (bass)

"Say quickly without lee." (quick)

"Say before without for." (be)

"Say chimney without knee." (chim)

4. Initial syllable adding.

What to say to the student: "Now let's add syllables (or parts) to words."
EXAMPLE: " Add '_____'" (stimulus syllable) "to the beginning of '_____.'" (stimulus syllable) (e.g., "Add 'pot' to the beginning of 'full.'") (potful)

> *NOTE: Use pictured items and/or manipulatives if necessary. Use any of the following stimulus words and/or others you select from the story. Correct answers are in parentheses.*

Stimulus items:

"Add mis- to the beginning of -ter." (mister)

"Add be to the beginning of for." (before)

"Add to to the beginning of -gether." (together)

"Add din- to the beginning of -er." (dinner)

"Add blaze the beginning of -ing." (blazing)

"Add sup to the beginning of -er." (supper)

"Add re- to the beginning of plied." (replied)

"Add gar- to the beginning of den." (garden)

"Add bun to the beginning of dull." (bundle)

"Add seck- to the beginning of -unds." (seconds)

5. Final syllable adding.

What to say to the student: "Now let's add syllables (or parts) to words."

EXAMPLE: "Add '_____'" (stimulus syllable) "to the end of '_____.'" (stimulus syllable) (e.g., "Add 'deed' to the end of 'in.'") (indeed)

> **NOTE:** *Use pictured items and/or manipulatives if necessary. Use any of the following stimulus words and/or others you select from the story. Correct answers are in parentheses.*

Stimulus items:

"Add -ul to the end of ap-." (apple)

"Add oh to the end of tommor-." (tomorrow)

"Add place to the end of fire." (fireplace)

"Add -und the end of seck-." (second)

"Add -er to the end of watt." (water)

"Add -ing to the end of climb." (climbing)

"Add knee to the end of chim-." (chimney)

"Add den to the end of gar." (garden)

"Add -er to the end of sup-" (supper)

"Add -ree to the end of ang-." (angry)

6. Syllable substituting.

What to say to the student: "Let's make up some new words."
EXAMPLE: "Say '_____.'" (stimulus word) "Instead of '_____'" (stimulus syllable) "say '_____.'" (stimulus syllable) (e.g., "Say 'into.' Instead of 'to' say 'stead.' The new word is 'instead.'")

> *NOTE: Use pictured items and/or manipulatives if necessary. Use any of the following stimulus words and/or others you select from the story. Correct answers are in parentheses.*

Stimulus items:

"Say potful. Instead of pot say mouth." (mouthful)

"Say chimney Instead of chim- say brown." (brownie)

"Say angry. Instead of ang- say hung." (hungry)

"Say before. Instead of for say hind." (behind)

"Say bundle. Instead of bun say han-." (handle)

"Say chinny. Instead of chin say skin." (skinny)

"Say frightened. Instead of fright say tight." (tightened)

"Say morning. Instead of morn say blaze." (blazing)

"Say replied. Instead of plied say do." (redo)

"Say indeed. Instead of deed say side." (inside)

PHONOLOGICAL AWARENESS ACTIVITIES AT THE PHONEME LEVEL

1. Counting sounds.

What to say to the student: "We're going to count sounds in words."
EXAMPLE: "How many sounds do you hear in this word? 'pig.'" (3)

> *NOTE: Use pictured items and/or manipulatives if necessary. Use any of the following stimulus words and/or others you select from the story. Be sure to give the letter sound and not the letter name. Use any group of 10 stimulus items you select per teaching set.*

Stimulus words with two sounds: by, to, go, me, know, no, sow, he, way, we, she, the, you, an, as, at, ate, eat, I'll, in, is, it, of, off, on, up

Stimulus words with three sounds: pig, pot, put, back, been, blew, blow, bought, but, time, took, tree, did, door, down, came, could, keep, get, got, chin, churn, man, met, much, nice, not, once, said, same, seek, some, soon, fair, far, fell, five, four, full, had, hair, have, hide, hill, him, his, home, house, huff, ran, right, roof, let, load, was, well, what, where, while, will, with, thing, third, thought, three, threw, throw, that, their, them then, there, this, those, tree, yes, your, and, apple, ever, old, over

Stimulus words with four sounds: pigs, please, boiled, build, butter, told, turned, dinner, climb, cover, great, chinny, just, merry, money, knocked, sent, six, straw, supper, farm, field, first, hard, ready, rolled, round, last, later, little, lived, water, went, wolf, after, again, along, apples, into, upon

Stimulus words with five sounds: Mr., bricks, bundle, chimney, jumped, next, Smith's, sticks, stopped, happened, wanted, another, around, indeed, o'clock

2. Sound categorization or identifying rhyme oddity.

What to say to the student: "Guess which word I say does not rhyme with the other three words."

EXAMPLE: "Tell me which word does not rhyme with the other three. '_____, _____, _____, _____.'" (stimulus words) (e.g., "bricks, ticks, door, licks. Which word doesn't rhyme?") (door)

NOTE: *Use pictured items if necessary. Use any of the following stimulus words and/or others you select from the story. Correct answers are in parentheses.*

Stimulus items:

puffed, huffed, first, cuffed (first)

their, pigs, hair, fair (pigs)

old, told, built, sold (built)

bought, thought, caught, sent (sent)

apple, six, bricks, sticks (apple)

climb, chin, time, dime (chin)

load, hill, will, chill (load)

churn, burn, learn, farm (farm)

five, blew, threw, two (five)

load, road, toad, wolf (wolf)

3. Matching rhyme.

What to say to the student: "We're going to think of rhyming words."
EXAMPLE: "Which word rhymes with '_____'?" (stimulus word) (e.g., "Which word rhymes with 'straw'? 'law, bundle, cover, sticks.'") (law)

> *NOTE: Use pictured items if necessary. Use any of the following stimulus words and/or others you select from the story. Correct answers are in parentheses.*

Stimulus items:

bundle: bought, trundle, told, door (trundle)

pot: came, hill, put, thought (thought)

house: mouse, load, chin, ever (mouse)

puff: blew, pigs, huff, wolf (huff)

bricks: build, churn, tricks, back (tricks)

blow: please, garden, turnips, throw (throw)

hide: cover, ride, water, field (ride)

please: road, apple, fleas, rolled (fleas)

dinner: boiled, butter, winner, straw (winner)

blazing: keep, turned, hill, grazing (grazing)

4. Producing rhyme.

What to say to the student: "Now we'll say rhyming words."
EXAMPLE: "Tell me a word that rhymes with '_____.'" (stimulus word) (e.g., "Tell me a word that rhymes with 'bricks.' You can make up a word if you want.") (ticks)

> *NOTE: Use pictured items if necessary. Use any of the following stimulus words and/or others you select from the story, i.e., you say a word from the list below and the student is to think of a rhyming word. Use any group of 10 stimulus items you select per teaching set.*

Stimulus items:

/p/: pig, pigs, please, pot, potful, put

/b/: back, basket, been, before, blazing, blew, blow, boiled, bought, bricks, build, bundle, but, butter, by

/t/: time, told, took, turned, turnips, two

/d/: did, dinner, door, down

/k/: came, climb, climbing, coming, could, cover, keep, quickly

/g/: garden, get, go, going, got, great

/ch/: chimney, chin, chinny, churn

/dz/: (as 1st sound in jelly): jumped, just

/m/: man, me, merry, met, money, morning, Mr., much, my

/n/: knocked, know, next, nice, no, not

/s/: said, same, second, seek, sent, six, Smith's, so, some, soon, sow, sticks, stopped, straw, supper,

/f/: fair, far, farm, fell, field, first, five, for, frightened, full

/v/: very

/h/: had, hair, happened, happily, hard, have, he, hide, hill, him, his, house, huff, huffed, hung

/r/: ran, ready, replied, right, rolled, roof, round

/l/: last, later, let, little, lived, load

/w/, /wh/: once, wanted, was, water, was, way, we, well, went, what, where, while, will, with, wolf

/sh/: she

/voiceless th/: thing, third, thought, three, threw, throw

/voiced th/: that, the, them, then, there, this, those

/y/ (as 1st sound in yellow): yes, you, yours

vowels: a, after, again, along, an, and, angry, another, apple, around, as, asked, at, ate, eat, ever, I, I'll, in, into, is, it, of, off, oh, old, on, over, up

5. Sound matching (initial).

What to say to the student: "Now we'll listen for the first sound in words."
EXAMPLE: "Listen to this sound: / /." (stimulus sound). "Guess which word I say begins with that sound. '_____, _____, _____, _____.'" (stimulus words) (e.g., "Listen to this sound /b/. Guess which word I say begins with that sound: 'pig, cover, bricks, field.'") (bricks)

NOTE: *Give letter sound not letter name. Use pictured items if necessary. Use any of the following stimulus words and/or others you select from the story. Correct answers are in parentheses.*

Stimulus items:

/g/: chin, climb, garden, nice (garden)

/d/: dinner, load, bricks, pigs (dinner)

/s/: blew, tree, great, straw (straw)

/ch/: apple, sticks, hair, churn (churn)

/f/: very, fair, little, into (fair)

/t/: house, farm, turnips, supper (turnips)

/b/: please, cover, pot, bundle (bundle)

/h/: last, house, wolf, third (house)

/k/: climbing, chimney, knocked, sent (climbing)

/m/: pot, keep, money, hide (money)

6. Sound matching (final).

What to say to the student: "Now we'll listen for the last sound in words."
EXAMPLE: "Listen to this sound: / /" (stimulus sound). "Guess which word I say ends with that sound '_____, _____, _____, _____.'" (stimulus words) (e.g., "Listen to this sound /n/. Guess which word I say ends with that sound: home, great, hide, chin.") (chin)

> ***NOTE:*** *Give letter sound not letter name. Use pictured items if necessary. Use any of the following stimulus words and/or others you select from the story. Correct answers are in parentheses.*

Stimulus items:

/k/: huffed, o'clock, field, apple (o'clock)

/r/: supper, house, pig, puff (supper)

/m/: fortune, bundle, much, farm (farm)

/l/: blew, bundle, load, hair (bundle)

/z/: pigs, six, climb, seek (pigs)

/d/: great, rolled, pick, down (rolled)

/ch/: old, time, much, please (much)

/f/: lived, home, man, wolf (wolf)

/t/: third, built, lived, fair (built)

/long E/: sticks, over, happily, little (happily)

7. Identifying initial sound in words.

What to say to the student: "I'll say a word two times. Tell me what sound is missing the second time. '______, _______.'" (stimulus words)

EXAMPLE: "What sound do you hear in '_____'" (stimulus word) "that is missing in '_____'?" (stimulus word) (e.g., "What sound do you hear in 'blow,' that is missing in 'low'?") (/b/)

> *NOTE: Give letter sound not letter name. Use pictured items and/or manipulatives if necessary. Use any of the following stimulus words and/or others you select from the story. Correct answers are in parentheses.*

Stimulus items:

"door, or. What sound do you hear in door that is missing in or?" (/d/)

"brick, Rick. What sound do you hear in brick that is missing in Rick?" (/b/)

"climb, lime. What sound do you hear in climb that is missing in lime?" (/k/)

"chin, in. What sound do you hear in chin that is missing in in?" (/ch/)

"while, I'll. What sound do you hear in while that is missing in I'll?" (/w/)

"hill, ill. What sound do you hear in hill that is missing in ill?" (/h/)

"told, old. What sound do you hear in told that is missing in old?" (/t/)

"stopped, topped. What sound do you hear in stopped that is missing in topped?" (/s/)

"fair, air. What sound do you hear in fair that is missing in air?" (/f/)

"sticks, ticks. What sound do you hear in sticks that is missing in ticks?" (/s/)

8. Identifying final sound in words.

What to say to the student: "I'll say a word two times. Tell me what sound is missing the second time. '______, _______.'" (stimulus words)

EXAMPLE: "What sound do you hear in '_____'" (stimulus word) "that is missing in '_____'?" (stimulus word) (e.g., "What sound do you hear in 'great' that is missing in 'grey'?") (/t/)

> *NOTE: Give letter sound not letter name. Use pictured items and/or manipulatives if necessary. Use any of the following stimulus words and/or others you select from the story. Correct answers are in parentheses.*

Stimulus items:

"told, toll. What sound do you hear in told that is missing in toll?" (/d/)

"keep, key. What sound do you hear in keep that is missing in key?" (/p/)

"chinny, chin. What sound do you hear in chinny that is missing in chin?" (/long E/)

"field, feel. What sound do you hear in field that is missing in feel?" (/d/)

"knocked, knock. What sound do you hear in knocked that is missing in knock?" (/t/)

"farm, far. What sound do you hear in farm that is missing in far?" (/m/)

"hide, high. What sound do you hear in hide that is missing in high?" (/d/)

"bricks, brick. What sound do you hear in bricks that is missing in brick" (/s/)

"house, how. What sound do you hear in house that is missing in how?" (/s/)

"wolf, wool. What sound do you hear in wolf that is missing in wool?" (/f/)

9. Segmenting initial sound in words.

What to say to the student: "Listen to the word I say and tell me the first sound you hear."

EXAMPLE: "What's the first sound in '_____'?" (stimulus word) (e.g., "What's the first sound in 'butter'?") (/b/)

> **NOTE:** *Give letter sound not letter name. Use pictured items and/or manipulatives if necessary. Use any of the following stimulus words and/or others you select from the story. Use any group of 10 stimulus items you select per teaching set.*

Stimulus items:

/p/: pig, pigs, please, pot, potful, put

/b/: back, basket, been, before, blazing, blew, blow, boiled, bought, bricks, build, bundle, but, butter, by

/t/: time, together, told, tomorrow, took, turned, turnips, two

/d/: did, dinner, door, down

/k/: came, climb, climbing, coming, could, cover, keep, quickly

/g/: garden, get, go, going, got, great

/ch/: chimney, chin, chinny, churn

/dz/: (as 1st sound in jelly): jumped, just

/m/: man, me, merry, met, money, morning, Mr., much, my

/n/: knocked, know, next, nice, no, not

/s/: said, same, second, seek, sent, six, Smith's, so, some, soon, sow, sticks, stopped, straw, supper

/f/: fair, far, farm, fell, field, fireplace, first, five, for, fortune, four, frightened, full

/v/: very

/h/: had, hair, happened, happily, hard, have, he, hide, hill, him, his, house, huff, huffed, hung

/r/: ran, ready, replied, right, rolled, roof, round

/l/: last, later, let, little, lived, load

/w/, /wh/: once, wanted, was, water, was, way, we, well, went, what, where, while, will, with, wolf

/sh/: she

/voiceless th/: thing, third, thought, three, threw, throw

/voiced th/: that, the, them, then, there, this, those

/y/ (as 1st sound in yellow): yes, you, yours

vowels: a, after, again, along, an, and, angry, another, apple, apples, around, as, asked, at, ate, eat, ever, I, I'll, in, indeed, into, is, it, o'clock, of, off, oh, old, on, over, up, upon

10. Segmenting final sound in words.

What to say to the student: "Listen to the word I say and tell me the last sound you hear."

EXAMPLE: "What's the last sound in the word '_____'?" (stimulus word) (e.g., "What's the last sound in the word 'took'?") (/k/)

> *NOTE: Give letter sound not letter name. Use pictured items and/or manipulatives if necessary. Use any of the following stimulus words and/or others you select from the story. Use any group of 10 stimulus items you select per teaching set.*

Stimulus items:

/p/: keep, up

/t/: asked, at, ate, basket, bought, built, but, eat, first, get, got, great, huffed, it, jumped, just, knocked, last, let, met, next, not, pot, puffed, put, sent, stopped, that, thought, tight, went, what

/d/: and, around, boiled, build, could, did, field, frightened, had, happened, heard, hide, indeed, lived, load, old, replied, rolled, round, said, second, third, turned, wanted

/k/: back, o'clock, pick, seek, took

/g/: pig

/ch/: much

/m/: came, climb, come, farm, him, home, same, some, them, time

/n/: again, an, been, chin, churn, down, fortune, garden, in, man, ran, soon, then, upon

/ng/: along, blazing, climbing, going, hung, morning, thing

/s/: bricks, fireplace, house, nice, once, six, Smith's, sticks, this, turnips, yes

/z/: apples, as, his, is, pigs, please, those, was

/f/: huff, off, puff, wolf

/v/: five, give, have, of

/r/: after, another, are, before, butter, cover, dinner, door, ever, fair, far, four, hair, later, Mr., over, supper, their, there, together, water, where, your

/l/: apple, bundle, fell, full, hill, I'll, little, potful, well, while, will

/long A/: way

/long E/: angry, chimney, chinny, he, me, merry, money, quickly, ready, she, three, tree, very, we

/long I/: by, my

/long O/: blow, go, know, so, throw, tomorrow

/oo/: blew, into, threw, to, two, you

/ah/: straw

/ow/: sow

11. Generating words from the story beginning with a particular sound.

What to say to the student: "Let's think of words **from the story** that start with certain sounds."

EXAMPLE: "Tell me a word **from the story** that starts with / /." (stimulus sound) (e.g., "the sound /l/)" (load)

NOTE: *Give letter sound not letter name. Use pictured items if necessary. Use any of the following stimulus words and/or others you select from the story. You say the sound (e.g., a voiceless /p/ sound) and the student is to say a word from the story that begins with that sound. Use any group of 10 stimulus items you select per teaching set.*

Stimulus items:

/p/: pig, pigs, please, pot, potful, put

/b/: back, basket, been, before, blazing, blew, blow, boiled, bought, bricks, build, bundle, but, butter, by

/t/: time, together, told, tomorrow, took, tree, turned, turnips, two

/d/: did, dinner, door, down

/k/: came, climb, climbing, coming, could, cover, keep, quickly

/g/: garden, get, go, going, got, great

/ch/: chimney, chin, chinny, churn

/dz/: (as 1st sound in jelly): jumped, just

/m/: man, me, merry, met, money, morning, Mr., much, my

/n/: knocked, know, next, nice, no, not

/s/: said, same, second, seek, sent, six, Smith's, so, some, soon, sow, sticks, stopped, straw, supper,

/f/: fair, far, farm, fell, field, fireplace, first, five, for, fortune, four, frightened, full

/v/: very

/h/: had, hair, happened, happily, hard, have, he, hide, hill, him, his, house, huff, huffed, hung

/r/: ran, ready, replied, right, rolled, roof, round

/l/: last, later, let, little, lived, load

/w/, /wh/: once, wanted, was, water, was, way, we, well, went, what, where, while, will, with, wolf

/sh/: she

/voiceless th/: thing, third, thought, three, threw, throw

/voiced th/: that, the, their, them, then, there, this, those

/y/ (as 1st sound in yellow): yes, you, yours

vowels: a, after, again, along, an, and, angry, another, apple, apples, around, as, asked, at, ate, eat, ever, I, I'll, in, indeed, into, is, it, o'clock, of, off, oh, old, on, over, up, upon

12. Blending sounds in monosyllabic words divided into onset-rime beginning with two consonant cluster + rime.

What to say to the student: "Now we'll put sounds together to make words."
EXAMPLE: "Put these sounds together to make a word (/ / + / /)." (stimulus sounds) "What's the word?" (e.g., "gr + ate: What's the word?") (great)

> *NOTE: Give letter sound not letter name. Use pictured items and/or manipulatives if necessary. Use any of the following stimulus words and/or others you select from the story. Correct answers are in parentheses.*

Stimulus items:

bl + ow (blow)

tr +ee (tree)

st + icks (sticks)

th + ought (thought)

pl + ease (please)

bl + aze (blaze)

cl + ime (climb)

br + icks (bricks)

st + raw (straw)

th + rew (threw)

13. Blending sounds in monosyllabic words divided into onset-rime beginning with single consonant + rime.

What to say to the student: "Let's put sounds together to make words."
EXAMPLE: "Put these sounds together to make a word (/ / + / /)." (stimulus sounds) "What's the word?" (e.g., "/t/ + old: what's the word?") (told)

> *NOTE: Give letter sound not letter name. Use pictured items and/or manipulatives if necessary. Use any of the following stimulus words and/or others you select from the story. Correct answers are in parentheses.*

Stimulus items:

/t/ + ime (time)

/w/ + ulf (wolf)

/f/ + air (fair)

/p/ + ought (pot)

/b/ + illed (build)
/s/ + icks (six)
/p/ + igs (pigs)
/b/ + ack (back)
/n/ + ice (nice)
/ch/ + urn (churn)

14. Blending sounds to form a monosyllabic word beginning with a continuant sound.

What to say to the student: "We'll put sounds together to make words."
EXAMPLE: "Put these sounds together to make a word (/ / + / / + / /)." (stimulus sounds) (e.g., "/m/ /short U/ /ch/.") (much)

> ***NOTE:*** *Give letter sound not letter name. Use pictured items and/or manipulatives if necessary. Use any of the following stimulus words and/or others you select from the story. Correct answers are in parentheses.*

Stimulus items:

/s/ /t/ /r/ /ah/ (straw)
/m/ /short A/ /n/ (man)
/l/ /long O/ /d/ (load)
/r/ /oo/ /f/ (roof)
/s/ /long A/ /m/ (same)
/h/ /long O/ /m/ (home)
/s/ /long E/ /k/ (seek)
/h/ /short I/ /l/ (hill)
/th/ /r/ /long E/ (three)
/f/ /ah/ /r/ /m/ (farm)

15. Blending sounds to form a monosyllabic word beginning with a noncontinuant sound.

What to say to the student: "We'll put sounds together to make words."
EXAMPLE: "Put these sounds together to make a word (/ / + / / + / /)." (stimulus sounds) (e.g., "/t/ /long O/ /l/ /d/.") (told)

> ***NOTE:*** *Give letter sound not letter name. Use pictured items and/or manipulatives if necessary. Use any of the following stimulus words and/or others you select from the story. Correct answers are in parentheses.*

Stimulus items:

/ch/ /short I/ /n/ (chin)
/k/ /l/ /long I/ /m/ (climb)
/p/ /short U/ /f/ (puff)
/k/ /w/ /short I/ /k/ (quick)

/b/ /l/ /oo/ (blew)
/p/ /short I/ /g/ (pig)
/ch/ /r/ /n/ (churn)
/b/ /r/ /short I/ /k/ /s/ (bricks)
/t/ /long I/ /m/ (time)
/b/ /short I/ /l/ /d/ (build)

16. Substituting initial sound in words.

What to say to the student: "We're going to change beginning/first sounds in words." *EXAMPLE:* "Say '_____.'" (stimulus word) "Instead of / /" (stimulus sound) "say / /." (stimulus sound) (e.g., Say 'pot.' Instead of /p/ say /k/. What's your new word?") (caught)

> ***NOTE:*** *Give letter sound not letter name. Use pictured items and/or manipulatives if necessary. Use any of the following stimulus words and/or others you select from the story. Correct answers are in parentheses.*

Stimulus items:

"Say churn. Instead of /ch/ say /b/." (burn)

"Say blow. Instead of /b/ say /g/." (glow)

"Say huff. Instead of /h/ say /p/." (puff)

"Say fair. Instead of /f/ say /h/." (hair)

"Say rolled. Instead of /r/ say /t/." (told)

"Say three. Instead of /voiceless th/ say /f/." (free)

"Say farm. Instead of /f/ say /ch/." (charm)

"Say bricks. Instead of /b/ say /t/." (tricks)

"Say water. Instead of /w/ say /d/." (daughter)

"Say chin. Instead of /ch/ say /voiceless th/." (thin)

17. Substituting final sound in words.

What to say to the student: "We're going to change ending/last sounds in words." *EXAMPLE:* "Say '_____.'" (stimulus word) "Instead of / /" (stimulus sound) "say / /." (stimulus sound) (e.g., "Say 'churn.' Instead of /n/ say /p/. What's your new word?") (chirp)

> ***NOTE:*** *Give letter sound not letter name. Use pictured items and/or manipulatives if necessary. Use any of the following stimulus words and/or others you select from the story. Correct answers are in parentheses.*

Stimulus items:

"Say ate. Instead of /t/ say /p/." (ape)

"Say great. Instead of /t/ say /p/." (grape)

"Say pigs. Instead of /z/ say /long E/."(piggy)

"Say off. Instead of /f/ say /n/." (on)

"Say nice. Instead of /s/, say /f/." (knife)

"Say huff. Instead of /f/ say /t/." (hut)

"Say load. Instead of /d/ say /n/." (loan)

"Say back. Instead of /k/ say /ch/." (batch)

"Say home. Instead of /m/ say /p/." (hope)

"Say boiled. Instead of /d/ say /z/." (boils)

18. Segmenting middle sound in monosyllabic words.

What to say to the student: "Tell me the middle sound in the word I say."
EXAMPLE: "What's the middle sound in the word '_____'?" (stimulus word) (e.g., "What's the middle sound in the word 'ran'?") (/short A/)

> ***NOTE:*** *Give letter sound not letter name. Use pictured items and/or manipulatives if necessary. Use any of the following stimulus words and/or others you select from the story. Correct answers are in parentheses.*

Stimulus items:

met (/short E/)

chin (/short I/)

roof (/oo/)

pot (/ah/)

seek (/long E/)

those (/long O/)

tree (/r/)

time (/long I/)

home (/long O/)

back (/short A/)

19. Substituting middle sound in words.

What to say to the student: "We're going to change the middle sound in words."
EXAMPLE: "Say '_____.'" (stimulus word) "Instead of / /" (stimulus sound) "say / /." (stimulus sound)(e.g., "Say 'pig.' Instead of /short I/ say /short U/. What's your new word?") (pug)

> **NOTE:** *Give letter sound not letter name. Use pictured items and/or manipulatives if necessary. Use any of the following stimulus words and/or others you select from the story. Correct answers are in parentheses.*

Stimulus items:

"Say went. Instead of /short E/ say /ah/." (want)

"Say sticks. Instead of /short I/ say /short A/." (stacks)

"Say hill. Instead of /short I/ say /ah/."(hall)

"Say boil. Instead of /oi/ say /ah/." (ball)

"Say chin. Instead of /short I/, say /short A/." (chan)

"Say huff. Instead of /short U/ say /short A/." (half)

"Say built. Instead of /short I/ say /long O/." (bolt)

"Say seek. Instead of /long E/ say /short I/." (sick)

"Say please. Instead of /long E/ say /long A/." (plays)

"Say fell. Instead of /short E/, say /ah/." (fall)

20. Identifying all sounds in monosyllabic words.

What to say to the student: "Now tell me all the sounds you hear in the word I say."
EXAMPLE: "What sounds do you hear in the word '_____'?" (stimulus word) (e.g., "What sounds do you hear in the word 'sent'?") (/s/ /short E/ /n/ /t/)

> **NOTE:** *Give letter sound not letter name. Use pictured items and/or manipulatives if necessary. Use any of the following stimulus words and/or others you select from the story. Correct answers are in parentheses.*

Stimulus items:

pig (/p/ /short I/ /g/)

blow (/b/ /l/ /long O/)

roof (/r/ /oo/ /f/)

ran (/r/ /short A/ /n/)

hide (/h/ /long I/ /d/)

three (/th/ /r/ /long E/)

seek (/s/ /long E/ /k/)

field (/f/ /long E/ /l/ /d/)

churn (/ch/ /r/ /n/)

great (/g/ /r/ /long A/ /t/)

21. Deleting sounds within words.

What to say to the student: "We're going to leave out sounds in words."

EXAMPLE: "Say '_____'" (stimulus word) "without / /." (stimulus sound) (e.g., "Say 'blew' without /l/.") (boo) "The word that was left, 'boo,' is a real word. Sometimes the word won't be a real word."

> ***NOTE:*** *Give letter sound not letter name. Use pictured items and/or manipulatives if necessary. Use any of the following stimulus words and/or others you select from the story. Correct answers are in parentheses.*

Stimulus items:

"Say please without /l/." (peas)

"Say tree without /r/." (tea)

"Say and without /n/." (ad)

"Say great without /r/." (gate)

"Say place without /l/." (pace)

"Say sticks without /t/." (sicks)

"Say fright without /r/." (fight)

"Say blow without /l/." (bow)

"Say bricks without /r/." (bicks)

"Say quick without /w/." (kick)

22. Substituting consonant in words having a two-sound cluster.

What to say to the student: "We're going to substitute sounds in words."

EXAMPLE: "Say '_____'" (stimulus word). "Instead of / /" (stimulus sound) "say / /" (stimulus sound) (e.g., "Say 'quick.' Instead of /w/ say /l/." (click). Say "Sometimes the new word will be a made-up word.")

> ***NOTE:*** *Give letter sound not letter name. Use pictured items and/or manipulatives if necessary. Use any of the following stimulus words and/or others you select from the story. Correct answers are in parentheses.*

Stimulus items:

"Say blow. Instead of /b/ say /g/." (glow)

"Say replied. Instead of /l/ say /r/." (repried)

"Say blazing. Instead of /l/ say /r/." (braising)

"Say blew. Instead of /l/ say /r/." (brew)

"Say sticks. Instead of /t/ say /l/."(slicks)

"Say climb. Instead of /l/ say /r/." (crime)

"Say stopped. Instead of /t/ say /l/." (slopped)

"Say please. Instead of /l/ say /r/." (preaze)

"Say heard. Instead of /d/ say /t/" (hurt)

"Say bricks. Instead of /b/ say /t/." (tricks)

23. Phoneme reversing.

What to say to the student: "We're going to say words backward."

EXAMPLE: "Say the word '_____'" (stimulus word) "backward." (e.g., "If we say 'but' backward, the word is 'tub.'")

> ***NOTE:*** *This is a difficult phoneme-level task and should only be done with older students. Give letter sound not letter name. Use pictured items and/or manipulatives if necessary. Use any of the following stimulus words and/or others you select from the story. Correct answers are in parentheses.*

Stimulus items:

right	(tire)	back	(cab)
time	(might)	did	(did)

let	(tell)	some	(muss)
door	(road)	chin	(niche)
pot	(top)	keep	(peek)

24. Phoneme switching.

What to say to the student: "We're going to switch the first sounds in two words."
EXAMPLE: "Switch the first sounds in '_____' and '_____.'" (stimulus words) (e.g., "Switch the first sounds in 'huffed puffed.'") (puffed huffed)

> ***NOTE:*** *This is a difficult phoneme-level task and should only be done with older students. Give letter sound not letter name. Use pictured items and/or manipulatives if necessary. Use any of the following stimulus words and/or others you select from the story. Correct answers are in parentheses.*

Stimulus items:

some turnips	(tum surnips)
little pig	(pittle lig)
butter churn	(chutter burn)
no money	(moe nunny)
my chinny	(chy minny)
for dinner	(dor finner)
back down	(dack bown)
merry garden	(gary marden)
wolf huffed	(holf wuffed)
ran home	(han rome)

25. Pig latin.

What to say to the student: "We're going to talk in a secret language using words from the story. In pig latin, you take off the first sound of a word, put it at the end of the word, and add a long A sound."
EXAMPLE: "Say chin in pig latin." (inchay)

> ***NOTE:*** *This is a difficult phoneme-level task and should only be done with older students. Use pictured items and/or manipulatives if necessary. Use any of the following stimulus words and/or others you select from the story. Correct answers are in parentheses.*

Stimulus items:

man	(anmay)
pig	(igpay)
farm	(armfay)
house	(ousehay)
turnips	(urnipstay)
little	(ittlelay)
second	(eckondsay)
chimney	(imneychay)
butter	(utterbay)
wolf	(olfway)

CHAPTER

PHONOLOGICAL AWARENESS ACTIVITIES TO USE WITH *THE SNOWY DAY*

Text version used for selection of stimulus items:
Keats, E.J. (1986). *The snowy day*. New York: Puffin Books.

PHONOLOGICAL AWARENESS ACTIVITIES AT THE WORD LEVEL

1. Counting words.

What to say to the student: "We're going to count words."

EXAMPLE: "How many words do you hear in this sentence (or phrase)? 'woke up.'" (2)

> ***NOTE:*** *Use pictured items and/or manipulatives if necessary. Use any of the following stimulus phrases or sentences and/or others you select from the story. Correct answers are in parentheses.*

Stimulus items:

big boys (2)

wet socks (2)

warm house (2)

his feet sank (3)

his warm house (3)

to make a path (4)

his dream was gone (4)

that made a new track (5)

he called to his friend (5)

slid all the way down (5)

2. Identifying missing word from list.

What to say to the student: "Listen to the words I say. I'll say them again. You tell me which word I leave out."

EXAMPLE: "Listen to the words I say: 'stick, wet, top.' I'll say them again. Tell me which one I leave out: 'stick, wet.'" (top)

> ***NOTE:*** *Use pictured items and/or manipulatives if necessary. Use any of the following stimulus words and/or others you select from the story. Correct answers are in parentheses.*

Stimulus set #1	**Stimulus set #2**
dream, plop	dream (plop)
socks, track	track (socks)
piled, warm, boys	piled, boys (warm)
toes, deep, house	toes, deep (house)
crunch, snowy, feet	snowy, feet (crunch)
climber, pocket, friend	pocket, friend (climber)
firm, woke, day, tall	firm, woke, tall (day)
top, bed, deep, ran	top, bed, ran (deep)
high, old, big, pot	high, old, big (pot)
tree, winter, hall, fun	winter, hall, fun (tree)

3. Identifying missing word in phrase or sentence.

What to say to the student: "Listen to the sentence I read. Tell me which word is missing the second time I read the sentence."

EXAMPLE: "'His warm house.' Listen again and tell me which word I leave out. 'His____ house.'" (warm)

NOTE: Use pictured items and/or manipulatives if necessary. Use any of the following stimulus sentences and/or others you select from the story. Correct answers are in parentheses.

Stimulus items:

Snowy day. Snowy_____. (day)

Wet socks. ____ socks. (Wet)

Handful of snow. Handful of ______. (snow)

He made angels. He made______. (angels)

Snow covered tree. Snow ____ tree. (covered)

A path for walking. A _____ for walking. (path)

Looked out the window. Looked out the _____. (window)

He dragged his feet slowly. He _____ his feet slowly. (dragged)

Melted all the snow away. Melted all the_____ away. (snow)

He looked in his pocket. He _____ in his pocket. (looked)

4. Supplying missing word as adult reads.

What to say to the student: "I want you to help me read the story. You fill in the words I leave out."

EXAMPLE: "New snow was ____." (falling)

NOTE: Use pictured items and/or manipulatives if necessary. Use any of the following stimulus sentences and/or others you select from the story. Correct answers are in parentheses.

Stimulus items:

Made a new _____. (track)

The snow was piled _____. (up)

He picked up a _____. (handful)

She took off his _____ socks. (wet)

Down fell the _____, plop. (snow)

He made a _____ snowman. (smiling)

His pocket was _____. (empty)

He packed it _____ and firm. (round)

When he woke up his _____ was gone. (dream)

It would be fun to join the big _____. (boys)

5. Rearranging words.

What to say to the student: "I'll say some words out of order. You put them in the right order so they make sense."

EXAMPLE: "'up climbed.' Put those words in the right order." (climbed up)

> *NOTE: Use pictured items and/or manipulatives if necessary. Use any of the following stimulus words and/or others you select from the story. Correct answers are in parentheses. This word-level activity can be more difficult than some of the syllable- or phoneme-level activities because of the memory load. If your students are only able to deal with two or three words to be rearranged, add more two- and three-word samples from the story and omit the four-word level until a later time.*

Stimulus items:

boys big (big boys)

house warm (warm house)

down slid (slid down)

walking path for (path for walking)

falling was snow (snow was falling)

morning winter one (one winter morning)

way down all the (all the way down)

snow mountain of heaping (heaping mountain of snow)

falling was snow new (new snow was falling)

slowly feet dragged his (dragged his feet slowly)

PHONOLOGICAL AWARENESS ACTIVITIES AT THE SYLLABLE LEVEL

1. Syllable counting.

What to say to the student: "We're going to count syllables (or parts) of words."

EXAMPLE: "How many syllables do you hear in '_____'?" (stimulus word) (e.g., "How many syllables in 'snow'?") (1)

NOTE: Use pictured items and/or manipulatives if necessary. Use any of the of the following stimulus words and/or others you select from the story. Use any group of 10 stimulus items you select per teaching set.

Stimulus items:

One-syllable words: path, picked, plop, pot, put, be, bed, big, boys, but, tall, to, toes, told, took, top, track, tracks, day, deep, down, dragged, dreamed, called, climbed, could, crunch, gone, got, great, just, made, make, knew, night, not, sad, sank, see, slept, slid, snow, so, socks, stick, still, street, sun, far, feet, fell, felt, fight, firm, for, found, friend, from, fun, very, had, hall, he, head, high, his, house, ran, right, round, like, liked, looked, one, walked, warm, was, way, went, wet, when, while, with, woke, would, she, thought, that, the, their, them, then, there, they, this, yet, a, all, and, as, in, it, of, off, old, on, out, up

Two-syllable words: Peter, pocket, pointing, before, breakfast, during, climber, covered, melted, morning, mother, mountain, slowly, smacking, smiling, snowball, snowman, snowy, snowsuit, something, sticking, fallen, falling, very, handful, heaping, walking, window, winter, across, after, along, angels, empty, enough, into, outside

Three-syllable words: pretended, together, tomorrow, adventures

2. Initial syllable deleting.

What to say to the student: "We're going to leave out syllables (or parts of words)."
EXAMPLE: "Say '_____.'" (stimulus word) "Say it again without '_____.'" (stimulus syllable) (e.g., "Say 'empty' without 'emp.'") (tee)

NOTE: Use pictured items and/or manipulatives if necessary. Use any of the following stimulus words and/or others you select from the story. Correct answers are in parentheses.

Stimulus items:

"Say snowball without snow." (ball)

"Say something without some." (thing)

"Say handful without hand." (full)

"Say window without win." (doe)

"Say breakfast without breck." (fist)

"Say fallen without fall." (-en)

"Say snowman without snow." (man)

"Say across without a." (cross)

"Say outside without out." (side)

"Say snowsuit without snow." (suit)

3. Final syllable deleting.

What to say to the student: "We're going to leave out syllables (or parts of words)." ***EXAMPLE:*** "Say '_____.'" (stimulus word) "Say it again without '_____.'" (stimulus syllable) (e.g., "Say 'before' without 'for.'") (be)

> ***NOTE:*** *Use pictured items and/or manipulatives if necessary. Use any of the following stimulus words and/or others you select from the story. Correct answers are in parentheses.*

Stimulus items:

"Say snowman without man." (snow)

"Say winter without -ter." (win)

"Say melted without -ed." (melt)

"Say smiling without -ing." (smile)

"Say into without to." (in)

"Say smacking without -ing." (smack)

"Say mountain without -en (or in)." (mount)

"Say after without -er." (aft)

"Say outside without side." (out)

"Say pocket without -ket." (paw)

4. Initial syllable adding.

What to say to the student: "Now let's add syllables (or parts) to words." ***EXAMPLE:*** " Add '_____'" (stimulus syllable) "to the beginning of '_____.'" (stimulus syllable) (e.g., "Add 'some' to the beginning of 'thing.'") (something)

> ***NOTE:*** *Use pictured items and/or manipulatives if necessary. Use any of the following stimulus words and/or others you select from the story. Correct answers are in parentheses.*

Stimulus items:

"Add emp- to the beginning of tee." (empty)

"Add snow to the beginning of ball." (snowball)

"Add pre- to the beginning of tended." (pretended)

"Add heap to the beginning of -ing." (heaping)

"Add out to the beginning of side." (outside)

"Add snow to the beginning of man." (snowman)

"Add ad to the beginning of ventures. (adventures)

"Add slow to the beginning of lee." (slowly)

"Add to to the beginning of morrow." (tomorrow)

"Add hand to the beginning of full." (handful)

5. Final syllable adding.

What to say to the student: "Now let's add syllables (or parts) to words."
EXAMPLE: "Add '_____'" (stimulus syllable) "to the end of '_____.'" (stimulus syllable) (e.g., "Add 'suit' to the end of 'snow.'") (snowsuit)

> *NOTE:* *Use pictured items and/or manipulatives if necessary. Use any of the following stimulus words and/or others you select from the story. Correct answers are in parentheses.*

Stimulus items:

"Add -ed to the end of pretend." (pretended)

"Add -ing to the end of stick." (sticking)

"Add full to the end of hand." (handful)

"Add -er to the end of Pete." (Peter)

"Add side to the end of out." (outside)

"Add to to the end of in." (into)

"Add thing to the end of every." (everything)

"Add -ing to the end of smile." (smiling)

"Add -ted to the end of mel." (melted)

"Add man to the end of snow." (snowman)

6. Syllable substituting.

What to say to the student: "Let's make up some new words."
EXAMPLE: "Say '_____.'" (stimulus word) "Instead of '_____'" (stimulus syllable) "say '_____.'" (stimulus syllable) (e.g., "Say 'outside.' Instead of 'out' say 'in.' The new word is 'inside.'")

> *NOTE: Use pictured items and/or manipulatives if necessary. Use any of the following stimulus words and/or others you select from the story. Correct answers are in parentheses.*

Stimulus items:

"Say snowman. Instead of man say suit." (snowsuit)

"Say heaping. Instead of heap say stick." (sticking)

"Say something. Instead of thing say one." (someone)

"Say into. Instead of in say on." (onto)

"Say handful. Instead of hand say pot." (potful)

"Say before. Instead of fore say side." (beside)

"Say across. Instead of cross say bout." (about)

"Say snowball. Instead of snow say foot." (football)

"Say outside. Instead of side say line." (outline)

"Say window. Instead of doe say -ter." (winter)

PHONOLOGICAL AWARENESS ACTIVITIES AT THE PHONEME LEVEL

1. Counting sounds.

What to say to the student: "We're going to count sounds in words."
EXAMPLE: "How many sounds do you hear in this word? 'deep.'" (3)

> *NOTE: Use pictured items and/or manipulatives if necessary. Use any of the following stimulus words and/or others you select from the story. Be sure to give the letter sound and not the letter name. Use any group of 10 stimulus items you select per teaching set.*

Stimulus words with two sounds: be, to, day, new, see, so, he, high, way, she, the, they, all, as, in, of, off, on, out, up

Stimulus words with three sounds: path, pot, put, bed, big, boys, but, tall, toes, took, top, deep, down, could, gone, got, join, made, make, night, not, sad, snow, sun, far, feet, fell, fight, firm, for, fun, had, hall, head, his, house, ran, right, like, wet, when, while, with, woke, would, thought, that, their, them, then, there, this, yet, and, away, old

Stimulus words with four sounds: Peter, picked, piled, plop, told, track, dream, great, just, sank, slid, snowy, socks, still, fallen, felt, found, from, very, round, liked, looked, walked, warm, went, about, after, enough, into

Stimulus words with five sounds: pocket, before, tracks, dragged, dreamed, climbed, covered, crunch, slept, slowly, sticks, street, friend, window, winter, across, another, empty, outside

2. Sound categorization or identifying rhyme oddity.

What to say to the student: "Guess which word I say does not rhyme with the other three words."

EXAMPLE: "Tell me which word does not rhyme with the other three. '_____, _____, _____, _____.'" (stimulus words) (e.g., "would, could, should, angels. Which word doesn't rhyme?") (angels)

> ***NOTE:*** *Use pictured items if necessary. Use any of the following stimulus words and/or others you select from the story. Correct answers are in parentheses.*

Stimulus items:

fun, sun, one, big (big)

top, plop, tub, shop (tub)

head, toes, bed, red (toes)

street, piled, feet, neat (piled)

right, fight, night, deep (deep)

socks, took, shook, cook (socks)

hall, high, tall, all (high)

mother, brother, other, like (like)

felt, thought, got, pot (felt)

crunch, bunch, lunch, snow (snow)

3. Matching rhyme.

What to say to the student: "We're going to think of rhyming words."
EXAMPLE: "Which word rhymes with '_____'?" (stimulus word) (e.g., "Which word rhymes with 'day'? 'tree, dream, way, ran.'") (way)

> *NOTE: Use pictured items if necessary. Use any of the following stimulus words and/or others you select from the story. Correct answers are in parentheses.*

Stimulus items:

snow: down, go, socks, still (go)

fight: empty, fell, night, slept (night)

wet: yet, deep, slid, street (yet)

head: far, church, stick, bed (bed)

sank: track, tank, big, woke (tank)

boys: angels, toes, toys, ran (toys)

tall: high, hall, while, path (hall)

walking: snowy, great, along, talking (talking)

mountain: snowman, firm, fountain, join (fountain)

slept: gone, kept, dragged, toes (kept)

4. Producing rhyme.

What to say to the student: "Now we'll say rhyming words."
EXAMPLE: "Tell me a word that rhymes with '_____.'" (stimulus word) (e.g., "Tell me a word that rhymes with 'big.' You can make up a word if you want.") (wig)

> *NOTE: Use pictured items if necessary. Use any of the following stimulus words and/or others you select from the story, i.e., you say a word from the list below and the student is to think of a rhyming word. Use any group of 10 stimulus items you select per teaching set.*

Stimulus items:

/p/: path, Peter, picked, piled, plop, pocket, pointing, pot, pretended, put

/b/: be, bed, before, big, boys, breakfast, but

/t/: tall, to, toes, together, told, took, top, track, tracks, tree

/d/: day, deep, down, dragged, dream, dreamed, during

/k/: called, climbed, climber, could, covered, crunch

/g/: gone, got, great

/dz/: (as 1st sound in jelly): just

/m/: made, make, melted, morning, mother, mountain

/n/: new, night, not

/s/: sad, sank, see, slept, slid, slowly, smacking, smiling, snow, snowball, snowman, snowsuit, snowy, so, socks, something, stick, sticking, still, street, sun

/f/: fallen, falling, far, feet, fell, felt, fight, firm, for, found, friend, from, fun

/v/: very

/h/: had, hall, handful, he, head, heaping, high, his, house

/r/: ran, right, round

/l/: like, liked, looked

/w/, /wh/: one, walked, walking, warm, was, way, went, wet, when, while, window, winter, with, woke, would

/sh/: she

/voiceless th/: thought

/voiced th/: that, the, their, them, then, there, they, this

/y/ (as 1st sound in yellow): yet

vowels: a, about, across, adventures, after, all, along, and, angels, another, as, away, empty, enough, everything, everywhere, in, into, of, off, old, on, out, outside, up

5. Sound matching (initial).

What to say to the student: "Now we'll listen for the first sound in words."

EXAMPLE: "Listen to this sound: / /." (stimulus sound). "Guess which word I say begins with that sound. '_____, _____, _____, _____.'" (stimulus words) (e.g., "Listen to this sound /p/. Guess which word I say begins with that sound: 'gone, path, deep, join.'") (path)

> ***NOTE:*** *Give letter sound not letter name. Use pictured items if necessary. Use any of the following stimulus words and/or others you select from the story. Correct answers are in parentheses.*

Stimulus items:

/h/: firm, house, round, slept (house)

/d/: dream, mother, toes, big (dream)

/s/: night, ran, snowy, feet (snowy)

/m/: fight, plop, dragged, melted (melted)

/f/: friend, top, boys, took (friend)

/t/: piled, tracks, during, felt (tracks)

/p/: right, pocket, found, tree (pocket)

/b/: boys, slowly, wet, dream (boys)

/k/: head, stick, made, crunch (crunch)

/w/: handful, away, winter, like (winter)

6. Sound matching (final).

What to say to the student: "Now we'll listen for the last sound in words."
EXAMPLE: "Listen to this sound: / /" (stimulus sound). "Guess which word I say ends with that sound '_____, _____, _____, _____.'" (stimulus words) (e.g., "Listen to this sound /n/. Guess which word I say ends with that sound: 'sun, up, snow, street.'") (sun)

> ***NOTE:*** *Give letter sound not letter name. Use pictured items if necessary. Use any of the following stimulus words and/or others you select from the story. Correct answers are in parentheses.*

Stimulus items:

/t/: pocket, dragged, plop, woke (pocket)

/n/: house, boys, mountain, big (mountain)

/m/: sun, far, hall, firm (firm)

/z/: tracks, angels, friend, house (angels)

/d/: night, sank, melted, dream (melted)

/r/: Peter, across, fallen, along (Peter)

/ch/: top, walked, crunch, head (crunch)

/p/: deep, liked, stick, tall (deep)

/l/: piled, warm, snow, hall (hall)

/s/: round, join, socks, covered (socks)

7. Identifying initial sound in words.

What to say to the student: "I'll say a word two times. Tell me what sound is missing the second time. '______, _______.'" (stimulus words)

EXAMPLE: "What sound do you hear in '_____'" (stimulus word) "that is missing in '_____'?" (stimulus word) (e.g., "What sound do you hear in 'tall,' that is missing in 'all'?" (/t/)

> *NOTE: Give letter sound not letter name. Use pictured items and/or manipulatives if necessary. Use any of the following stimulus words and/or others you select from the story. Correct answers are in parentheses.*

Stimulus items:

"gone, on. What sound do you hear in gone that is missing in on?" (/g/)

"slid, lid. What sound do you hear in slid that is missing in lid?" (/s/)

"feet, eat. What sound do you hear in feet that is missing in eat?" (/f/)

"climb, lime. What sound do you hear in climb that is missing in lime?" (/k/)

"thought, ought. What sound do you hear in thought that is missing in ought?" (/voiceless th/)

"bed, Ed. What sound do you hear in bed that is missing in Ed?" (/b/)

"track, rack. What sound do you hear in track that is missing in rack?" (/t/)

"street, treat. What sound do you hear in street that is missing in treat?" (/s/)

"snow, no. What sound do you hear in snow that is missing in no?" (/s/)

"while, I'll. What sound do you hear in while that is missing in I'll?" (/w/)

8. Identifying final sound in words.

What to say to the student: "I'll say a word two times. Tell me what sound is missing the second time. '______, _______.'" (stimulus words)

EXAMPLE: "What sound do you hear in '_____'" (stimulus word) "that is missing in '_____'?" (stimulus word) (e.g., "What sound do you hear in 'firm' that is missing in 'fir'?") (/m/)

> *NOTE: Give letter sound not letter name. Use pictured items and/or manipulatives if necessary. Use any of the following stimulus words and/or others you select from the story. Correct answers are in parentheses.*

Stimulus items:

"picked, pick. What sound do you hear in picked that is missing in pick?" (/t/)

"warm, war. What sound do you hear in warm that is missing in war?" (/m/)

"great, gray. What sound do you hear in great that is missing in gray?" (/t/)

"felt, fell. What sound do you hear in felt that is missing in fell?" (/t/)

"window, wind. What sound do you hear in window that is missing in wind?" (/long O/)

"made, may. What sound do you hear in made that is missing in may?" (/d/)

"boys, boy. What sound do you hear in boys that is missing in boy?" (/z/)

"told, toll. What sound do you hear in told that is missing in toll?" (/d/)

"right, rye. What sound do you hear in right that is missing in rye?" (/t/)

"socks, sock. What sound do you hear in socks that is missing in sock?" (/s/)

9. Segmenting initial sound in words.

What to say to the student: "Listen to the word I say and tell me the first sound you hear."

EXAMPLE: "What's the first sound in '_____'?" (stimulus word) (e.g., "What's the first sound in 'woke?'") (/w/)

> ***NOTE:*** *Give letter sound not letter name. Use pictured items and/or manipulatives if necessary. Use any of the following stimulus words and/or others you select from the story. Use any group of 10 stimulus items you select per teaching set.*

Stimulus items:

/p/: path, Peter, picked, piled, plop, pocket, pointing, pot, pretended, put

/b/: be, bed, before, big, boys, breakfast, but

/t/: tall, to, toes, together, told, tomorrow, took, top, track, tracks, tree

/d/: day, deep, down, dragged, dream, dreamed, during

/k/: called, climbed, climber, could, covered, crunch

/g/: gone, got, great

/dz/: (as 1st sound in jelly): just

/m/: made, make, melted, morning, mother, mountain

/n/: new, night, not

/s/: sad, sank, see, slept, slid, slowly, smacking, smiling, snow, snowball, snowman, snowsuit, snowy, so, socks, something, stick, sticking, still, street, sun

/f/: fallen, falling, far, feet, fell, felt, fight, firm, for, found, friend, from, fun

/v/: very

/h/: had, hall, handful, he, head, heaping, high, his, house

/r/: ran, right, round

/l/: like, liked, looked

/w/, /wh/: one, walked, walking, warm, was, wasn't, way, went, wet, when, while, window, winter, with, woke, would

/sh/: she

/voiceless th/: thought

/voiced th/: that, the, their, them, then, there, they, this

/y/ (as 1st sound in yellow): yet

vowels: a, about, across, adventures, after, all, along, and, angels, another, as, away, empty, enough, everything, everywhere, in, into, of, off, old, on, out, outside, up

10. Segmenting final sound in words.

What to say to the student: "Listen to the word I say and tell me the last sound you hear."

EXAMPLE: "What's the last sound in the word '_____'?" (stimulus word) (e.g., "What's the last sound in the word 'angels'?") (/z/)

> **NOTE:** *Give letter sound not letter name. Use pictured items and/or manipulatives if necessary. Use any of the following stimulus words and/or others you select from the story. Use any group of 10 stimulus items you select per teaching set.*

Stimulus items:

/p/: deep, plop, top, up

/t/: about, breakfast, but, feet, felt, fight, got, great, it, just, liked, looked, night, not, out, picked, pocket, pot, put, right, slept, snowsuit, street, that, thought, walked, wasn't, went, wet, yet

/d/: and, bed, called, climbed, could, covered, dragged, dreamed, found, friend, had, head, made, melted, old, outside, piled, pretended, round, sad, slid, told, would

/k/: like, make, sank, stick, took, track, woke

/g/: big

/ch/: crunch

/m/: dream, firm, from, them, warm

/n/: down, fallen, fun, gone, in, join, mountain, on, one, ran, snowman, sun, then, when

/ng/: along, during, everything, falling, heaping, morning, pointing, smacking, smiling, something, sticking, walking

/s/: across, house, socks, this, tracks

/z/: adventures, angels, as, boys, his, toes

/f/: enough, off

/v/: of

/r/: after, another, before, climber, everywhere, far, for, mother, Peter, their, there, together, winter

/l/: all, fell, hall, handful, snowball, still, tall, while

/voiceless th/: earth, with

/long A/: away, day, they, way

/long E/: be, empty, he, see, she, slowly, snowy, tree, very

/long I/: high

/long O/: so, tomorrow, window

/oo/: into, knew, new, to

11. Generating words from the story beginning with a particular sound.

What to say to the student: "Let's think of words **from the story** that start with certain sounds."

EXAMPLE: "Tell me a word **from the story** that starts with / /." (stimulus sound) (e.g., "the sound /p/") (path)

> **NOTE:** *Give letter sound not letter name. Use pictured items if necessary. Use any of the following stimulus words and/or others you select from the story. You say the sound (e.g., a voiceless /p/ sound) and the student is to say a word from the story that begins with that sound. Use any group of 10 stimulus items you select per teaching set.*

Stimulus items:

/p/: path, Peter, picked, piled, plop, pocket, pointing, pot, pretended, put

/b/: be, bed, before, big, boys, breakfast, but

/t/: tall, to, toes, together, told, tomorrow, took, top, track, tracks, tree

/d/: day, deep, down, dragged, dream, dreamed, during

/k/: called, climbed, climber, could, covered, crunch

/g/: gone, got, great

/dz/: (as 1st sound in jelly): just

/m/: made, make, melted, morning, mother, mountain

/n/: knew, night, not

/s/: sad, sank, see, slept, slid, slowly, smacking, smiling, snow, snowball, snowman, snowsuit, snowy, so, socks, something, stick, sticking, still, street, sun

/f/: fallen, falling, far, feet, fell, felt, fight, firm, for, found, friend, from, fun

/v/: very

/h/: had, hall, handful, he, head, heaping, high, his, house

/r/: ran, right, round

/l/: like, liked, looked

/w/, /wh/: one, walked, walking, warm, was, wasn't, way, went, wet, when, while, window, winter, with, woke, would

/sh/: she

/voiceless th/: thought

/voiced th/: that, the, their, them, then, there, they, this

/y/ (as 1st sound in yellow): yet

vowels: a, about, across, adventures, after, all, along, and, angels, another, as, away, empty, enough, everything, everywhere, in, into, of, off, old, on, out, outside, up

12. Blending sounds in monosyllabic words divided into onset-rime beginning with two consonant cluster + rime.

What to say to the student: "Now we'll put sounds together to make words."
EXAMPLE: "Put these sounds together to make a word (/ / + / /)." (stimulus sounds) "What's the word?" (e.g., "pl + op: What's the word?") (plop)

NOTE: Give letter sound not letter name. Use pictured items and/or manipulatives if necessary. Use any of the following stimulus words and/or others you select from the story. Correct answers are in parentheses.

Stimulus items:

cl + ime (climb)

cr + unch (crunch)

dr + ag (drag)

gr + ate (great)

sl + oh (slow)

fr + end (friend)

sl + ept (slept)

tr + ack (track)

st + ick (stick)

sn + oh (snow)

13. Blending sounds in monosyllabic words divided into onset-rime beginning with single consonant + rime.

What to say to the student: "Let's put sounds together to make words."
EXAMPLE: "Put these sounds together to make a word (/ / + / /)." (stimulus sounds) "What's the word?" (e.g., "/d/ + ay: what's the word?") (day)

NOTE: Give letter sound not letter name. Use pictured items and/or manipulatives if necessary. Use any of the following stimulus words and/or others you select from the story. Correct answers are in parentheses.

Stimulus items:

/d/ + eep (deep)

/f/ + eat (feet)

/b/ + ig (big)

/s/ + ocks (socks)

/p/ + ath (path)

/s/ + ank (sank

/m/ + elt (melt)

/g/ + on (gone)

/n/ + ite (night

/t/ + oes (toes)

14. Blending sounds to form a monosyllabic word beginning with a continuant sound.

What to say to the student: "We'll put sounds together to make words."
EXAMPLE: "Put these sounds together to make a word (/ / + / / + / /)." (stimulus sounds) (e.g., "/m/ /long A/ /k/.") (make)

NOTE: Give letter sound not letter name. Use pictured items and/or manipulatives if necessary. Use any of the following stimulus words and/or others you select from the story. Correct answers are in parentheses.

Stimulus items:

/f/ /r/ /m/ (firm)
/n/ /long I/ /t/ (night)
/th/ /ah/ /t/ (thought)
/m/ /long A/ /d/ (made)
/f/ /long E/ /t/ (feet)
/s/ /ah/ /k/ /s/ (socks)
/f/ /r/ /short E/ /n/ /d/ (friend)
/w/ /short E/ /t/ (wet)
/s/ /t/ /r/ /long E/ /t/ (street)
/r/ /ow/ /n/ /d/ (round)

15. Blending sounds to form a monosyllabic word beginning with a noncontinuant sound.

What to say to the student: "We'll put sounds together to make words."
EXAMPLE: "Put these sounds together to make a word (/ / + / / + / /)." (stimulus sounds) (e.g., "/p/ /long I/ /l/.") (pile)

NOTE: Give letter sound not letter name. Use pictured items and/or manipulatives if necessary. Use any of the following stimulus words and/or others you select from the story. Correct answers are in parentheses.

Stimulus items:

/d/ /r/ long E/ /m/ (dream)
/t/ /ah/ /p/ (top)
/dz/ /short U/ /s/ /t/ (just)
/p/ /l/ /ah/ /p/ (plop)
/g/ /r/ /long A/ /t/ (great)
/t/ /long O/ /z/ (toes)
/b/ /short E/ /d/ (bed)
/d/ /long E/ /p/ (deep)
/p/ /ah/ /t/ (pot)
/t/ /r/ /short A/ /k/ /s/ (tracks)

16. Substituting initial sound in words.

What to say to the student: "We're going to change beginning/first sounds in words."
EXAMPLE: "Say '_____.'" (stimulus word) "Instead of / /" (stimulus sound) "say / /." (stimulus sound) (e.g., Say 'bed.' Instead of /b/ say /sh/. What's your new word?") (shed)

***NOTE:** Give letter sound not letter name. Use pictured items and/or manipulatives if necessary. Use any of the following stimulus words and/or others you select from the story. Correct answers are in parentheses.*

Stimulus items:

"Say tall. Instead of /t/ say /m/." (mall)

"Say Peter. Instead of /p/ say /l/." (liter)

"Say right. Instead of /r/ say /n/." (night)

"Say join. Instead of /dz/ say /k/." (coin)

"Say pocket. Instead of /p/ say /s/." (socket)

"Say socks. Instead of /s/ say /t/." (talks)

"Say took. Instead of /t/ say /sh/." (shook)

"Say sun. Instead of /s/ say /f/." (fun)

"Say deep. Instead of /d/ say /ch/." (cheap)

"Say path. Instead of /p/ say /b/." (bath)

17. Substituting final sound in words.

What to say to the student: "We're going to change ending/last sounds in words."
EXAMPLE: "Say '_____.'" (stimulus word) "Instead of / /" (stimulus sound) "say / /." (stimulus sound) (e.g., "Say 'gone.' Instead of /n/ say /t/. What's your new word?") (got)

***NOTE:** Give letter sound not letter name. Use pictured items and/or manipulatives if necessary. Use any of the following stimulus words and/or others you select from the story. Correct answers are in parentheses.*

Stimulus items:

"Say great. Instead of /t/ say /p/." (grape)

"Say night. Instead of /t/ say /f/." (knife)

"Say slid. Instead of /d/ say /k/."(slick)

"Say stick. Instead of /k/ say /f/." (stiff)

"Say tall. Instead of /l/ say /p/." (top)

"Say tree. Instead of /long E/ say /long A/." (tray)

"Say climber. Instead of /r/ say /d/." (climbed)

"Say right. Instead of /t/ say /m/." (rhyme)

"Say could. Instead of /d/ say /k/." (cook)

"Say snowy. Instead of /long E/ say /d/." (snowed)

18. Segmenting middle sound in monosyllabic words.

What to say to the student: "Tell me the middle sound in the word I say."
EXAMPLE: "What's the middle sound in the word '_____'?" (stimulus word) e.g., "What's the middle sound in the word 'feet'?" (/long E/)

> ***NOTE:*** *Give letter sound not letter name. Use pictured items and/or manipulatives if necessary. Use any of the following stimulus words and/or others you select from the story. Correct answers are in parentheses.*

Stimulus items:

sad (/short A/)	old (/l/)
night (/long I/)	head (/short E/)
sun (/short U/)	make (/long A/)
feet (/long E/)	big(/short I/)
gone (/ah/)	snow (/n/)

19. Substituting middle sound in words.

What to say to the student: "We're going to change the middle sound in words."
EXAMPLE: "Say '_____.'" (stimulus word) "Instead of / /" (stimulus sound) "say / /." (stimulus sound) (e.g., "Say 'bed.' Instead of /short E/ say /short A/. What's your new word?") (bad)

> ***NOTE:*** *Give letter sound not letter name. Use pictured items and/or manipulatives if necessary. Use any of the following stimulus words and/or others you select from the story. Correct answers are in parentheses.*

Stimulus items:

"Say woke. Instead of /long O/ say /long A/." (wake)

"Say heaping. Instead of /long E/ say /long O/." (hoping)

"Say melt. Instead of /short E/ say /ah/."(malt)

"Say socks. Instead of /ah/ say /short A/." (sacks)

"Say great. Instead of /long A/, say /long E/." (greet)

"Say slid. Instead of /short I/ say /short E/." (sled)

"Say pocket. Instead of /ah/ say /short A/." (packet)

"Say deep. Instead of /long E/ say /short I/." (dip)

"Say liked. Instead of /long I/ say /short I/." (licked)

"Say track. Instead of /short A/, say /short U/." (truck)

20. Identifying all sounds in monosyllabic words.

What to say to the student: "Now tell me all the sounds you hear in the word I say."
EXAMPLE: "What sounds do you hear in the word '_____'?" (stimulus word) (e.g., "What sounds do you hear in the word 'top'?") (/t/ /ah/ /p/)

> ***NOTE:*** *Give letter sound not letter name. Use pictured items and/or manipulatives if necessary. Use any of the following stimulus words and/or others you select from the story. Correct answers are in parentheses.*

Stimulus items:

snow (/s/ /n/ /long O/)

toes (/t/ /long O/ /z/)

slid (/s/ /l/ /short I/ /d/)

deep (/d/ /long E/ /p/)

wet (/w/ /short E/ /t/)

socks (/s/ /ah/ /k/ /s/)

track (/t/ /r/ /short A/ /k/)

melt (/m/ /short E/ /l/ /t/)

fun (/f/ /short U/ /n/)

stick (/s/ /t/ /short I/ /k/)

21. Deleting sounds within words.

What to say to the student: "We're going to leave out sounds in words."

EXAMPLE: "Say '_____'" (stimulus word) "without / /." (stimulus sound) (e.g., "Say 'plop' without /l/.") (pop) "The word that was left, 'pop,' is a real word. Sometimes the word won't be a real word."

> *NOTE: Give letter sound not letter name. Use pictured items and/or manipulatives if necessary. Use any of the following stimulus words and/or others you select from the story. Correct answers are in parentheses.*

Stimulus items:

"Say told without /l/." (toad)

"Say great without /r/." (gate)

"Say and without /n/." (ad)

"Say stick without /t/." (sick)

"Say melt without /l/." (met)

"Say smack without /m/." (sack)

"Say from without /r/." (fum)

"Say tree without /r/." (tea)

"Say snow without /n/." (so)

"Say track without /r/." (tack)

22. Substituting consonant in words having a two-sound cluster.

What to say to the student: "We're going to substitute sounds in words."

EXAMPLE: "Say '_____'" (stimulus word). "Instead of / /" (stimulus sound) "say / /" (stimulus sound) (e.g., "Say 'stick.' Instead of /t/ say /l/.") (slick). Say "Sometimes the new word will be a made-up word."

> *NOTE: Give letter sound not letter name. Use pictured items and/or manipulatives if necessary. Use any of the following stimulus words and/or others you select from the story. Correct answers are in parentheses.*

Stimulus items:

"Say tracks. Instead of /k/ say /p/." (traps)

"Say climb. Instead of /l/ say /r/." (crime)

"Say slid. Instead of /l/ say /k/." (skid)

"Say smacking. Instead of /m/ say /l/." (slacking)

"Say plop. Instead of /l/ say /r/."(prop)

"Say slept. Instead of /l/ say /t/." (stepped)

"Say smiling. Instead of /m/ say /t/." (styling)

"Say tree. Instead of /t/ say /f/." (free)

"Say friend. Instead of /f/ say /t/" (trend)

"Say snow. Instead of /n/ say /t/." (stow)

23. Phoneme reversing.

What to say to the student: "We're going to say words backward."

EXAMPLE: "Say the word '_____'" (stimulus word) "backward." (e.g., "If we say 'tall' backward, the word is 'lot.'")

> ***NOTE:*** *This is a difficult phoneme-level task and should only be done with older students. Give letter sound not letter name. Use pictured items and/or manipulatives if necessary. Use any of the following stimulus words and/or others you select from the story. Correct answers are in parentheses.*

Stimulus items:

bed	(Deb)	big	(gib)
right	(tire)	got	(tog)
pot	(top)	but	(tub)
gone	(nog)	like	(Kyle)
make	(came)	fun	(nough)

24. Phoneme switching.

What to say to the student: "We're going to switch the first sounds in two words."

EXAMPLE: "Switch the first sounds in '_____' and '_____.'" (stimulus words) (e.g., "Switch the first sounds in 'feet sank.'") (seet fank)

> *NOTE: This is a difficult phoneme-level task and should only be done with older students. Give letter sound not letter name. Use pictured items and/or manipulatives if necessary. Use any of the following stimulus words and/or others you select from the story. Correct answers are in parentheses.*

Stimulus items:

very sad	(sery vad)
wet socks	(set walks)
winter morning	(minter warning)
warm house	(horm wouse)
toes pointing	(poes tointing)
just right	(rust jight)
down fell	(fown dell)
heaping mountain	(meaping hountain)
found something	(sound fumthing)
Peter's head	(heaters ped)

25. Pig latin.

What to say to the student: "We're going to talk in a secret language using words from the story. In pig latin, you take off the first sound of a word, put it at the end of the word, and add a long A sound."

EXAMPLE: "Say sank in pig latin." (anksay)

> *NOTE: This is a difficult phoneme-level task and should only be done with older students. Use pictured items and/or manipulatives if necessary. Use any of the following stimulus words and/or others you select from the story. Correct answers are in parentheses.*

Stimulus items:

feet	(eatfay)
winter	(interway)
Peter	(eterpay)
handful	(andfulhay)

melted	(eltedmay)
mountain	(ountainmay)
tomorrow	(omorrowtay)
night	(ightnay)
pocket	(ocketpay)
deep	(eepday)

CHAPTER

13

PHONOLOGICAL AWARENESS ACTIVITIES TO USE WITH *THE VERY HUNGRY CATERPILLAR*

Text version used for selection of stimulus items:
Carle, E., G. (1969). *The very hungry caterpillar.* New York: Philomel Books.

PHONOLOGICAL AWARENESS ACTIVITIES AT THE WORD LEVEL

1. Counting words.

What to say to the student: "We're going to count words."
EXAMPLE: "How many words do you hear in this sentence (or phrase)? 'two weeks.'" (2)

> ***NOTE:*** *Use pictured items and/or manipulatives if necessary. Use any of the following stimulus phrases or sentences and/or others you select from the story. Correct answers are in parentheses.*

Stimulus items:

three plums (2)

swiss cheese (2)

in the light (3)
the next day (3)
his way out (3)
out of the egg (4)
one nice green leaf (4)
he felt much better (4)
he built a small house (5)
he ate through one piece (5)

2. Identifying missing word from list.

What to say to the student: "Listen to the words I say. I'll say them again. You tell me which word I leave out."

EXAMPLE: "Listen to the words I say: 'cheese, cocoon, green.' I'll say them again. Tell me which one I leave out: 'cheese, green.'" (cocoon)

> ***NOTE:*** *Use pictured items and/or manipulatives if necessary. Use any of the following stimulus words and/or others you select from the story. Correct answers are in parentheses.*

Stimulus set #1	Stimulus set #2
salami, nice	salami (nice)
egg, lollipop	lollipop (egg)
hungry, plums, cone	hungry, cone (plums)
tiny, leaf, watermelon	leaf, watermelon (tiny)
oranges, two, pickle	oranges, two (pickle)
around, built, pears	around, pears (built)
cocoon, more, through, slice	more, through, slice (cocoon)
swiss, Friday, three, butterfly	swiss, three, butterfly (Friday)
pushed, felt, himself, stayed	pushed, felt, stayed (himself)
beautiful, out, nibbled, pop	beautiful, nibbled, pop (out)

3. Identifying missing word in phrase or sentence.

What to say to the student: "Listen to the sentence I read. Tell me which word is missing the second time I read the sentence.

EXAMPLE: "'He was a big fat caterpillar.' Listen again and tell me which word I leave out. 'He was a big fat ____.'" (caterpillar)

> ***NOTE:*** *Use pictured items and/or manipulatives if necessary. Use any of the following stimulus sentences and/or others you select from the story. Correct answers are in parentheses.*

Stimulus items:

One lollipop. One _____. (lollipop)

Little caterpillar. _____caterpillar. (Little)

He stayed inside. He _____ inside. (stayed)

One ice-cream cone. One ice-cream _____. (cone)

One slice watermelon. _____ slice watermelon. (One)

More than two weeks. More than _____ weeks. (two)

He built a small house. He built a ____ house. (small)

He nibbled a hole. He _____ a hole. (nibbled)

He was a beautiful butterfly. He was a _____ butterfly. (beautiful)

The warm sun came up. The _____ sun came up. (warm)

3. Supplying missing word as adult reads.

What to say to the student: "I want you to help me read the story. You fill in the words I leave out."

EXAMPLE: "A very hungry ______." (caterpillar)

> ***NOTE:*** *Use pictured items and/or manipulatives if necessary. Use any of the following stimulus sentences and/or others you select from the story. Correct answers are in parentheses.*

Stimulus items:

He felt much _____. (better)

He nibbled a _____. (hole)

One Sunday _____. (morning)

A _____ butterfly. (beautiful)

He started to look for some _____. (food)

The next _____ was Sunday again. (day)

One _____ green leaf. (nice)

He built a small _____. (house or cocoon)

But he was still _____. (hungry)

He wasn't a little _____ anymore. (caterpillar)

5. Rearranging words.

What to say to the student: "I'll say some words out of order. You put them in the right order so they make sense."

EXAMPLE: "'out way.' Put those words in the right order." (way out)

> ***NOTE:*** *Use pictured items and/or manipulatives if necessary. Use any of the stimulus words and/or others you select from the story. Correct answers are in parentheses. This word-level activity can be more difficult than some of the syllable- or phoneme-level activities due to the memory load. If your students are only able to deal with two or three words to be rearranged, add more two- and three-word samples from the story and omit the four-word level items.*

Stimulus items:

caterpillar little (little caterpillar)

house small (small house)

cake chocolate (chocolate cake)

of piece one (one piece of)

morning Sunday one (one Sunday morning)

through ate he (he ate through)

much felt better (felt much better)

slice one of watermelon (one slice of watermelon)

was he still hungry (he was still hungry)

through strawberries four ate (ate through four strawberries)

PHONOLOGICAL AWARENESS ACTIVITIES AT THE SYLLABLE LEVEL

1. Syllable counting.

What to say to the student: "We're going to count syllables (or parts) of words."

EXAMPLE: "How many syllables do you hear in '_____'?" (stimulus word) (e.g., "How many syllables in 'cherry'?") (2)

> *NOTE: Use pictured items and/or manipulatives if necessary. Use any of the following stimulus words and/or others you select from the story. Use any group of 10 stimulus items you select per teaching set.*

Stimulus items:

One-syllable words: pears, pie, piece, plums, pop, pushed, big, built, but, two, day, cake, came, cone, cream, green, cheese, moon, more, much, next, nice, night, now, slice, small, some, still, sun, swiss, fat, felt, five, food, four, he, his, hole, house, lay, leaf, light, look, one, warm, was, way, weeks, three, through, than, that, the, then, a, and, ate, egg, ice, in, on, out, up

Two-syllable words: pickle, better, tiny, Tuesday, cocoon, cupcake, cherry, Monday, morning, nibbled, sausage, started, Sunday, Friday, Wednesday, very, himself, hungry, little, Thursday, after, again, any, apple, around, inside

Three-syllable words: beautiful, butterfly, chocolate, salami, Saturday, stomachache, strawberries, lollipop, oranges

Four-syllable words: caterpillar, watermelon

2. Initial syllable deleting.

What to say to the student: "We're going to leave out syllables (or parts of words)."
EXAMPLE: "Say '_____.'" (stimulus word) "Say it again without '_____.'" (stimulus syllable) (e.g., "Say 'Sunday.' Say it again without 'sun.'") (day)

> *NOTE: Use pictured items and/or manipulatives if necessary. Use any of the stimulus words and/or others you select from the story. Correct answers are in parentheses.*

Stimulus items:

"Say chocolate without choc-." (-olate)

"Say sausage without sauce." (-age)

"Say himself without him." (self)

"Say Friday without fry." (day)

"Say strawberries without straw." (berries)

"Say cupcake without cup." (cake)
"Say inside without in." (side)
"Say around without a." (round)
"Say better without bet" (-er)
"Say Tuesday without Tues-." (day)

3. Final syllable deleting.

What to say to the student: "We're going to leave out syllables (or parts of words)."
EXAMPLE: "Say '_____.'" (stimulus word) "Say it again without '_____.'" (stimulus syllable) (e.g., "Say 'around' without 'round.'") (a)

> ***NOTE:*** *Use pictured items and/or manipulatives if necessary. Use any of the stimulus words and/or others you select from the story. Correct answers are in parentheses.*

Stimulus items:

"Say butterfly without fly." (butter)
"Say stomachache without ache." (stomach)
"Say cupcake without cake." (cup)
"Say lollipop without pop." (lolli)
"Say hungry without -ree." (hung)
"Say Sunday without day."(sun)
"Say morning without -ing." (morn)
"Say started without -ed." (start)
"Say after without -er." (aft)
"Say inside without side." (in)

4. Initial syllable adding.

What to say to the student: "Now let's add syllables (or parts) to words."
EXAMPLE: " Add '_____'" (stimulus syllable) "to the beginning of '_____.'" (stimulus syllable) (e.g., "Add 'twos' to the beginning of 'day.'") (Tuesday)

> ***NOTE:*** *Use pictured items and/or manipulatives if necessary. Use any of the following stimulus words and/or others you select from the story. Correct answers are in parentheses.*

Stimulus items:

"Add sauce to the beginning of age." (sausage)

"Add cat to the beginning of -erpillar." (caterpillar)

"Add cuh- to the beginning of coon." (cocoon)

"Add cup to the beginning of cake." (cupcake)

"Add straw to the beginning of berries." (strawberries)

"Add but to the beginning of -erfly." (butterfly)

"Add him to the beginning of self." (himself)

"Add watt to the beginning of -ermelon." (watermelon)

"Add morn to the beginning of -ing." (morning)

"Add Thurs- to the beginning of day." (Thursday)

5. Final syllable adding.

What to say to the student: "Now let's add syllables (or parts) to words."
EXAMPLE: "Add '_____'" (stimulus syllable) "to the end of '_____.'" (stimulus syllable) (e.g., "Add 'day' to the end of 'Satur-.'") (Saturday)

> ***NOTE:*** *Use pictured items and/or manipulatives if necessary. Use any of the following stimulus words and/or others you select from the story. Correct answers are in parentheses.*

Stimulus items:

"Add ache to the end of stomach." (stomachache)

"Add pop to the end of lolli-." (lollipop)

"Add -ple to the end of ap-." (apple)

"Add -ful to the end of beauti-." (beautiful)

"Add day to the end of mun-." (Monday)

"Add cake to the end of cup." (cupcake)

"Add -est to the end of soapy." (soapiest)

"Add -er to the end of aft-." (after)

"Add fly to the end of butter." (butterfly)

"Add let to the end of chocko-." (chocolate)

6. Syllable substituting.

What to say to the student: "Let's make up some new words."
EXAMPLE: "Say '_____.'" (stimulus word) "Instead of '_____'" (stimulus syllable) "say '_____.'" (stimulus syllable) (e.g., "Say 'Sunday.' Instead of 'day' say 'burn.' The new word is 'sunburn.'"

NOTE: Use pictured items and/or manipulatives if necessary. Use any of the following stimulus words and/or others you select from the story. Correct answers are in parentheses.

Stimulus items:

"Say Tuesday. Instead of Tues- say Thurs-." (Thursday)

"Say started. Instead of -ed say -ing." (starting)

"Say around. Instead of round say -bout." (about)

"Say cupcake. Instead of cake say -ful." (cupful)

"Say butterfly. Instead of fly say spread." (butterspread)

"Say strawberries. Instead of straw say blue." (blueberries)

"Say inside. Instead of in say out." (outside)

"Say better. Instead of bet say late." (later)

"Say himself. Instead of him say her." (herself)

"Say morning. Instead of more say eve." (evening)

PHONOLOGICAL AWARENESS ACTIVITIES AT THE PHONEME LEVEL

1. Counting sounds.

What to say to the student: "We're going to count sounds in words."
EXAMPLE: "How many sounds do you hear in this word? 'lay.'" (2)

NOTE: Use pictured items and/or manipulatives if necessary. Use any of the following stimulus words and/or others you select from the story. Be sure to give the letter sound and not the letter name. Use any group of 10 stimulus items you select per teaching set.

Stimulus words with two sounds: pie, two, day, now, he, lay, one, way, the, ate, egg, ice, in, on, out, up

Stimulus words with three sounds: piece, pop, big, but, cake, came, cone, cheese, moon, more, much, nice, night, some, sun, fat, five, food, four, his, hole, house, leaf, light, look, was, three, through, than, that, then, and, any, apple

Stimulus words with four sounds: pears, pickle, pushed, better, built, tiny, called, cream, green, cherry, slice, small, stayed, still, swiss, felt, very, little, warm, weeks, after

Stimulus words with five sounds: Tuesday, cocoon, next, nibbled, plums, sausage, Sunday, Friday, hungry, Thursday, around

2. Sound categorization or identifying rhyme oddity.

What to say to the student: "Guess which word I say does not rhyme with the other three words."

EXAMPLE: "Tell me which word does not rhyme with the other three. '_____, _____, _____, _____.'" (stimulus words) (e.g., "'cake, lake, cheese, bake.' Which word doesn't rhyme?") (cheese)

> ***NOTE:*** *Use pictured items if necessary. Use any of the following stimulus words and/or others you select from the story. Correct answers are in parentheses.*

Stimulus items:

cherry, slice, berry, fairy (slice)

green, scene, nibbled, sheen (nibbled)

weeks, leeks, squeeks, cone (cone)

leaf, thief, warm, chief (warm)

weeks, five, thrive, chive (weeks)

hole, three, mole, coal (three)

swiss, miss, chocolate, kiss (chocolate)

through, better, chew, knew (better)

scream, cream, dream, oranges (oranges)

better, pickle, tickle, nickle (better)

3. Matching rhyme.

What to say to the student: "We're going to think of rhyming words."

EXAMPLE: "Which word rhymes with '_____'?" (stimulus word) (e.g., "Which word rhymes with 'day?' 'big, pop, plums, say.'") (say)

NOTE: Use pictured items if necessary. Use any of the following stimulus words and/or others you select from the story. Correct answers are in parentheses.

Stimulus items:

moon: cherry, night, cheese, loon (loon)

house: mouse, four, hungry, warm (mouse)

plum: pie, green, thumb, sausage (thumb)

cheese: please, salami, nibble, butterfly (please)

look: Friday, small, hungry, took (took)

after: tiny, laughter, morning, slice (laughter)

still: stomachache, food, will, started (will)

built: quilt, cone, sausage, cupcake (quilt)

better: came, chocolate, wetter, nibbled (wetter)

tiny: green, himself, Wednesday, shiny (shiny)

4. Producing rhyme.

What to say to the student: "Now we'll say rhyming words."

EXAMPLE: "Tell me a word that rhymes with '_____.'" (stimulus word) (e.g., "Tell me a word that rhymes with 'more.') You can make up a word if you want." (four)

NOTE: Use pictured items if necessary. Use any of the following stimulus words and/or others you select from the story (i.e., you say a word from the list below and the student is to think of a rhyming word.) Use any group of 10 stimulus items you select per teaching set.

Stimulus items:

/p/: pears, pickle, pie, piece, plums, pop

/b/: beautiful, better, big, built, butterfly, but

/t/: tiny, Tuesday, two

/d/: day

/k/: cake, called, came, caterpillar, cocoon, cone, cream, cupcake

/g/: green

/ch/: cheese, cherry, chocolate

/n/: next, nibbled, nice, night, now

/s/: salami, Saturday, sausage, slice, small, some, started, stayed, still, stomachache, strawberries, sun, Sunday, swiss

/f/: fat, felt, five, food, four, Friday

/v/: very

/h/: he, himself, his, hole, house, hungry

/l/: lay, leaf, light, little, lollipop, look

/w/, /wh/: one, warm, was, watermelon, way, Wednesday, weeks

/voiceless th/: three, through, Thursday

/voiced th/: than, that, the, then

vowels: a, after, again, and, any, apple, around, ate, egg, ice, in, inside, on, oranges, out, up

5. Sound matching (initial).

What to say to the student: "Now we'll listen for the first sound in words."
EXAMPLE: "Listen to this sound: / /." (stimulus sound). "Guess which word I say begins with that sound. '_____, _____, _____, _____.'" (stimulus words) (e.g., "Listen to this sound /p/. Guess which word I say begins with that sound: 'leaf, cupcake, pear, slice.'") (pear)

> **NOTE:** *Give letter sound not letter name. Use pictured items if necessary. Use any of the following stimulus words/or others you select from the story. Correct answers are in parentheses.*

Stimulus items:

/k/: nibbled, Monday, caterpillar, light (caterpillar)

/s/: salami, Tuesday, warm, cheese (salami)

/b/: cocoon, around, chocolate, butterfly (butterfly)

/ch/: sausage, cherry, stomachache, weeks (cherry)

/f/: night, beautiful, Friday, cupcake (Friday)

/h/: hungry, Thursday, started, built (hungry)

/l/: better, Saturday, lollipop, moon (lollipop)

/t/: oranges, strawberries, cream, tiny (tiny)

/n/: green, cupcake, nibbled, himself (nibbled)

/w/: around, butterfly, light, watermelon (watermelon)

6. Sound matching (final).

What to say to the student: "Now we'll listen for the last sound in words."

EXAMPLE: "Listen to this sound: / /" (stimulus sound). "Guess which word I say ends with that sound '_____, _____, _____, _____.'" (stimulus words) (e.g., "Listen to this sound /k/. Guess which word I say ends with that sound: 'day, pushed, look, Thursday.'") (look)

> ***NOTE:*** *Give letter sound not letter name. Use pictured items if necessary. Use any of the following stimulus words and/or others you select from the story. Correct answers are in parentheses.*

Stimulus items:

/long A/: cheese, Tuesday, slice, tiny (Tuesday)

/z/: lollipop, stayed, cheese, caterpillar (cheese)

/p/: food, stomachache, cream, lollipop (lollipop)

/ng/: morning, ice, butterfly, apple (morning)

/d/: egg, sausage, around, beautiful (around)

/m/: cocoon, plum, chocolate, again (plum)

/f/: himself, watermelon, night, lollipop (himself)

/d/: look, swiss, caterpillar, food (food)

/l/: Wednesday, piece, pickle, himself (pickle)

/long E/: strawberry, five, morning, hole (strawberry)

7. Identifying initial sound in words.

What to say to the student: "I'll say a word two times. Tell me what sound is missing the second time. '_______, _______.'" (stimulus words)

EXAMPLE: "What sound do you hear in '_____'" (stimulus word) "that is missing in '_____'?" (stimulus word) (e.g., "What sound do you hear in 'cake,' that is missing in '-ache'?") (/k/)

NOTE: Give letter sound not letter name. Use pictured items and/or manipulatives if necessary. Use any of the following stimulus words and/or others you select from the story. Correct answers are in parentheses.

Stimulus items:

"small, mall. What sound do you hear in small that is missing in mall?" (/s/)

"cheese, ease. What sound do you hear in cheese that is missing in ease?" (/ch/)

"four, or. What sound do you hear in four that is missing in or?" (/f/)

"around, round. What sound do you hear in around that is missing in round?" (/a/)

"pie, I. What sound do you hear in pie that is missing in I?" (/p/)

"now, ow. What sound do you hear in now that is missing in ow?" (/n/)

"still, till. What sound do you hear in still that is missing in till?" (/s/)

"cone, own. What sound do you hear in cone that is missing in own?" (/k/)

"more, or. What sound do you hear in more that is missing in or?" (/m/)

"fat, at. What sound do you hear in fat that is missing in at" (/f/)

8. Identifying final sound in words.

What to say to the student: "I'll say a word two times. Tell me what sound is missing the second time. '_______, _______.'" (stimulus words)

EXAMPLE: "What sound do you hear in '_____'" (stimulus word) "that is missing in '_____'?" (stimulus word) (e.g., "What sound do you hear in 'ice' that is missing in 'I'?") (/s/)

NOTE: Give letter sound not letter name. Use pictured items and/or manipulatives if necessary. Use any of the following stimulus words and/or others you select from the story. Correct answers are in parentheses.

Stimulus items:

"pickle, pick. What sound do you hear in pickle that is missing in pick?" (/l/)

"leaf, Lee. What sound do you hear in leaf that is missing in Lee?" (/f/)

"built, bill. What sound do you hear in built that is missing in bill?" (/t/)

"felt, fell. What sound do you hear in felt that is missing in fell?" (/t/)

"cake, Kay. What sound do you hear in cake that is missing in Kay?" (/k/)

"warm, war. What sound do you hear in warm that is missing in war?" (/m/)

"house, how. What sound do you hear in house that is missing in how?" (/s/)

"slice, sly. What sound do you hear in slice that is missing in sly?" (/s/)

"cherry, chair. What sound do you hear in cherry that is missing in chair?" (/long E/)

"light, lie. What sound do you hear in light that is missing in lie?" (/t/)

9. Segmenting initial sound in words.

What to say to the student: "Listen to the word I say and tell me the first sound you hear."

EXAMPLE: "What's the first sound in '_____'?" (stimulus word) (e.g., "What's the first sound in 'cocoon'?") (/k/)

> ***NOTE:*** *Give letter sound not letter name. Use pictured items and/or manipulatives if necessary. Use any of the following stimulus words and/or others you select from the story. Use any group of 10 stimulus items you select per teaching set.*

Stimulus items:

/p/: pears, pickle, pie, piece, plums, pop

/b/: beautiful, better, big, built, butterfly, but

/t/: tiny, Tuesday, two

/d/: day

/k/: cake, called, came, caterpillar, cocoon, cone, cream, cupcake

/g/: green

/ch/: cheese, cherry, chocolate

/n/: next, nibbled, nice, night, now

/s/: salami, Saturday, sausage, slice, small, some, started, stayed, still, stomachache, strawberries, sun, Sunday, swiss

/f/: fat, felt, five, food, four, Friday

/v/: very

/h/: he, himself, his, hole, house, hungry

/l/: lay, leaf, light, little, lollipop, look

/w/, /wh/: one, warm, was, watermelon, way, Wednesday, weeks

/voiceless th/: three, through, Thursday

/voiced th/: than, that, the, then

vowels: a, after, again, and, any, apple, around, ate, egg, ice, in, inside, on, oranges, out, up

10. Segmenting final sound in words.

What to say to the student: "Listen to the word I say and tell me the last sound you hear." ***EXAMPLE:*** "What's the last sound in the word '_____'?" (stimulus word) (e.g., "What's the last sound in the word 'egg'?" (/g/)

> ***NOTE:*** *Give letter sound not letter name. Use pictured items and/or manipulatives if necessary. Use any of the following stimulus words and/or others you select from the story. Use any group of 10 stimulus items you select per teaching set.*

Stimulus items:

/p/: lollipop, pop, up

/t/: ate, built, but, chocolate, fat, felt, light, next, night, out, pushed, that

/d/: and, around, food, inside, started, stayed

/k/: cake, cupcake, look, stomachache

/g/: big, egg

/dz/: (as 1st sound in jelly): orange, sausage

/ch/: much

/m/: came, cream, plum, some, warm

/n/: again, cocoon, cone, green, in, moon, one, sun, than, then, watermelon, on

/ng/: morning

/s/: house, ice, nice, piece, slice, swiss, weeks

/z/: cheese, his, was

/f/: himself, leaf

/v/: five

/r/: after, better, caterpillar, four, more, pear

/l/: apple, beautiful, call, hole, little, nibble, pickle, small, still

/long A/: day, Friday, Monday, Saturday, Sunday, Thursday, Tuesday, way, Wednesday

/long E/: any, cherry, he, hungry, salami, strawberry, three, tiny, very

/long I/: butterfly, pie

11. Generating words from the story beginning with a particular sound.

What to say to the student: "Let's think of words **from the story** that start with certain sounds."

EXAMPLE: "Tell me a word **from the story** that starts with / /." (stimulus sound) (e.g., "the sound /f/.") (five)

> ***NOTE:*** *Give letter sound not letter name. Use pictured items if necessary. Use any of the following stimulus words and/or others you select from the story. You say the sound (e.g., a voiceless /p/ sound) and the student is to say a word from the story that begins with that sound. Use any group of 10 stimulus items you select per teaching set.*

Stimulus items:

/p/: pears, pickle, pie, piece, plums, pop

/b/: beautiful, better, big, built, butterfly, but

/t/: tiny, Tuesday, two

/d/: day

/k/: cake, called, came caterpillar, cocoon, cone, cream, cupcake

/g/: green

/ch/: cheese, cherry, chocolate

/n/: next, nibbled, nice, night, now

/s/: salami, Saturday, sausage, slice, small, some, started, stayed, still, stomachache, strawberries, sun, Sunday, swiss

/f/: fat, felt, five, food, four, Friday

/v/: very

/h/: he, himself, his, hole, house, hungry

/l/: lay, leaf, light, little, lollipop, look

/w/, /wh/: one, warm, was, watermelon, way, Wednesday, weeks

/voiceless th/: three, through, Thursday

/voiced th/: than, that, the, then

vowels: a, after, again, and, any, apple, around, ate, egg, ice, in, inside, on, oranges, out, up

12. Blending sounds in monosyllabic words divided into onset-rime beginning with two consonant cluster + rime.

What to say to the student: "Now we'll put sounds together to make words."
EXAMPLE: "Put these sounds together to make a word (/ / + / /)." (stimulus sounds) "What's the word?" (e.g., "th + roo. What's the word?") (through)

> *NOTE: Give letter sound not letter name. Use pictured items and/or manipulatives if necessary. Use any of the following stimulus words and/or others you select from the story. Correct answers are in parentheses.*

Stimulus items:

st + ill (still)	st + raw (straw)
cr + eam (cream)	sw + iss (swiss)
sl + ice (slice)	pl + um (plum)
gr + een (green)	ch + eez (cheese)
th + ree (three)	st + art (start)

13. Blending sounds in monosyllabic words divided into onset-rime beginning with single consonant + rime.

What to say to the student: "Let's put sounds together to make words."
EXAMPLE: "Put these sounds together to make a word (/ / + / /)." (stimulus sounds) "What's the word?" (e.g., "/k/ + ache: what's the word?") (cake)

> *NOTE: Give letter sound not letter name. Use pictured items and/or manipulatives if necessary. Use any of the following stimulus words and/or others you select from the story. Correct answers are in parentheses.*

Stimulus items:

p + I (pie)	s + un (sun)
n + ice (nice)	h + ole (hole)

k + own (cone)
p + eece (piece)
f + at (fat)
w + eek (week)
f + elt (felt)
h + ouse (house)

14. Blending sounds to form a monosyllabic word beginning with a continuant sound.

What to say to the student: "We'll put sounds together to make words."
EXAMPLE: "Put these sounds together to make a word (/ / + / / + / /)." (stimulus sounds) (e.g., "/m/ /oo/ /n/.") (moon)

> ***NOTE:*** *Give letter sound not letter name. Use pictured items and/or manipulatives if necessary. Use any of the following stimulus words and/or others you select from the story. Correct answers are in parentheses.*

Stimulus items:

/n/ /long I/ /t/ (night)
/s/ /l/ /long I/ /s/ (slice)
/f/ /short A/ /t/ (fat)
/s/ /w/ /short I/ /s/ (swiss)
/f/ /long I/ /v/ (five)
/voiceless th/ /r/ /long E/ (three)
/l/ /long E/ /f/ (leaf)
/f/ /oo/ /d/ (food)
/s/ /m/ /ah/ /l/ (small)
/m/ /short U/ /ch/ (much)

15. Blending sounds to form a monosyllabic word beginning with a noncontinuant sound.

What to say to the student: "We'll put sounds together to make words."
EXAMPLE: "Put these sounds together to make a word (/ / + / / + / /)." (stimulus sounds) e.g., "/p/ /short O/ /p/." (pop)

> ***NOTE:*** *Give letter sound not letter name. Use pictured items and/or manipulatives if necessary. Use any of the following stimulus words and/or others you select from the story. Correct answers are in parentheses.*

Stimulus items:

/ch/ /long E/ /z/ (cheese)
/p/ /long I/ (pie)
/k/ /long A/ /k/ (cake)
/k/ /r/ /long E/ /m/ (cream)
/t/ /oo/ (two)
/k/ /long O/ /n/ (cone)

/b/ /short I/ /l/ /t/ (built)
/p/ /long E/ /s/ (piece)
/p/ /l/ /short U/ /m/ (plum)
/g/ /r/ /long E/ /n/ (green)

16. Substituting initial sound in words.

What to say to the student: "We're going to change beginning/first sounds in words." *EXAMPLE:* "Say '_____.'" (stimulus word) "Instead of / /" (stimulus sound) "say / /." (stimulus sound) (e.g., "Say 'tiny.' Instead of /t/ say /sh/. What's your new word?") (shiny)

> ***NOTE:*** *Give letter sound not letter name. Use pictured items and/or manipulatives if necessary. Use any of the following stimulus words and/or others you select from the story. Correct answers are in parentheses.*

Stimulus items:

"Say weeks. Instead of /w/ say /s/." (seeks)

"Say house. Instead of /h/ say /m/." (mouse)

"Say cream. Instead of /k/ say /d/." (dream)

"Say cone. Instead of /k/ say /f/." (phone)

"Say piece. Instead of /p/ say /l/." (lease)

"Say pickle. Instead of /p/ say /t/." (tickle)

"Say pear. Instead of /p/ say /f/." (fair)

"Say much. Instead of /m/ say /s/." (such)

"Say Sunday. Instead of /s/ say /m/." (Monday)

"Say more. Instead of /m/ say /f/." (four)

17. Substituting final sound in words.

What to say to the student: "We're going to change ending/last sounds in words." *EXAMPLE:* "Say '_____.'" (stimulus word) "Instead of / /" (stimulus sound) "say / /." (stimulus sound) (e.g., "Say 'cheese.' Instead of /z/ say /p/. What's your new word?") (cheap)

> ***NOTE:*** *Give letter sound not letter name. Use pictured items and/or manipulatives if necessary. Use any of the following stimulus words and/or others you select from the story. Correct answers are in parentheses.*

Stimulus items:

"Say came. Instead of /m/ say /p/." (cape)

"Say slice. Instead of /s/ say /m/." (slime)

"Say ate. Instead of /t/ say /p/." (ape)

"Say nice. Instead of /s/ say /t/." (night)

"Say green. Instead of /n/ say /s/." (grease)

"Say five. Instead of /v/ say /t/." (fight)

"Say swiss. Instead of /s/ say /m/." (swim)

"Say ice. Instead of /s/ say /m/." (I'm)

"Say cone. Instead of /n/ say /t/." (coat)

"Say some. Instead of /m/ say /n/." (sun)

18. Segmenting middle sound in monosyllabic words.

What to say to the student: "Tell me the middle sound in the word I say."
EXAMPLE: "What's the middle sound in the word '_____'?" (stimulus word) (e.g., "What's the middle sound in the word 'leaf'?" (/long E/)

> ***NOTE:*** *Give letter sound not letter name. Use pictured items and/or manipulatives if necessary. Use any of the following stimulus words and/or others you select from the story. Correct answers are in parentheses.*

Stimulus items:

swiss (/short I/)

cheese (/long E/)

pop (/ah/)

much (/short U/)

house (/ow/)

sun (/short U/)

hole (/long O/)

moon (/oo/)

leaf (long /E/)

cone (long /O/)

19. Substituting middle sound in words.

What to say to the student: "We're going to change the middle sound in words."
EXAMPLE: "Say '_____.'" (stimulus word) "Instead of / /" (stimulus sound) "say / /." (stimulus sound) (e.g., "Say 'pop.' Instead of /ah/ say /short U/. What's your new word?") (pup)

> ***NOTE:*** *Give letter sound not letter name. Use pictured items and/or manipulatives if necessary. Use any of the following stimulus words and/or others you select from the story. Correct answers are in parentheses.*

Stimulus items:

"Say cone. Instead of /long O/ say /long A/." (cane)

"Say green. Instead of /long E/ say /short I/." (grin)

"Say leaf. Instead of /long E/ say /long O/."(loaf)

"Say moon. Instead of /oo/ say /long E/." (mean)

"Say men. Instead of /short E/ say /short A/." (man)

"Say piece. Instead of /long E/ say /long A/." (pace)

"Say weeks. Instead of /long E/ say /short I/." (wicks)

"Say cheese. Instead of /long E/ say /long O/." (chose)

"Say pear. Instead of /long A/ say /long O/." (pour)

"Say ache. Instead of /k/ say /p/." (ape)

20. Identifying all sounds in monosyllabic words.

What to say to the student: "Now tell me all the sounds you hear in the word I say."
EXAMPLE: "What sounds do you hear in the word '_____'?" (stimulus word) (e.g., "What sounds do you hear in the word 'cake'?") (/k/ /long A/ /k/)

> ***NOTE:*** *Give letter sound not letter name. Use pictured items and/or manipulatives if necessary. Use any of the following stimulus words and/or others you select from the story. Correct answers are in parentheses.*

Stimulus items:

cheese (/ch /long E/ /z/)
plum (/p/ /l/ /short U/ /m/)
nice (/n/ /long I/ /s/)
cream (/k/ /r/ /long E/ /m/)
built (/b/ /short I/ /l/ /t/)
slice (/s/ /l/ /long I/ /s/)
house (/h/ /ow/ /s/)
night (/n/ /long I/ /t/)
green (/g/ /r/ /long E/ /n/)
swiss (/s/ /w/ /short I/ /s/)

21. Deleting sounds within words.

What to say to the student: "We're going to leave out sounds in words."
EXAMPLE: "Say '_____'" (stimulus word) "without / /." (stimulus sound) e.g., "Say 'plum' without /l/."(pum). " 'Pum,' is a made-up word. Sometimes the word will be a real word and sometimes it will be a made-up word."

> ***NOTE:*** *Give letter sound not letter name. Use pictured items and/or manipulatives if necessary. Use any of the following stimulus words and/or others you select from the story. Correct answers are in parentheses.*

Stimulus items:

"Say weeks without /k/." (wees)

"Say stay without /t/." (say)

"Say pushed without /sh/."(put)

"Say slice without /l/." (sice)

"Say cream without /r/." (keem)

"Say still without /t/." (sill)

"Say swiss without /w/." (sis)

"Say green without /r/." (geen)

"Say next without /k/." (nest)

"Say built without /l/." (bit)

22. Substituting consonant in words having a two-sound cluster.

What to say to the student: "We're going to substitute sounds in words."
EXAMPLE: "Say '_____'" (stimulus word). "Instead of / /" (stimulus sound) "say / /" (stimulus sound) (e.g., "Say 'quick.' Instead of /w/ say /l/.") (click). Say; "Sometimes the new word will be a made-up word."

> ***NOTE:*** *Give letter sound not letter name. Use pictured items and/or manipulatives if necessary. Use any of the following stimulus words and/or others you select from the story. Correct answers are in parentheses.*

Stimulus items:

"Say slice. Instead of /l/ say /p/." (spice)

"Say green. Instead of /r/ say /l/." (glean)

"Say cream. Instead of /k/ say /d/." (dream)

"Say still. Instead of /t/ say /p/." (spill)

"Say felt. Instead of /t/ say /d/."(felled)

"Say small. Instead of /m/ say /t/." (stall)

"Say plums. Instead of /z/ say /p/." (plump)

"Say warm. Instead of /m/ say /p/." (warp)

"Say weeks. Instead of /k/ say /t/" (wheats)

"Say three. Instead of /th/ say /t/." (tree)

23. Phoneme reversing.

What to say to the student: "We're going to say words backward."
EXAMPLE: "Say the word '_____'" (stimulus word) "backward." e.g., "Say 'piece' backward." (seep)

> *NOTE: This is a difficult phoneme-level task and should only be done with older students. Give letter sound not letter name. Use pictured items and/or manipulatives if necessary. Use any of the following stimulus words and/or others you select from the story. Correct answers are in parentheses.*

Stimulus items:

but	(tub)	ice	(sigh)
day	(aid)	still	(lits)
came	(make)	cake	(cake)
much	(chum)	more	(roam)
leaf	(feel)	pop	(pop)

24. Phoneme switching.

What to say to the student: "We're going to switch the first sounds in two words."
EXAMPLE: "Switch the first sounds in '_____' and '_____.'" (stimulus words) (e.g., "Switch the first sounds in 'very hungry.'") (hairy vungry)

NOTE: This is a difficult phoneme-level task and should only be done with older students. Give letter sound not letter name. Use pictured items and/or manipulatives if necessary. Use any of the following stimulus words and/or others you select from the story. Correct answers are in parentheses.

Stimulus items:

some food	(fum sood)
chocolate cake	(cockolate chake)
one pickle	(pun wickle)
two weeks	(woo teeks)
one sausage	(sun wausage)
little caterpillar	(kittle laterpillar)
big fat	(fig bat)
next day	(dext nay)
Sunday morning	(munday sorning)
cherry pie	(perry chy)

25. Pig latin.

What to say to the student: "We're going to talk in a secret language using words from the story. In pig latin, you take off the first sound of a word, put it at the end of the word, and add a long A sound."

EXAMPLE: "Say sun in pig latin." (unsay)

NOTE: This is a difficult phoneme-level task and should only be done with older students. Use pictured items and/or manipulatives if necessary. Use any of the following stimulus words and/or others you select from the story. Correct answers are in parentheses.

Stimulus items:

cheese	(eesechay)
tiny	(inytay)
watermelon	(ahtermelonway)
food	(oodfay)
chocolate	(ocolatechay)

weeks	(eeksway)
salami	(alamisay)
night	(ightnay)
little	(ittlelay)
Sunday	(undaysay)

REFERENCES

California State Department of Education. (1998). *California language arts content standards.* Sacramento: California State Department of Education.

Farnham-Diggory, S. (1990). Foreword. In R. B. Spalding & W. T. Spalding (Eds.), *The writing road to reading* (pp. 1–12). New York: Quill William Morrow.

Frith, U. (1986). A developmental framework for developmental dyslexia. *Annals of Dyslexia, 36,* 69–81.

Goldsworthy, C. (1996). *Developmental reading disabilities: A language-based treatment approach.* San Diego: Singular Publishing Group.

Goldsworthy, C. (1998). *Sourcebook of phonological awareness activities: Children's classic literature.* San Diego: Singular Publishing Group.

Hodson, B. W., & Edwards, M .L. (1997). *Perspectives in applied phonology*. Gaithersburg, MD: Aspen.

Lance, D. M., Swanson, L. A., & Peterson, H. A. (1997). A validity study of an implicit phonological awareness paradigm. *Journal of Speech, Language, and Hearing Research, 40,* 1002–1010.

Moats, L. C., Furry, A. R., & Brownell, N. (1998). *Learning to read: Components of beginning reading instruction K–8.* Sacramento: California State Board of Education.

Perfetti, C. A. (1991). Representations and awareness in the acquisition of reading competence. In L. Rieben & C. A. Perfetti (Eds.), *Learning to read: Basic research and its implications* (pp. 33–46). Hillsdale, NJ: Lawrence Erlbaum.

National Center on Education and the Economy. (1999). *Primary literacy standards.* Washington, DC: National Center on Education and the Economy.

Snow, C. E., Burns, M. S., & Griffin, P. (1998). *Preventing reading difficulties in young children.* Washington, DC: National Academy Press.

Stackhouse, J. (1997). Phonological awareness: Connecting speech and literacy problems. In B. W. Hodson & M. L. Edwards (Eds.), *Perspectives in applied phonology* (pp. 157–196). Gaithersburg, MD: Aspen.

APPENDIX

FORMS FOR TRACKING STUDENT PERFORMANCE

RECORD SHEET #1

Record Sheet #1 is suggested as one way of tracking a student's performance on the various phonological awareness activities. A check off mark (✓), date, and/or percent accuracy can be recorded in the box intersecting a particular story with activity.

STUDENT: ______________________

STORIES:	Blueberries for Sal	Corduroy	Happy BD Moon	Harry & Terrible Whatzit	Harry the Dirty Dog	Stone Soup	The Hungry Thing	The Little Red Hen	The Three Little Pigs	The Snowy Day	The Very Hungry Caterpillar
ACTIVITIES:											
WORD LEVEL:											
1. Counting words											
2. ID missing words											
3. ID missing words phrase/sentence											
4. Supplying word											
5. Rearranging words											
SYLLABLE LEVEL:											
1. Counting syllables											
2. Initial syllable deleting											
3. Final syllable deleting											
4. Initial syllable adding											
5. Final syllable adding											
6. Syllable substituting											

(continued)

(continued)

STORIES:	Blueberries for Sal	Corduroy	Happy BD Moon	Harry & Terrible Whatzit	Harry the Dirty Dog	Stone Soup	The Hungry Thing	The Little Red Hen	The Three Little Pigs	The Snowy Day	The Very Hungry Caterpillar
ACTIVITIES:											
PHONEME LEVEL:											
1. Counting sounds											
2. Sound categorization											
3. Matching rhyme											
4. Producing rhyme											
5. Initial sound matching											
6. Final sound matching											
7. ID initial sound											
8. ID final sound											
9. Seg. initial sound											
10. Seg. final sound											
11. Generating words											
12. Blending sds: onset-rime 2- cons. beg.											
13. Blending sds: onset-rime single cons. beg.											

(continued)

STORIES:	Blueberries for Sal	Corduroy	Happy BD Moon	Harry & Terrible Whatzit	Harry the Dirty Dog	Stone Soup	The Hungry Thing	The Little Red Hen	The Three Little Pigs	The Snowy Day	The Very Hungry Caterpillar
ACTIVITIES:											
14. Blending sds. beg. with continuant sd.											
15. Blending sds. beg. with noncontinuant sd.											
16. Substituting initial sound											
17. Substituting final sound											
18. Segmenting middle sound											
19. Substituting middle sound											
20. ID all sounds											
21. Deleting sounds within words											
22. Substituting consonant in 2-sd. cluster											
23. Phoneme reversing											
24. Phoneme switching											
25. Pig Latin											

RECORD SHEET #2

Record Sheet #2 is suggested as one way of tracking a student's performance on the various phonological awareness activities. A check off mark (✓), date, percent accuracy, and/or specific notes can be recorded on the lines next to activities.

STUDENT: ______________________ **STORY:** ______________________

PHONOLOGICAL AWARENESS ACTIVITIES AT THE WORD LEVEL

1. Counting words: ______________________
2. Identifying missing word from list: ______________________
3. Identifying missing word in phrase or sentence: ______________________
4. Supplying missing word as adult reads: ______________________
5. Rearranging words: ______________________

PHONOLOGICAL AWARENESS ACTIVITIES AT THE SYLLABLE LEVEL

1. Syllable counting: ______________________
2. Initial syllable deleting: ______________________
3. Final syllable deleting: ______________________
4. Initial syllable adding: ______________________
5. Final syllable adding: ______________________
6. Syllable substituting: ______________________

PHONOLOGICAL AWARENESS ACTIVITIES AT THE PHONEME LEVEL

1. Counting sounds: ______________________
2. Sound categorization or identifying rhyme oddity: ______________________
3. Matching rhyme: ______________________
4. Producing rhyme: ______________________
5. Sound matching (initial): ______________________
6. Sound matching (final): ______________________
7. Identifying initial sound in words: ______________________
8. Identifying final sound in words: ______________________
9. Segmenting initial sound in words: ______________________

10. Segmenting final sound in words:____
11. Generating words from the story beginning with a particular sound:____
12. Blending sounds in monosyllabic words divided into onset-rime beginning with two consonant cluster + rime:____
13. Blending sounds in monosyllabic words divided into onset-rime beginning with single consonant + rime:____
14. Blending sounds to form a monosyllabic word beginning with a continuant sound:____
15. Blending sounds to form a monosyllabic word beginning with a noncontinuant sound:____
16. Substituting initial sound in words:____
17. Substituting final sound in words:____
18. Segmenting middle sound in monosyllabic words:____
19. Substituting middle sound in words:____
20. Identifying all sounds in monosyllabic words:____
21. Deleting sounds within words:____
22. Substituting consonant in words having a two-sound cluster____
23. Phoneme reversing:____
24. Phoneme switching:____
25. Pig Latin:____